Contents

Foreword   7

Introduction   9

Chapter 1   **Different Perspectives**   11

Part 1   What is a Sports Therapist and What Knowledge, Skills,
Expertise and Personal Qualities Must They Possess
That Identifies Them From Other Professionals Working
in the Health Care Field?   11

Part 2   Sporting Mentality   14

Part 3   Anatomical, Physiological and Pathological Considerations   17

Part 4   A Practical Journey Around the Lower and Upper Limb,
Trunk and Spine   40

Part 5   Sports Injuries – Research/Epidemiology, Classification,
Causes and Risk Reduction   55

Part 6   Special Interest/Age Groups Involved in Sport   92

Part 7   Working Relationships – P Principles   111

Chapter 2   **Exercise, Training, Fitness and Performance**   119

Part 1   What is Exercise?   119

Part 2   The Case For and Against Exercise   120

Part 3   Exercise and the Immune System – the Overuse/
Overtraining/Under-performance Syndrome   124

Part 4   Exercise – Some of its Uses in Treatment,
Training and Rehabilitation   127

Part 5   Some Factors to Consider when Developing an Exercise   129

Part 6   Training and Training Principles   130

| Part 7 | Fitness Testing | 133 |
| Part 8 | Factors Affecting and Improvement of Performance | 136 |

| **Chapter 3** | **Injury, Inflammation, Healing and Repair** | **149** |

Part 1	Tissue Fluid Dynamics	149
Part 2	Structural Changes and Affectation to Flow	150
Part 3	Soft and Bony Tissues – Injury, Repair and Treatment Implications	151
Part 4	Factors Affecting, Influencing and Delaying Healing and Repair	171
Part 5	Complications of Injury	174
Part 6	Swellings, Lumps and Bumps	178

| **Chapter 4** | **Examination, Assessment and Diagnosis** | **185** |

Part 1	An Overview of First Aid and the Immediate Care of the Sports Person in the Sporting Environment	185
Part 2	Principles, Procedures, Protocols and the Practice of Examination	188
Part 3	Hypermobility	202
Part 4	Gait Analysis in Walking and Running	204
Part 5	Postural Analysis	207
Part 6	Body Weight and Fat Assessment	210

| **Chapter 5** | **Treatment** | **215** |

Part 1	Aims, Objectives, Priorities, Principles, Procedures, Protocols and Practicalities	215
Part 2	Improving Effectiveness	219
Part 3	The Pain Factor	228
Part 4	The Role of Soft Tissue Manipulation in the Care and Treatment of Sports People	244
Part 5	Mechanical Massagers	255
Part 6	Bandaging, Strapping and Taping	257
Part 7	Electrotherapy and Thermal Treatment	266

| **Chapter 6** | **Rehabilitation** | **281** |

| Part 1 | Aims, Objectives, Principles and Practicalities | 281 |
| Part 2 | The Role of Proprioception in Treatment and Rehabilitation | 287 |

SPORTS THERAPY

Theoretical and Practical Thoughts and Considerations

James Briggs

CORPUS PUBLISHING

First published in collaboration with the Northern Institute of Massage in 2001 by
Corpus Publishing Limited
9 Roman Way, Fishbourne, Chichester, PO19 3QN

Author's note

During the course of this book the term athletes is not gender specific and refers to all kinds of people involved in any sporting activity.

Disclaimer

This publication is intended as an informational guide. The techniques described are a supplement, and not a substitute for professional tuition. Whilst the information herein is supplied in good faith, no responsibility is taken by either the publisher or the author for any damage, injury or loss, however caused, which may arise from the use of the information provided.

British Library Cataloguing in Publication Data
A CIP record for this book is available from the British Library
ISBN 1 903333 04 0

Acknowledgements

Due acknowledgement is made to Andrew Martin and Johanne Carter for their help, advice and artistic skills regarding illustrative material. To Ann for her lightening fast fingers on the keyboard in trying to put my thoughts and considerations into print. To Graham for the foreword and Alison for the hours spent proofing, and to Clive Warden for proofing Chapter 3. Also, to Verna and Frank for starting me off on the journey. To Dee for always believing and being there and Tim, my always supporting, best mate! To the many students who not only provide me with an audience and a challenge but also those who acted as models. Finally, to all my educators, family and friends who have always provided me with a never ending source of inspiration, encouragement and support.

The publisher would like to acknowledge Bill Tancred, whose nomograms were used in Appendix 5. His permission was sought through the original publisher, but we were unable to obtain full permission from the author.

Models Tristan Boyd, Australian Beach Volleyball World Series Player, and Jane Vanstone
Drawings Simon Golding (non-anatomical). Michael Courtnage (anatomical)
Text and Cover Design Sara Howell
Printed and bound in Great Britain by Bell & Bain Ltd., Glasgow
Distributed throughout the world by Human Kinetics – www.humankinetics.com – or:

USA
P O Box 5076, Champaign, IL 61825-5076, T: 1-800-747-4457, F: 217-351-1549

Canada
475 Devonshire Road, Unit 100, Windsor, ON N8Y 2L5, T: 1-800-465-7301, F: 519-971-9797

Australia
P O Box 80, Torrens Park, S. Australia 5062, T: (08) 8277-1555, F: (08) 8277-1566

UK and Europe
Units C2-C3 Wira Business Park, West Park Ring Road, Leeds, LS16 6EB, UK
T: +44 (0) 113 278 1708. F: +44 (0) 113 278 1709

New Zealand
P O Box 105-231, Auckland Central, T: (09) 523-3462, F: (09) 523-5462

Part 3	The Psychology of Injury and Rehabilitation	293
Part 4	The Role of Nutrition in Rehabilitation	296

Chapter 7	**Legal, Professional, Ethical, Moral and Practice Management Issues**	**299**

Part 1	The Compensation Culture	299
Part 2	Terminology and Practical Issues	301
Part 5	The Importance of Record Keeping	312
Part 4	Referrals and Reports	316
Part 5	Advertising and Attracting Patients	318
Part 6	Insurance and Sport	319

Chapter 8	**Final Thoughts and Considerations**	**321**

Part 1	The Drugs/Cheating Issue – Sports Nutrition, Supplementation, Performance Enhancement, Alcohol, Smoking and Caffeine	321
Part 2	The Sports Injury Clinic	336
Part 3	Travelling with the Teams	338

Glossary of Terms	**353**

Useful Addresses	**363**

Appendices	**369**

Appendix 1	How Good a Communicator are you?	369
Appendix 2	Common Injuries of the Lower Limb and Upper Limb, Trunk and Spine	370
Appendix 3	Training Regimes	372
Appendix 4	Record Keeping	374
Appendix 5	Body Fat Assessment	380

Index	**381**

Foreword

It is with very great pleasure that I write the foreword for Sports Therapy – Theoretical and Practical Thoughts and Considerations. As a fellow professional I have long been witness to the professionalism and dedication of James Briggs, educator and sports therapist. As a close personal friend I have also endured and enjoyed his humour and wit. All of these facets are to be found within this book.

Whilst Mr Briggs brings his own unique and indomitable personality to the tome, it is much more than a collection of humorous stories. James writes with an easy and informal style, but expertly combines this with the serious investigation of many issues prevalent in contemporary sports therapy. This is a very interesting book, offering insight into the world of the sports therapist. Yet, it is intended not only for the qualified sports therapists, but also for all of those who claim an interest (however remote) in the burgeoning worlds of the professional and amateur sporting arena.

Each of the eight chapters offers insightful understanding of the basics of sports therapy. The whole ethos is to introduce the reader to a new approach to the subject, whilst stimulating the thought processes. The text is intelligently written and interspersed with excellent illustrations. Throughout there is clearly presented and detailed information, beginning with Different Perspectives, which sees James launch headlong (in his own undaunted and unique way) into the minefield of 'What is a sport therapist'. What an opener!

As both professional and amateur sports people expect more from their therapist and with the expectation that all practice is underpinned by research-based evidence, the education and expertise of professionals is open to scrutiny. Thus knowledge through extensive reading and continued learning is essential. This book does not claim to have all the answers. However, it does admit to the provision of a sound foundation upon which to build a working knowledge of many aspects of sports therapy. The proviso is that the reader will continue to learn and also to develop their understanding. The need for continuing education and professional development is of paramount importance in the sporting arena.

Read the book, reach your own conclusions, but most of all learn and enjoy.

Graham N. Smith

GradDipPhys MCSP DipTP CertED SRP
Chartered Physiotherapist
Rehabilitation and Sports Injury Consultant

Introduction

Today, much precocious talent is being identified by adults at a younger and younger age. My involvement and success in sport started as most people of my generations did, at primary school, when I found that sports day proved fruitful for my ego, winning most things that involved getting from A to B in the quickest time. At that time in my education just taking part and being successful was the thrill and winning at all costs wasn't an issue. Manipulation was something that entered my life much later and even then it had nothing to do with winning and 'bending the rules'. At secondary school I found myself representing not only school but also town and county at football and athletics. My first serious injury was not until my early 20's when I injured my shoulder lifting a gymnast up onto the rings – it was only then that I sought the help of a physiotherapist. Up until that time I thought only my doctor dealt with everything and anything to do with illness and injury. Since then I have broadened my horizons a little and realised that there are many complementary and allopathic practitioners offering to treat a multitude of ailments related to this phenomenon we call the human body.

Declining a career in football, my early training as a physical education teacher, coach and then manual therapist introduced me to the notion of having separate titles for all things related to sport – injuries, cream, massage, mentality etc. However, prior to 1989 I was not aware of the term 'sports therapist' and it was not a term that readily rolled off everyone's lips. In fact it was only when Mr. Graham N. Smith, suggested the idea of a Society of Sports Therapists, in the late 80's – early 90's did the term enter my memory bank.

In a relatively short space of time, sport and exercise medicine has become growth medicine and sports therapy has equally grown with courses on the subject being offered from a few hours to many years, leading to degree and masters degree status. Exercise is now being given on prescription. Doctors are being encouraged to attend postgraduate sport and exercise medicine courses. Continuing professional development has now become a major issue (Dr. N. Webborn, 2000).

Professional and retired professionals are jumping on the bandwagon. Both allopathic and complementary medicines are addressing key issues. Everyone is getting involved. Titles are becoming protected.

Most sportsmen and women regularly involved in exercise related activities would suggest this as no bad thing. The more people involved in looking after our welfare the better. However, this resultant boom has coincided with a closer scrutiny of all things coming under the educational banner related to sport, with 'quality control' involved in the training of such people needing careful appraisal. Does everyone get a diploma who have put their gluteus maximus on a seat or just the ones who have achieved the required/acceptable standard? The issue of what is required and acceptable has now become 'the issue'. Setting the high jump to 7 feet will make it difficult for only those capable of overcoming the obstacle but lowering the bar to 2 feet ensures that almost everyone is successful. Also the question arises of who oversees such quality control, the educational, medical or sporting establishment? The mere mention of sports injury clinics and even the use of the term sport therapist cause some individuals/groups to go apoplectic.

I am aware that by putting thoughts into print I am leaving myself open to close scrutiny and of course you are never going to please everyone all of the time. It depends on whose or from which perspective the scrutiny comes. I was once informed on a management course that to get a unanimous decision, don't put more than one person on the committee. Many bodies and groups involved in the welfare of sports people have an invested interest in wanting their say in the process. But having attended many courses, workshops and conferences on the subject, as well as having taught and tutored on such courses, there definitely appeared to be a need for a text that addressed the topic of sports therapy from a non-medical perspective. Having written an update of an existing sports therapy course for the Northern Institute of Massage, I was sufficiently motivated and then subsequently encouraged to write this book.

This book is an honest attempt to tackle many of the issues that confront not only sport in general but also consider such issues from the point of view of sports therapy. The following does not purport to be definitive and is written in good faith.

It is intended to be a thought provoking, tongue in cheek, humorous and at times a cynical view of sport. However, it is one that will provide not only theoretical and practical thoughts and considerations but also a solid foundation for the sports therapist on which to build further knowledge, skills and expertise on the subject of sports therapy. It initially addresses the key issue of what must a sports therapist know to be a safe, effective, efficient, competent, problem-solving practitioner. Remembering that expertise is a never-ending process of learning modification and change. This then provides the basis for the rest of the chapters in the book.

James Briggs 2001

Chapter 1
Different Perspectives

"A little learning is a dangerous thing!"
Alexander Pope

Part 1

What is a Sports Therapist and What Knowledge, Skills, Expertise and Personal Qualities Must They Possess That Identifies Them From Other Professionals Working in the Health Care Field?

"A sports therapist might be someone capable of offering advice on exercise – or someone who delivers massage before and after a sporting event – or a highly trained practitioner able to recognise common orthopaedic conditions and soft tissue injuries as well as being able to complete a progressive and effective rehabilitation programme of treatment and rehabilitation."
Hudson, M., 1998

Whilst this definition at least attempts to outline and justify the role of the sports therapist, encompassing the various levels of training on offer at present, i.e. clinical/medical, massage and exercise-orientated, it is vague and generalised containing phrases/words such as, 'might be' and 'or'. It does, however, highlight the fact that going into the twenty-first century, although increasing in its usage, the term is still lacking specificity, having something to do with sport and something to do with therapy. This in itself causes other professionals working in this field to become sceptical and cynical. A sports therapist in essence acquires an identity that differentiates them from others working in the health care field because of not only what knowledge, skills and expertise they **SHOULD** and **MUST** possess by training specifically with sport in general in mind but by the fact they have an interest in sport, whether directly or indirectly.

Other therapists may have specialised knowledge in a particular field to which the sports therapist can and may refer but may not initially train for working in sport, i.e. physiotherapist, doctor, consultant, masseur/masseuse, podiatrist/chiropodist, osteopath, chiropractic, etc. However, postgraduate training may follow. These people may not even have any personal interest or involvement in sport and in some cases may have a particular bias against sport in general. This is in no way meant to denigrate or infer that their dedication and professionalism is compromised but just a statement of fact. Sports therapists deal with sports people with a problem not just the problem. This is the excitement of sports therapy. The **PERSON** is the central core of their work. The periphery, the injury, the medicine, the technology, etc. is considered in relation to this. Not secondary to but in relation to it. This makes their work highly individualised, as no two people are the same. It requires a great deal of understanding, empathy, compassion and flexibility, as to why sports people do what they do.

What Must the Sports Therapist Know?

"Give me the facts but above all give me the understanding."
Solomon

WHAT I HEAR...

...I FORGET

WHAT I SEE...

...I REMEMBER

WHAT I DO...

...I UNDERSTAND

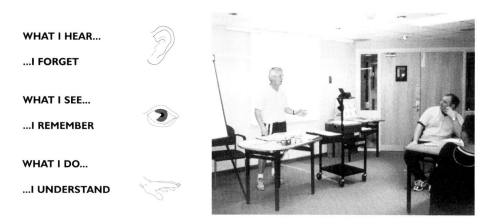

▲ *Figure 1. What must a sports therapist know? A little learning is a dangerous thing!*

The quest for **KNOWLEDGE** is all about what:

- **COULD** you know, which is never ending and constantly changing.
- **LIKE** to know, which is dependent on who wants to know.
- **MUST** you know, which is necessary on any course to attain the required standard. This can be considered the minimum amount of knowledge, skills and expertise to be safe and effective.
- **NEED** to know, which also relates to must.

- **SHOULD** you know, which is dependent on who is setting the standard and what particular invested interest they have and/or who do they represent.

Unfortunately, as mentioned in the introduction, the issue for **COULD** and **MUST** is one of 'quality control' and who oversees and assesses such quality. In these days of accountability and litigation, **QUALITY** of training needs to be weighed against **QUANTITY**, not only in terms of numbers of students and their relevance to funding and jobs but also what to include in the relevant curriculum. The latter again is dependent on which professional body is developing it. As soon as definitive/prescriptive documentation appears, criteria for pass and fail can ensure the curriculum becomes very insular and focused, but sometimes not for the right reason, i.e. position in a league table.

Finally, one can never escape the 'political in-fighting' related to who is the chief and who are the Indians.

- **DECLARATIVE KNOWLEDGE** can be considered as making statements of known facts, whilst;
- **PROCEDURAL KNOWLEDGE** is showing that what is known can be put into practice. **ALL GOOD SAFE, EFFECTIVE PRACTITIONERS SHOULD POSSESS BOTH AS SOUND THEORY UNDERPINS GOOD PRACTICE.**

All clinical decisions are based on probability theory using declarative and procedural knowledge, experience and professional interaction to help make the correct decisions. More knowledge is more useful than less knowledge. All practitioners, not only sports therapists, should also be able to answer the following questions.

What Are You Doing and Why Are You Doing That?

If they can't, then they should not be putting their 'hands-on' and can be deemed not safe and/or effective. Practitioners should be assisting the body's natural processes, not interfering with them.

To be safe and effective and to provide the best possible healthcare for any individual at that moment in time a good sports therapist needs to be aware of, have knowledge of, familiarity with, reflect on and be informed by:

- **Not only their own sport but all other sports and all that this involves, i.e. sporting mentality, role conflict, physical and mental demands, risks and social culture.**
- **Anatomy, physiology, pathology, biochemistry, physics, biomechanics etc.**

- What constitutes individuality in a performer/athlete.
- Training, treatment and rehabilitation principles and protocols both on and off the field of play/competition arena.
- The objective and subjective clinical perspectives, which very much relates to the examination, assessment and diagnosis.
- All forms of evidence, including research, e.g. sports science and medical advances.

Obviously the level and depth to which this knowledge goes depends upon many variables. One of the aims of this book is to identify such knowledge and what **MUST** be known in each area and not **CAN** be known.

Part 2

Sporting Mentality

In essence, an understanding of all sports and the people who participate in it must be an integral part of any person's armoury when working in sports medicine. Training and professional development in a particular therapy can then be allied to this knowledge.

Understanding sporting mentality, or as some people would intimate, lack of, is one such area that is vital to the knowledge of a sports therapist. People who participate in sport do so for a variety of reasons. For children it can be pleasure, fun, enjoyment, belonging to, acceptance, a sense of achievement, mastery, competence, excellence, responsibility, freedom, health and fitness. For adults it can be to improve health and welfare, a way of improving social life, fulfilling an ambition, to prove a point. Each individual will have their particular reason/hidden agenda. A Baltimore conference on medical aspects of sport concluded:

> "Sport promotes mental health and peace of mind....and can relieve natural hostilities, aggressiveness and competitiveness."
> *Jon Zneimer, 2000*

The way that some sportsmen and women behave these days, this conclusion needs redefining.

Understanding Sporting Mentality

Instinctively successful sports people have an in-built need and desire to be fully fit, mobile and involved in a competitive environment. In the main they are habitual, competitive, committed, dedicated, obsessed, goal-orientated animals, and whilst this is good for motivation and business it can be bad for image in terms of injury management and prevention. Researchers and epidemiologists find this an interesting area of study. Dr. Hamer (2000) postulates a genetic theory claiming that thirty per cent of people are genetically disposed to 'thrill seeking' with the need to go beyond what is expected as the norm to 'get their kicks' and this contains a self-destruct element. But not all feel the need to use it. Could it be that these thirty per cent gravitate towards certain sports?

Obviously this competitiveness and the resultant stresses this imposes are dependent on the level at which they participate and the rewards that are involved, i.e. professional, semi-professional, amateur, recreational, hobby, etc. Unfortunately these needs and desires can also become addictive and this addiction, material, chemical, pharmaceutical or otherwise, means that in essence some sports people will only stop when injuries force them to and will consider doing anything to win. Prior to this they generally ignore the body's warning sign – **PAIN** – seeing this as extra motivation to overcome. No pain, no gain!

It is at this stage, some would argue, that certain sports and those involved display a distinct lack of any mentality, never mind sporting (*see Chapter 1, Part 5*). It can also be observed that some sports take on an individualised, ritualised personality and associated behaviour patterns related to language and posture, with anyone entering such sports being initiated at a very early age into such customs (*see Chapter 4, Parts 4 and 5*). Some sports set a diabolical example to young, impressionable minds paying lip-service to the concept of fair play and enjoyment. Konrad Lorenz, a twentieth century German psychologist believes that most species cannot survive without aggression, which is learned through imitation and persists as long as the rewards outweigh the potential punishments.

These observed personality and behaviour patterns of aggression such as spitting, foul language, swearing, official abuse, monosyllabic communication and neolithic gait patterns are designed to communicate messages of a macho sport. However, to the uninitiated, they display signs of a childish, selfish, thug wanting his or her own way, possibly to mask skill mediocrity.

> **"Violence occurs when individuals know no other way to cope.
> It is the result of impotence."**
> *Jon Zneimer, 2000*

Or is it just frustration because they realise the odds are stacked against them?

"The.....team were much more serious and aggressive. If a mistake was made, they would shout things like, 'f....... hell'. They would work themselves up into a frenzy about being beaten.... Very seldom do we use the F-word, but in England its use is routine: everything is f..., f..., f... Every second word on the football pitch is f..., which at least makes it easier for foreigners to understand."

Lars Leese, 2000

To counteract this image, some sports have developed ritualised bonding to try and convey a more user-friendly image, which consists of kissing, cuddling and lying on top of each other. There is even user-friendly terminology that can be used when commentating on such sports and behaviour, with a ready-made excuse and justification for such actions. This personality and behaviour associated with some sports although providing the psychologist with a constant source of research material leads to mind-setting, cloning, in-breeding and a detectable, closed-shop mentality which is difficult to infiltrate unless one is prepared to accept and justify such behaviour. Rules are applied to sport to allow a fair and just competition between opponents and are also there to reduce the risk of injury during the contest. A foul is when the rules are broken and some kind of deterrent must be enforced to stop the contest becoming unfair and farcical.

But now some sports seem to want to differentiate between different kinds of foul. Is a professional foul one which means that only people who are paid can carry them out to stop a fair and just competition and in the act of doing so may actually cause injury? Or is it called a professional foul because those who are entitled to commit it have undergone some prolonged period of training and belong to a professional body? In which case, can professional fouls be committed by amateurs? The referee, the arbitrator in all this, is seen as some kind of ignorant, spoil sport who has very little, if any, right to enter the competitive arena especially if he or she dares to banish a player from the field of play for blatant, consistent infringement of the rules. After all what does he or she know? There are some involved in sport that argue making referees full-time professionals would solve some of the problems.

Is this in response to the professional foul? Glenn Hoddle, the ex-England football manager, suggested paying football referees £100,000 per annum which he feels would end the disciplinary chaos that soured the start of the 2000/2001 football season, where 71 yellow and 8 red cards were shown in the first week (*Peter Fitton, 27.8.00*).

But in some sports, where the agenda appears to have been decided in the dressing room before the game/competition even begins, the solutions, in the author's opinion, are not in the hands of the referees. After all if people didn't want to always try and break/manipulate the rules would we need so many? Two years previously, Philip Don, a Football Premiership Referee's Officer, reported in the *Daily Mail (24.10.98)*, that there were 340 assaults on park referees by the participants during the season ending 1998. In 1999 this figure was 465, give or take the odd punch! On 18.3.99 and 10.5.00, programmes on television called, *'Foul Play 1 and 2'*, gave us graphic illustrations of the levels to which sport can degenerate. Some sports people are even encouraged to make videos of their uncontrolled behaviour/antics and/or write about them in a book. At times the selection of our modern sporting heroes leaves plenty to be desired!

Many key issues coming under the umbrella of, 'winning at-all-costs', provides us with a never-ending source of topics for discussion (*see Chapter 8, Part 1*). Anyone entering sports therapy needs to address such issues.

A sports therapist needs to be able to communicate, empathise and, at times, condone what goes on in sport, otherwise they run the risk of rejection for a 'lack of understanding' from sport itself. How good a communicator are you? (*see Appendix 1*). Being a good communicator/active listener can be added to the list of qualities essential to a sports therapist.

Good communication requires a closed-loop where information/messages/questions are sent out and feedback returns data. Failure to obtain feedback leads to insufficient data retrieval, an open-loop and poor communication. The kind of feedback that is required depends on the reason for the communication. A positive interaction between both the sports therapist and the sports person is vital for a safe, effective outcome. Remember that team work/interaction is like a chain in that it is only as strong as the weakest link!

The X chromosome has been identified as being related to social skills. Women are identified in genetic terms as XX (two lots of social /interaction skill) whilst men are XY (only one lot!). Good communication also requires the participants to have an empathy and compassion with each other.

Part 3

Anatomical, Physiological and Pathological Considerations

There is a basic core of anatomical, physiological and pathological knowledge that sports therapists **MUST** familiarise themselves with in order to address the issues of **WHAT AM I DOING AND WHY AM I DOING IT?** An overview of such knowledge will provide such a core leaving further in-depth study from the numerous excellent texts written on the subjects, up to the individual.

Anatomy, physiology and pathology are subjects of continuous research and development and, as with all disciplines/professions, have their own peculiar vocabulary/terminology. This is necessary for the accurate understanding of the subject matter. Sometimes, however, such terminology can be the subject of much debate and conjecture.

> **"I know what's what and who's who but I have no idea why's why."**
> *Ashleigh Brilliant, 1977*

Anatomy

This can generally be defined as the study of the structure of the body and the relationship of various parts to one another. The word is derived from the Greek words *ana*, meaning 'up' and *temos* or *tomos*, meaning 'cutting'. Four types of anatomy can be considered in the work of the sports therapist.

1. **BOOK ANATOMY** is that found in the texts.
2. **FUNCTIONAL ANATOMY** is that found in reality, with everyone being different. You only find pictures and descriptions of people in books not real live bodies.
3. **TRAUMATIC ANATOMY** is that found when the body has been misused, overused and abused.
4. **DEVELOPMENTAL ANATOMY** can be considered and related to scientific progress as the latest research uncovers more and more fascinating, facts and figures.

Physiology

This is the study of the functioning of the body parts. Its Greek derivation also coming from two words – *physics*, meaning 'nature' and *logos*, which means 'science or study'.

Pathology

This is the study, by scientific methods, which deals with the causes of and changes produced in the body by disease. In simplicity it is physiology gone wrong. Disease is a process which can lead to death and therefore can be considered as disturbances to body homeostasis. Homeostatis (maintaining stability) and allostasis (maintaining stability through change) considers how the body adapts and adjusts to the resting and active states *(Sterling, P. and Eyer, J., 1988)*. It could be argued that participation in sport can often compromise such homeostasis, leading to too much compensation, with resultant problems later in life which may not have otherwise become obvious. Pain is indicative that the pathological disease process has started and therefore on this question of having to compensate, it is interesting to note that in sport we are encouraged to simply 'run it off'.

Surely an indicator of disease should not be glibly dismissed? Certain predisposing factors make the development of disease more likely and may put someone at more risk without actually being the cause of the disease, i.e. lifestyle, job, diet, age, posture, stress, environment, personality, somatotype, etc. Sometimes pre-existing conditions, other than heredity factors, may compromise the immune system making the person more susceptible to further complications, e.g. training with an illness.

Finally, it must be appreciated that structure and function are very much interrelated and although subjects are initially studied in isolation, each part is very much a segment of the whole picture. This is the treatment philosophy of wholistic/holistic medicine, whether that comes from a complementary or an allopathic perspective. But that is another story!

General Structure of the Human Body

Differing levels of organisation influence structure and function but we tend to view the body as a structural entity, compartmentalised and working in isolation instead of realising that it consists of many millions of smaller structures and interrelated processes. These structures can be viewed as working on the following levels:

CHEMICAL – ORGANELLE – CELLULAR – TISSUE – ORGANIC – SYSTEMATIC

Chemicals

Over one hundred different chemical building blocks called **ATOMS** combine to form **MOLECULES** that form **MACROMOLECULES**. The relationship of the chemicals provides us with the essential material of human life **ECTOPLASM**. Chemistry involves the study of these chemicals.

Organelles

These can be considered as collections of molecules organised in such a way as to perform an individual function. These can be found in cells. **MITOCHONDRIA** are barrel-like structures that are responsible for energy production. **MICROTUBULES** allow the passage of fluids in and out of cells.

Cells

These are the simplest forms of living matter that can maintain life and their own internal environment and are capable of both movement and replication. They are quite complex and have different functions, e.g. blood cells, muscle cells. Cytology is the study of cells. In simplicity, cells have a nucleus (centre), membrane (external barrier) and cytoplasm/ protoplasm that is the substance contained within the membrane. The nucleus contains forty-six chromosomes (genetic messengers), forty-four of which are paired female and male and two of which are either XX (female) or XY (male). DNA (deoxyribonucleic acid) is the genetic code of life.

Tissues

These are organisations of large numbers of similar cells with varying amounts of non-living substance between them (intercellular), performing a specific function. The main tissues are:

Epithelial Tissue

PROTECTS, SECRETES, ABSORBS and COVERS body surfaces, LINES body cavities and FORMS glands. It can be considered as:

SIMPLE	FUNCTION
Flat/squamous	Lining blood vessels/heart cavities.
Cuboidal	Lining glands and digestive tracts and are involved in secretion/absorption.
Columnar	Can be ciliated (covered in tiny hairs).

COMPOUND/ STRATIFIED (several layers)	FUNCTION
Squamous	These are single cells and are found in the oral cavity, anus and vagina. They protect against wear and tear.
Columnar	Lining reproductive tracts.
Transitional	Found in the bladder and kidneys and are capable of distension and contraction.

Histology is the study of tissues. GLANDS are groups of epithelial tissues that produce specialised secretions onto the epithelial surface of an organ directly or through a duct – EXOCRINE GLANDS. Or they become isolated from epithelial surfaces and discharge their secretions into the blood and lymph –

ENDOCRINE GLANDS (ductless). Their secretions are called **HORMONES** (chemical messengers).

Connective Tissue

Connective tissue is the most abundant tissue found in the body. It is made up of macrophages, fibroblast and mast cells surrounded by an extracellular ground matrix, which is a continuous medium that varies in density. The fibroblasts secrete the matrix gel. This viscous gel contains lots of water, parts of gases, food and nutrition. Connective tissue also contains collagen, reticulin (a thin type of collagen) and yellow elastin fibres. Elastin is yellow, strong, elastic tissue giving connective tissue fifty per cent of its length. It is therefore sometimes compared to spaghetti bolognaise with the sauce being the ground matrix and the fibres the spaghetti. Short sections of the fibres are called procollagen. Once outside the cell the procollagen molecules join together to form chains which become collagen fibres. Microscopically collagen is a triple helix bundle, cross-linked and joined by chemical bonds. This gives it great tensile strength and rigidity. Therefore its fibres are arranged along lines of stress. These cross-links increase with age producing lines and wrinkles.

Twenty-five per cent of all body protein is collagen. There are numerous types of collagen, Type 1 – skin, bone, tendons; Type 2 – cartilage etc.

Visco elasticity is the overall mechanical property of connective tissue. It consists of the elastic component, 'elastic spring' (stored elastic energy) and the hydraulic component, (viscous energy) which dampens the elastic component effect. The difference in the tissues classified as connective is determined by the ratio of collagen, elastin, reticulin and water. It can be considered as:

ORDINARY   loose, adipose, dense, elastic or reticular (this category includes; skin, fat, ligaments, tendons and fascia).

SPECIAL   haemopoietic (red marrow, yellow marrow and lymphoid tissue); supporting/sclerous – cartilage (hyaline, fibro and elastic); bone (compact/hard, cancellous/soft).

TENDONS from the Greek '*tendu*' – to stretch, possess a very parallel fibre arrangement with little or no give. They vary in length, width and thickness depending on where they are located. White, flattened tendons, which serve mainly to connect a muscle with the parts that it moves, are known as aponeurosis.

LIGAMENTS from the Latin *'ligare'* – to bind or tie, possess a fibre arrangement in different directions to allow multidirectional movement within limits. Not only are they used at joints where there is obvious movement but in many other parts of the body. The functions of ligaments are to:

- Join bone to bone.
- Determine the range of movement.
- Be non-contractile.
- Help to monitor proprioception.
- Be taut in various positions throughout full range of movement.

SKIN has a random fibre arrangement along lines of stress and is therefore very adaptable. Its functions include:

- Protection.
- Excretion/elimination.
- Sensation.
- Secretion.
- Absorption.
- Temperature regulation.

Connective tissue is adaptive and responsive to injury and its functions include support, structure separation, space mobility, stabilisation, binding and scar formation. In fact in terms of dysfunction it is one of the first to show signs of losing fluidity, as it can shorten and adhere causing binding and lesion. This restricts the range and ease of movement, which relates to **HOW FAR** and **HOW EASILY** movement is achieved. Its water-binding component (gelatin) is significant and effective for support and function.

If connective tissue is to stay soft, water must be added. This is another reason why it is important to drink plenty of water. It also possesses a slow 'synthesis rate' which is bad news for repair and a percentage will not repair. It is considered 'rigid' and can resist ballistic/elastic stretching although it yields to prolonged stress (i.e. end range for thirty seconds). Sapega, et al., 1987, inform us that resistance to stretch is by the extensive, connective framework and sheathing around the muscle (epimysium, perimysium and endomysium) and not the muscle itself. There also seems to be a piezoelectric property to collagen that affects it. In simplicity, mechanical stress/pressure energy is converted into electrical energy.

Fascia

In manual therapy much is said about the muscles, tendons and ligaments, etc. but not much emphasis is placed on fascia.

> **"Technically, the term fascia designates all fibrous connective tissue not otherwise specifically named."**
> *Alter, 1998*

This tissue is a very important component of the body in that postural fascia, which stabilise or permits upright posture, is one of the first tissues to show dysfunction after injury as well as being significant in treatment, e.g. stretching. Like all connective tissue it consists of cross-linked, waves of collagen fibres in a gelatinous matrix. We can consider three layers:

1. **SUPERFICIAL** is a loose knit, fibroelastic, areolar tissue containing adipose tissue found connected to the underside of the skin. Because of its loose knit nature, fluid and other metabolites can accumulate and because of this a potential space is sometimes described as layer two.
2. **DEEP** is a tougher more resilient, restraining, tighter and more compact tissue than superficial. It surrounds, separates and compartmentalises internal visceral organs and muscles contributing to the contours of the body. It possesses two layers and is the most extensive. The peritoneum, pericardium and pleura are specialised elements of deep fascia. Found within this type of fascia are fat, nervous tissue (especially the pacinian corpuscles and skin receptors related to the rate of movement and acceleration), veins, capillary and lymphatic channels. The outer layer usually contains the fat and varies in thickness whilst the inner layer is thin and elastic. Compartment syndromes refer to problems relating to structures within the fascia/compartments being compressed because of increased pressure caused by trauma and overuse.
3. **SUBSEROUS** is loose areolar tissue covering the internal, visceral organs beneath the serous membrane. It lubricates their surfaces and contains small circulating channels. In simplicity, fascia is like a body stocking, connecting, enveloping and investing all the inside and outside body parts, i.e. the muscle's connective tissue envelope.

Fascia, can be palpated in sheaths or planes running on the surface of the body (iliotibial band); perpendicular to the body or bone (linea alba and nuchal ligament) and horizontally (diaphragm and pelvic floor).

Fascial Functions

- Transmits the force created by muscle fibres to tendons.
- Serves as a storehouse for water and fat.
- Insulates against loss of heat.
- Provides mechanical protection from blows.
- Lubricates without drag allowing movement between structures without causing irritation, friction or inflammation/heat and provides pathways (fascial planes).
- Supports vessels and nerves as they pass through the body.
- Reduces the effects of pressure and friction by the formation of bursal sacs.
- Contributes to the contour and function of the body.
- Provides fluid nutrition.
- Covers and supports the viscera.
- Part of reflex mechanisms, i.e. the pacinian corpuscles in the superficial fascia relating to the rate of relay afferent (sensory) messages and accelerations of movement.
- Provides a continuous, integrated reporting network throughout the body.
- Mechanoreceptors and proprioceptors constantly report movement and positional sense to the spinal cord and brain. These are found in the fascia, tendons, muscles and ligaments. This information is then used to produce a combination of intended and actual movement. The cerebrum decides what movement is needed to carry out an action. The message is then relayed to the cerebellum. The kinaesthetic and proprioceptive mechanisms in and around the joints relay messages to the cerebellum as to their positional sense, state, and condition. The result of these two factors brings about actual modified movement as to what is actually possible.
- Can respond to **DEFORMATION** by contracting and relaxing because of its elastic properties.
- Possesses **PLASTIC** (permanent) and **ELASTIC** (temporary, recoverable, transient) stretch properties, which relate to its elastic, spring recoil, viscous and hydraulic capabilities.
- It is continuous with specialised elements of fascia such as ligaments and tendons.
- It 'creeps', i.e. when extended and loaded it relaxes and has less resistance to further loading.
- It is '**STRAIN RATE DEPENDENT**', i.e. the faster it is stretched the more tension it develops, e.g. speed fast – stiffer less pliable, less elastic; speed slow – increased elasticity, pliability.
- It possesses a property known as **HYSTERESIS** – when stressed it looses energy and changes. Known as the 'hysteresis loop', this is the difference in mechanical energy used to stretch and elongate it and the energy used to return the tissue to its original resting length, i.e. stretch phase v relaxation phase.

When stressed, certain responses occur:

- **INFLAMMATORY RESPONSE**, which is easily absorbed in superficial fascia but not so in deep fascia causing changes. This is **PALPABLE**.
- **BIOMECHANICALLY**, depending on the amount or type of load, the number and type of collagen and elastic fibres. Deformation is temporary or permanent.
- Connective tissue injury is related to the ability of the receptors to adapt and the central nervous system to adjust.
- **BIOCHEMICAL AND IMMUNOLOGICAL CHANGES** occur within the ground substance gelatin leading to scar tissue. This effects support, movement and lubrication which can have long-term consequences, e.g. whiplash. The topic of scar tissue will be dealt with in Chapter 3.

Cartilage and Bone

There are three kinds of cartilage:
1. **HYALINE**, which means *glass*, is transluscent with a pearl-bluish tint in appearance. It is very elastic, cushiony and the most common cartilage. It covers the articular ends of bones and is also found in rings of the trachea and bronchi. It helps reduce friction, wear and tear between bone surfaces, whilst considerably improving ease of movement. One of the effects of exercise is to thicken the hyaline cartilage so that greater forces can be tolerated by the joint.
2. **ELASTIC** contains elastic fibres as well as collagen fibres thus offering elasticity as well as firmness. It maintains the shape of certain organs, e.g. external ear – pinna.
3. **WHITE FIBROCARTILAGE** contains more collagen fibres than the other two kinds and is elastic, flexible and taut and has great tensile strength. Fibrocartilage is found in the intervertebral discs, the knee (menisci) and the symphysis pubis. It is laid down to give greater stability to incongruent joint surfaces. Fibrocartilage however, is physiologically weaker than hyaline cartilage. Unlike bone cartilage it is avascular and is therefore a poor healer. Oxygen and nutrients reach the chondrocytes via diffusion.

Bone (osseus) tissue is typical of other connective tissue in that it consists of cells, fibres and extracellular material or matrix. However, its matrix is calcified. Bone consists of approximately 45% minerals such as calcium, phosphorus and carbonates; 30% organic material, mainly collagen and 25% water. Bone is not a completely solid structure and this gives it its strength.

Engineers/constructional workers inform us that hollow tubes are stronger than solid rods. All bone has spaces and a **nutrient foramen**, in its hard composition that provides channels for blood vessels bringing nutrient to the bone cells. The blood supply to a typical long bone is via the **nutrient artery** with a periosteal supply and vascular circle to the bone ends, **epiphysis**. The shaft of a long bone is known as the **diaphysis** that if sectioned longitudinally consists of a **central medullary cavity**, which is lined with a thin epithelial membrane, **endosteum**, and filled with marrow. Red marrow, named for its function in the production of erythrocytes, is located mainly in the epyphysis and the yellow marrow is marrow that has become saturated with fat. In children the medullary cavity contains only red marrow.

Osteoblasts are bone-forming cells, **osteoclasts** bone reabsorbing cells and **osteocytes** are mature bone cells. All bones are enclosed in a dense, white fibrous covering called the **periosteum**. It consists of two layers, an outer fibrous layer of connective tissue containing blood vessels, lymph vessels and nerves which enter into the bone and the inner, or osteogenic layer, consisting of elastic fibres, blood vessels and osteoblasts. Although the periosteum does not cover the articular ends of the bone, epiphysis (cancellous/soft bone) it continues over the joint itself to form the joint capsule.

Types of Bone

Bones can be:
- Hard/compact.
- Soft, spongy, cancellous.
- Long.
- Short.
- Flat.
- Irregular.
- Sesamoid.

Some bones have characteristics of more than one type. Bones perform various functions each one aimed at maintaining body homeostasis:

- Blood cell formation in the red marrow.
- Mineral reservoir/haematopoiesis.
- Protection.
- Shape and support.
- Aid movement.

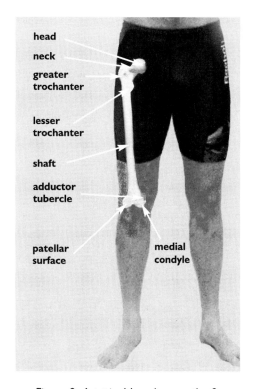

▲ *Figure 2. A typical long bone – the femur.*

Bone growth, development, healing and repair will be dealt with more in Chapter 3.

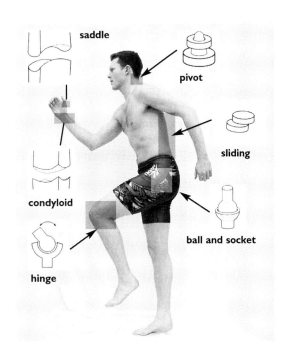

► *Figure 3.*
Different joints
found in the body.

Different Joints Found in the Body

1. Synarthrodial, fibrous or immovable joints, e.g. the sutures of the skull.
2. Amphiarthrosis, cartilaginous or partly movable joints, e.g. the lumbar vertebra.
3. Diathrosis, synovial or freely movable joints, e.g. the hip, the knee.

Classification of Synovial Joints

1. Plane or gliding joints, e.g. the carpals.
2. Saddle joints, e.g. the thumb.
3. Hinge joints, e.g. the knee.
4. Pivot joints, e.g. C1 and C2.
5. Ball and socket joints, e.g. the hip and the shoulder.
6. Condyloid or ellipsoid joints, e.g. the wrist.

Synovial Fluid and Lining

Synovial fluid is a transparent, viscous fluid, resembling the white of an egg, secreted by synovial membranes which acts as a lubricant for many joints, bursae and tendons. It contains mucin, albumin, fat and mineral salts. The synovial lining is thin, between one and three cells deep, highly vascular and rests on loose connective tissue, backed by muscle, fibrous capsule, tendon or fat. Eighty per cent of its surface is cellular with the remaining area, the interstitial space, being a highly permeable matrix.

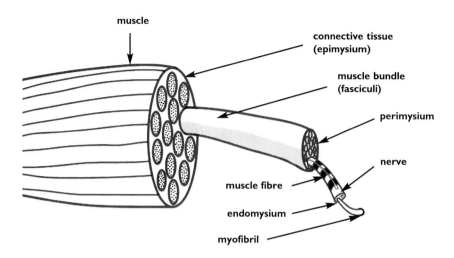

▲ *Figure 4. Cross-section of skeletal muscle.*

Contractile Tissue

There are three types of muscle tissue, the structure and function of which are the subject of a book on their own. Here and at various times throughout this book a little on the subject will be discussed.

1. **SKELETAL/STRIATED/VOLUNTARY** muscle is under the control of the will and is concerned with movement of the skeleton.
2. **INVOLUNTARY/SMOOTH/VISCERAL/UNSTRIATED** muscle is not under the direct control of the will and can be found in such places as the digestive, circulatory and respiratory tracts.
3. **HEART/CARDIAC/SLIGHTLY STRIATED/BRANCHED** muscle is highly specialised and can be found below the 3rd, 4th and 5th ribs on the left-hand side of the body.

Skeletal muscles have the ability to be:

*   **CONTRACTED**, they can only pull not push.
*   **EXTENDED**, as they are stretched because their partner is pulling.
*   **EXCITED** via a stimulus. A good blood and nerve supply is vital.
*   **RETURNED TO A NATURAL RESTING POSITION** because of their own and the connective tissue components elasticity.

Skeletal muscles work as groups and are controlled centrally not peripherally. The Central Nervous System (CNS) only responds to established **ENGRAM** patterns of movement. The motor system is a very complex, interactive system. It works:

- **AGONISTICALLY** to initiate movement.
- **SYNERGISTICALLY** to help and to control the agonist.
- **AS A FIXATOR** to hold in position or to fix unwanted movement, especially in biarticular muscles, which are more vulnerable to injury.
- **ANTAGONISTICALLY**, as one muscle or muscle group contracts (**AGONIST**) others allow the movement to take place and work as they are being stretched via the '**ALL OR NOTHING PRINCIPLE**'. This states that muscle fibres either contract totally or not at all. Not all fibres are contracted at once, as it depends on the workload.

The muscle belly fibres generate the force that is transmitted to the tendons via the fascial/connective tissue. The epimysium, perimysium and endomysium are the connective tissue element of muscles, which provides the resistance to stretch. Pre-stretching the muscle will pre-load it and takes up the slack. The cross-bridging of the **ACTIN** and **MYOSIN** increases with age therefore shortening the muscle.

When a muscle is stretched, the actin and myosin filaments are pulled apart and the overlap is reduced. If during movement a muscle is subjected to prolonged stretch or repeated stretching beyond its normal range, new actin and myosin filaments grow on the end of the muscle. This allows a greater overlap to be maintained. This is the **OVERLOAD PRINCIPLE OF TRAINING** (*see Chapter 2*).

Biarticular muscles act over more than one joint and are more prone to injury than monoarticular and demonstrate 'passive and active insufficiency'. This means that they cannot be actively contracted across both joints fully or stretched across both joints passively. Biceps and triceps brachii are biarticular muscles.

Isometric, Isotonic and Isokinetic Contraction

Continuing on from the 'all-or-nothing principle' we can start to consider how exercise, training and therapy regimes are developed related to our knowledge of how muscles work. These primarily are designed to improve **strength, suppleness/flexibility, stamina/endurance, speed/power, co-ordination, range/mobility of movement and cardiovascular fitness as well as assist the body to repair and recover after injury. They are also an integral part of examination and assessment. These areas are specialised areas of knowledge.**

Isometric Contraction (Active/Static)

A muscle does not need to alter its length when it contracts.

ISO – infers same/unchanged.
METRIC – refers to length.

Isometric contraction is when the overall length of the muscle stays the same. There is no movement at the joint but the muscle develops tension. This is very common and is seen when an attempt is made to move or lift an immovable object. The effort does not overcome the resistance/barrier. This is related to voluntary muscles working posturally to maintain position. This can be used to compare, assess and improve the tone and strength of muscles as well as help mobilising and improving the range and ease of movement.

In terms of rehabilitation after injury isometric contraction can be implemented early in the programme as this stimulates the nerve and blood supply without moving the joint therefore reducing the risk of further damage.

Isotonic Contraction (Active/Dynamic)

ISO – infers same/unchanged.
TONIC – means tone.

Isotonic contraction is when the length of a muscle does change and there is movement at the joint. The tone remains constant. In this type of contraction the muscle develops tension to overcome a resistance/barrier resulting in the moving of the body parts. It stimulates the Golgi tendon organ, a sensory nerve ending that is sensitive to both tension and excessive passive stretch of a skeletal muscle, better than isometric and comes in two forms:

1. **CONCENTRIC CONTRACTION.** The muscle actively shortens and thickens as the insertion moves towards the origin and the joint angle decreases. This is related to the agonist/prime mover. This kind of contraction can be considered as the accelerator.
2. **ECCENTRIC CONTRACTION.** The brake, the decelerator, because here the muscle is lengthening as it develops tension. The origin and insertion are pulled apart as the muscle resists and overcomes the movement/barrier. This is related to the antagonist and is brought about not because the muscles have been stimulated but partly because they have retained some contraction (muscle tone) and partly because of their recoil, elastic properties. This ensures a controlling effect (the brake) on agonist action. In concentric muscle action only about 25%

of the energy released via the oxidation process is converted into useful work. The rest, about 75%, raises muscle temperature. Whereas eccentrically, 90% is converted into useful work and only 10% converted into heat. This relates to voluntary muscles working phasically to take the joint into a position.

Isokinetic Contraction

ISO – infers same/unchanged.
KINETIC – is related to movement energy.

Isokinetic contraction is related to muscular contraction at a constant speed over the full range of movement. This requires machinery to apply the constant force/speed/resistance that matches that of the patient/athlete. The muscle tension remains high throughout. In isotonic contraction the force exerted by the patient/athlete varies throughout the full range of movement.

Range of Movement/Ease of Movement

As mentioned previously, these relate to **HOW FAR** and **HOW EASILY** and can be used in different contexts. Range of movement related to the musculoskeletal system is composed of three parts:

1. **FULL RANGE**. The muscle works from its extreme stretched position to its extreme contracted position.
2. **MID – INNER RANGE**. The muscle works from a position which is halfway between its two extremes of movement to its fullest contracted position. It is in this position that the muscles are working in their most contracted position which is the true position of strength. This is when body builders refer to 'bulking up'.
3. **OUTER RANGE**. The muscle works from its extreme stretched position to a point which is half way between its two extremes of movement. This doesn't so much strengthen as stretch/lengthen fibres which benefits overtight muscles. Overworking a muscle in this range may cause injury as it is usually at its most vulnerable in this position.

With relevance to rehabilitation after injury, the muscle work would involve:

- **ISOMETRICS**, so as not to aggravate the condition to improve tone.
- **ISOTONICS**, to improve the tensile strength of muscles.
- **ISOKINETICS**, if suitable equipment was available, to specifically target strengthening muscles through their full range.

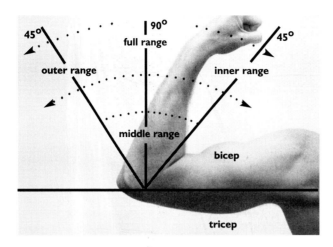

◀ *Figure 5.*
Range of
movement
related to the
musculoskeletal
system.

Ranges of Movement Related to Treatment

There are three generally accepted ranges of movement related to treatment:

1. **PAIN FREE.** Either the patient or therapist moves the joint and there is no resistance to such movement either because of 'blockages' or 'binding' or pain.
2. **STIFFNESS AND MINIMAL DISCOMFORT.** The joint is moved and such movement may cause minimal discomfort and feels restricted or 'stiff'.
3. **STIFFNESS AND PAIN.** The joint is moved and such movement feels stiff and in trying to overcome such stiffness definite pain is experienced.

To be safe and effective in sports therapy, (1) and (2) are acceptable; (3) is not. The challenge for the sports therapist is convincing the athlete that NO PAIN = MORE GAIN = YOUR GAIN.
Myk Hungerford, 1998

Ranges or Regions of Movements Related to the Myofascial Component

1. **TOE RANGE.** This is the pre-elastic, slack range. Taking out the 'kinks and curls' with no true elongation of collagen fibres.
2. **ELASTIC RANGE.** The physiological range. Creep deformation is transient. Stretch at the end of the elastic range will go into the plastic range because of the 'hysteresis loop', i.e. loading the tissue will change its properties.
3. **PLASTIC RANGE.** The anatomical range. Initially there is molecular displacement leading to micro tears and then to complete rupture. Once inside this range there is a loss of mechanical properties and any mechanical changes are irreversible. Elongation is permanent. It should now be seen how these different ranges of movement are interrelated and in what context they can be used in sports therapy.

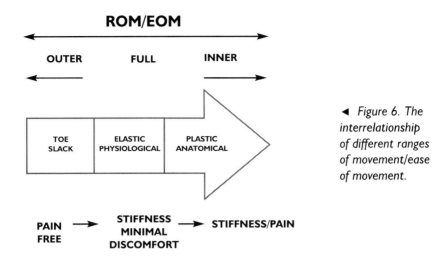

◄ Figure 6. The interrelationship of different ranges of movement/ease of movement.

Nervous Tissue

Co-ordinates and controls, together with the hormonal/endocrinal (chemical) system, bodily functions by initiating and transmitting nerve impulses. It possesses irritability and conductivity. The nervous system consists of the:

1. Central Nervous System (CNS) (brain and spinal cord) – grey matter (cell bodies), white matter (neurons).
2. Peripheral Nervous System – which can sometimes include the Autonomic Nervous System.
3. Sensory (afferent), motor (efferent) and mixed nerves.
4. Ganglia – a collection of cell bodies outside the CNS.
5. Plexus – a complete network of converging and diverging nerves, blood vessels and lymphatics.
6. Nerve endings – receptors.

A nerve cell is known as a **NEURON** that conducts impulses and **NEUROGLIA** are the special connecting and supporting cells related to the systems that do not conduct impulses. Morphology is the study/science of the structure and form of organisms.

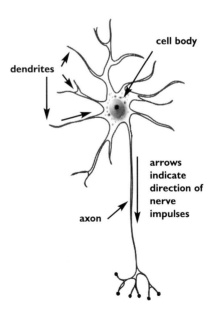

▲ Figure 7. A nerve cell is known as a neuron.

Cavities

The body is not a solid structure, but can be divided into cavities. There are three ventral cavities, i.e. in the front part of the body, and one dorsal cavity, i.e. in the back part of the body. These are sometimes sub-divided. The ventral cavities are:

Chest or Thoracic Cavity

This contains organs and vessels such as the lungs including left and right bronchus, left and right pleural cavities, the mediastinum in the mid portion containing the heart, the largest artery (aorta), and the two pericardial cavities, largest veins (venae cavae) the air pipe (trachea), and the food channel (oesophagus). There is also the thymus gland and various lymph nodes.

Abdominal Cavity

The **upper portion** contains the liver and its gall bladder, stomach, pancreas (sweetbread), spleen, kidneys and intestines.

The **lower portion** contains part of the large intestine and the reproductive organs according to gender. The cavity at the back part of the body, i.e. the dorsal cavity, may be considered as two compartments:

1. Cranial cavity, which lies in the skull and holds the brain.
2. Spinal cavity, which lies within the centre of the backbone or spine and contains the spinal cord.

Splanchnology is the study of the viscera and organs within the cavities of the body.

Membranes

These are made of either connective or epithelial tissue and line the cavities and hollow organs of the body. They also cover and protect body surfaces and anchor organs and structures to each other. Their cells form sheets that secrete fluid of varying viscosity and have various characteristics and functions. They can be classified as **connective**, which is the synovial membrane that secretes synovial fluid lining joints and cavities, and **epithelial** which are subdivided as:

1. **CUTANEOUS** or skin, one of the largest and most visible organs.
2. **SEROUS** which secretes serum fluid lining the heart and lungs. Parietal, is the actual wall-lining membrane that covers the cavity surface. Visceral refers to the thin membrane that covers the organ or viscera within a cavity.

3. **MUCOUS** which secretes mucous lining the oesophagus and trachea. Protects against mechanical or chemical abuse by cleaning, filtering and lubricating.

Membranes can be considered as selective or non-selective, permeable, or non-permeable, allowing or not allowing the process of **DIFFUSION** (passage of fluid/substance in and out of the cells). Membranes are subjected to all kinds of pressures and according to Dr. Dodds, 1989, diet can metabolically change the membrane over a three-month period, via fatty acid composition.

Systems

These are where organs of varying numbers and types are arranged to perform complex bodily functions. Various texts, publications and authorities, classify the systems according to a particular course of study. This means that the classifications may differ as several systems may be classed under one term. **However, it must be appreciated that whichever way they are classified, they do not work in isolation and are interrelated and interdependent.** For completeness an overview of the systems has been included to overcome any confusion. Obviously some systems are considered more important than others, but here the systems are listed in no order of priority/importance.

A. Skeletal

The skeletal system includes the bones of the body, their cartilages, the joints of the body and their ligaments. The scientific study of the bones is called osteology. The study of ligaments is called syndesmology and the meaning of this word has been extended to include the study of articulations and joints (arthrology) and so is sometimes referred to as the articulatory system.

B. Muscular

Muscular means all the muscles of the body. The study of muscles is called myology.

C. Respiratory

The respiratory system consists of the lungs and their air passages. Its function is to supply oxygen, remove carbon dioxide, and help to keep the blood in a very slightly alkaline condition i.e. regulate the acid – base balance of the body.

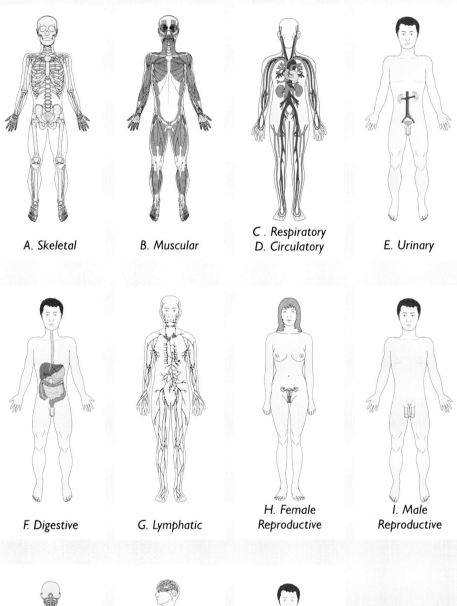

A. Skeletal

B. Muscular

C. Respiratory
D. Circulatory

E. Urinary

F. Digestive

G. Lymphatic

H. Female
Reproductive

I. Male
Reproductive

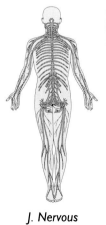

J. Nervous

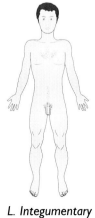

K. Endocrine

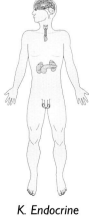

L. Integumentary

Figure 8.
The systems
of the body.

D. Circulatory (circulatory/cardiovascular)

The circulatory system is concerned with the heart (cardio-), the blood and lymph vessels (-vascular). Cardiology is the name given to the study of the heart and its functions. Angiology relates to the study of blood and lymph vessels. Haematology is the study of blood.

E. Excretory

The excretory system is the one whereby the body rids itself of gases, liquids and solids for which it has no further use, i.e. toxic waste material.

F. Digestive/Alimentary

The digestive/alimentary system is the one by which the food is changed physically and chemically for use by the cells. Strictly speaking it also relates to the elimination of waste by-products of digestion. The study of the stomach and intestines, in health and disease, is called gastroenterology. Nutrition involves ingestion, digestion, absorption, assimilation and elimination. **It is vital that the sports therapist appreciates the importance of nutrition in the healthy functioning of the human body and its significance in the fuelling of the athlete** (*see Chapter 1, Part 5; Chapter 2, Part 8; Chapter 3, Part 4 and Chapter 8, Part 1*).

G. Lymphatic

The lymphatic system is an extensive network of capillary vessels that transports the interstitial fluid of the body as lymph to the venous blood circulation. It plays a crucial role in maintaining appropriate fluid levels in the tissues as well as maintaining proper blood volume by ensuring that interstitial fluid is returned. This helps to keep the cardiovascular system working efficiently (*Wilmore, J., and Costill, D. L., 1994*).

H and I. Reproductive

The reproductive system consists of the male and female gonads, associated ducts and glands and the external genitalia that function in the procreation of offspring. In women these include the ovaries, fallopian tubes, uterus, vagina, clitoris and vulva. In men these include the testes, penis, prostrate gland, seminal vesicles, epididymis and vas deferens.

J. Nervous

The nervous system consists of the brain, spinal cord, nerves and the sense organs such as the ear. Neurology is the branch of medical science dealing with the nervous system both normal and in disease.

K. Hormonal

The hormonal/endocrine system consists of glands that produce chemical substances (hormones) which have a specific regulatory effect on the activity of certain cells or organs. The study of the endocrine system is called endocrinology.

L. Integumentary

The integumentary system provides and maintains the skin, its appendages and structures, e.g. hair, sweat oil (sebaceous) glands, eye, ear, mammary glands. The study of the diagnosis and treatment of skin disorders is called dermatology.

Anatomical Terminology

Position – Planes

In anatomy, the locations, positions, relationships and directions within the body are described in relation to the person, or subject, standing erect in a certain position, known as the **ANATOMICAL POSITION**. Left and right refer to the patient, not the observer (sports therapist). It is presumed that the subject is facing the observer with the arms by their side and the palms facing forward.

1. **ANTERIOR**. The front or near to the front view – sometimes known as **VENTRAL**.
2. **POSTERIOR**. The body back or near to the back view – sometimes known as **DORSAL/DORSUM**.

Terms of position and direction are usually along one of the major **BODY PLANES**.

3. **MEDIAN**. The midline dividing the body equally into left and right – sometimes known as **MIDSAGITTAL**.
4. **SAGITTAL**. Dividing the body into unequal left and right, parallel to the median plane.
5. **CORONAL/FRONTAL**. Dividing the body into equal/unequal front and back parts.
6. **TRANSVERSE**. Dividing the body into upper and lower body parts.

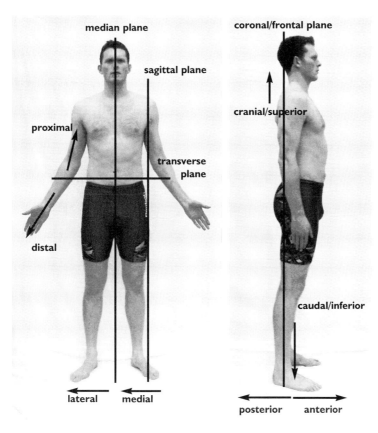

◄ *Figure 9.*
Anatomical
planes, directions
and positions.

Direction – Planes

Here are some more anatomical terms, together with, where applicable their opposites and reference to body planes:

1. **ANTERIOR OR VENTRAL, POSTERIOR OR DORSAL.** Usually used with reference to the coronal/frontal plane.
2. **SUPERIOR (CEPHALAD).** Towards the head. Mostly used in reference to structures of the trunk, e.g. the head is superior to the stomach.
3. **INFERIOR (CAUDAL/CAUDAD).** Towards the tail, away from the head. Again usually with reference to the trunk, e.g. the stomach is inferior to the head. The two are usually with reference to the transverse plane.
4. **MEDIAL.** Situated towards the midline of the body or a structure, e.g. the eyes are medial to the ears. Used with reference towards the midsagittal plane.
5. **LATERAL.** Situated away from the midline and is related to the side, e.g. the eyes are lateral to the nose. Used with reference away from the midsagittal plane. Both terms are usually used with reference to the sagittal plane.
6. **IPSILATERAL.** Situated on, or affecting the same side of the body, e.g. the left shoulder and heart can be considered as ipsilateral.

7. **CONTRALATERAL**. Situated on or affecting the opposite side of the body, e.g. the left and right shoulder are contralateral.

8. **PROXIMAL**. Nearer to the trunk or point of origin, e.g. the shoulder is proximal to the elbow.

9. **DISTAL**. Further from the trunk or point of origin, e.g. the hand is distal to the elbow.

10. **DEEP**. Towards the inside of a part, away from the surface, e.g. the muscles are deep to the skin.

11. **SUPERFICIAL**. Towards the outside of a part, peripheral, towards the surface, e.g. the skin is a superficial organ.

12. **PRONE**. Lying face down, a position of relative security.

13. **SUPINE**. Lying face up, a position of relative vulnerability.

Terminology Used When Describing/Relating to Bony Features

1. **BORDER**. A ridge of bone separating two surfaces. Usually provides muscle attachment.

2. **CANAL/MEATUS**. An opening or tunnel through any part of the body.

3. **SPINES/SPINOUS PROCESSES**. Sharp ridges, e.g. iliac crest.

4. **TROCHANTER/TUBEROSITY/TUBERCLE**. Broad roughened bony projections usually for the attachment of muscles or ligaments. Trochanters and tuberosites are larger, e.g. greater trochanter or femur, ischial/tibial tuberosity.

5. **FOSSA**. A depression.

6. **FORAMEN**. A hole through a bone, e.g. nutrient foramen. The small nutrient artery supplies the middle of the bone and passes through here.

7. **GROOVE**. Furrow on a bone eminence.

8. **CONDYLE**. Rounded bulging projection of bone which participates in a joint, e.g. tibial condyle.

9. **EPICONDYLE**. A blunt projection, lateral and medial from the condyles, e.g. medial epicondyle of femur.

10. **MALLEOLUS/MALLEOLI**. Rounded projections found at the distal end of the tibia and fibula.

Part 4

A Practical Journey Around the Lower and Upper Limb, Trunk and Spine

The following can be considered as a guideline to the minimum knowledge, skill and expertise that in the author's opinion, a sports therapist must know and possess in relation to practical issues.

Anatomical Areas of Special Consideration

There are areas of the body where nerves and blood vessels are relatively close to the skin surface and are not well protected by other tissues. Obviously a sports therapist needs to be aware of such sites when tissue handling during examination/assessment and treatment, e.g. deep massage to the areas could cause damage. Here are listed some such structures and areas in relation to the upper and lower limbs.

Lower Limb

- The popliteal artery/vein and common peroneal tibial nerve in the fossa at the back of the knee.
- The common peroneal nerve around the fibula head.
- The external iliac artery, femoral artery, great saphenous and femoral vein and femoral nerve located in the inguinal triangle.
- The sciatic nerve located in the sciatic notch ($^2/_3$ distance from PSIS to ischial tuberosity).
- Tibial artery and nerve located around posterior/inferior aspect of medial malleolus.
- The kidneys located in the thoracolumbar junction ($T_{12} - L_3$) either side of the spine.

Upper Limb

- The vagus nerve and nerves and vessels to the thyroid gland located in the anterior throat and sternal notch region.
- The carotid artery, jugular and vagus nerve located in the anterior triangle of the neck.
- The nerves of the brachial plexus, the brachiocephalic artery and vein (superior to the clavicle) and the subclavian arteries and vein, located in the posterior triangle of the neck.
- The cubital fossa bounded by the pronator teres, brachioradialis muscles. Its contents include the biceps tendon, brachial artery, median, radial/posterior interosseus nerves.
- McBurney's Point located in the right lower quadrant of the abdomen. An are associated with appendicitis and psoas spasm.
- The ulnar nerve of the medial epicondyle.
- The radial nerve at the lateral epicondyle.
- The brachial artery, axillary vein and artery, cephalic vein and nerves of the brachial plexus in the axillary region.
- The ulnar artery and nerve located in the Tunnel of Guyon.
- The median nerve located in the Carpal Tunnel.

Sports therapists must be able to locate and practically demonstrate a familiarity with bony points and soft tissues. This will enable them to acquire not only the necessary anatomical and theoretical knowledge but also the practical, tactile sensitivity that is vital when handling tissues during examination/assessments and treatment.

The Lower Limb – Bony Points/Ligaments

Lumbo/Sacral/Pelvic/Hip Region

1. Anterior superior iliac spine (ASIS).
2. Symphysis pubis.
3. Greater trochanter.
4. Ischial tuberosity.
5. Inguinal ligament.
6. Posterior superior iliac spine (PSIS).
7. Sacrum base and apex lumbosacral angle.

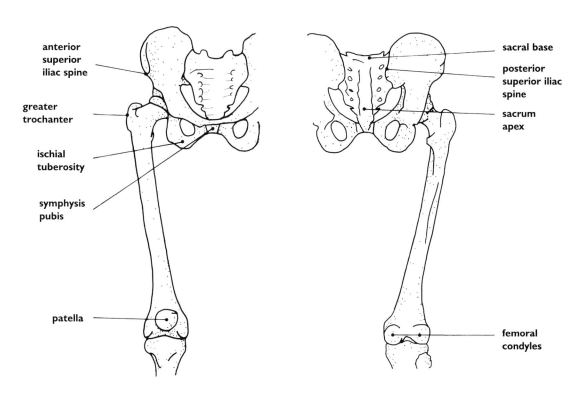

▲ Figure 10.   ▲ Figure 11.

Knee Region

1. Femoral condyles.
2. Patella.
3. Tibial condyles.
4. Edge of tibial plateau – knee joint line.
5. Head of fibula.
6. Medial collateral ligament.
7. Lateral collateral ligament.
8. Tibial tuberosity.

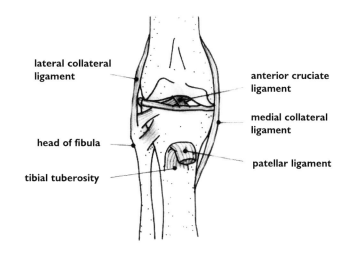

▴ *Figure 12.*

Lower Leg/ Ankle Region

1. Anterior border of tibia.
2. Medial border of tibia.
3. Calcaneus.
4. Medial malleolus.
5. Lateral malleolus.
6. Anterior talofibular ligament.
7. Calcaneofibular ligament.
8. Posterior talofibular ligament.
9. Deltoid ligament.

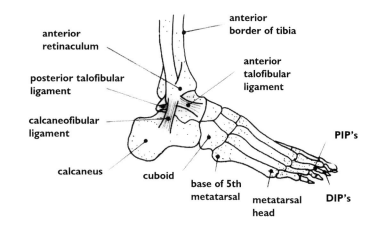

▴ *Figure 13.*

Foot

1. Base of 5th metatarsal.
2. Metatarsal heads.
3. Cuboid.
4. Distal and proximal interphalangeal joints (DIP's and PIP's).

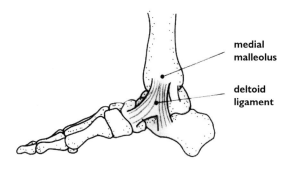

▴ *Figure 14.*

Surface Markings of Joints

Hip Joint

This is just inferior of the midpoint of the inguinal ligament (i.e. between the anterior superior iliac spine and pubic symphysis). The level of the greater trochanter is used to give an intersection on this line and a more accurate marking is a few centimetres inferior to this.

Knee Joint

The anterior margins of the tibial plateau are palpable. The joint line may be taken to be 1cm superior to the head of fibula and 2.5cm above the tibial tuberosity.

Ankle Joint and Foot

The anterior edge of the inferior articular surface is palpable. The joint line extends as a horizontal line drawn between a point 2.5cm above the tip of the lateral malleolus and 1cm above the tip of the medial malleolus. Interphalangeal joints of the foot – distal and proximal should be identified (DIP's and PIP's). Also the metatarsal phalangeal joints of the foot.

Range of Movement – Ease of Movement (Active, Passive and Resistive)

Sports therapists must be competent in moving and resisting limbs as they are going through their full range of movement and also in communicating to sports people what it is they want them to do in examination and treatment/rehabilitation. Getting sports people to do exactly what you want them to do and not what they think you want them to do is a skill in its own right. Movements possible at the:

Hip Joint

1. Flexion.
2. Extension.
3. Abduction.
4. Adduction.
5. Medial and lateral rotation.
6. Circumduction.

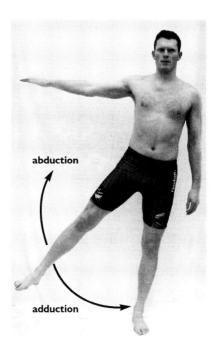

▲ *Figure 15. Range of movement of hip joint.*

Knee Joint

1. Flexion.
2. Extension.
3. Medial and lateral rotation as accessory movements caused by the foot when the knee is flexed.

Ankle Joint

1. Dorsiflexion.
2. Plantar flexion.

Subtalar Joint

1. Inversion.
2. Eversion.

Pronation and supination occur at the mid-foot and is a combined movement of plantar flexion, inversion and adduction and vice versa respectively. Abduction and adduction are secondary movements as a result of pronation and supination at the mid-foot.

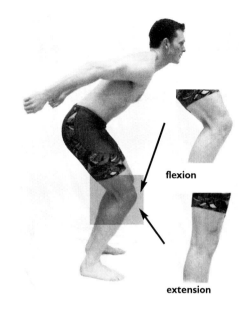

▲ Figure 16. Range of movement of knee joint.

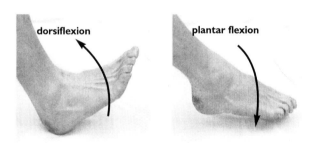

▲ Figure 17. Range of movement of ankle joint.

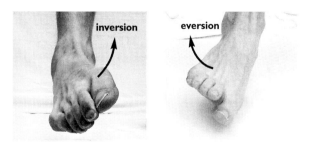

▲ Figure 18. Range of movement of subtalar joint.

Palpation of a Pulse

- Popliteal (difficult).
- Dorsalis pedis (difficult).
- Posterior tibial.
- Femoral.

The Upper Limb, Trunk and Spine – Bony Points/Ligaments

Shoulder Region

1. Greater tuberosity.
2. Coracoid process.
3. Clavicle – distal and proximal ends.
4. Acromion process.
5. The three parts of the sternum.
6. Xiphoid process/xiphisternum.
7. Sternal notch.
8. Sternal angle.
9. Inferior angle of scapula.
10. Spine of scapula.
11. Axillary and vertebral borders of the scapula. The ligaments related to the glenohumeral (G/H), acromioclavicular (A/C) and sternoclavicular (S/C) joints and the significance of the coracohumeral and glenohumeral ligaments in shoulder stability/instability.

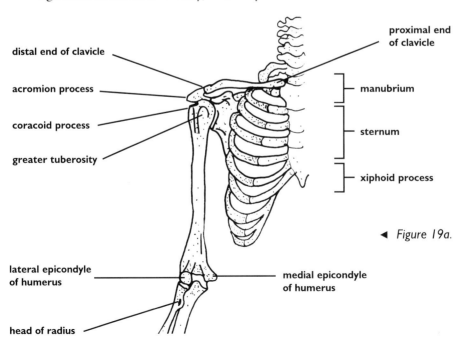

◄ Figure 19a.

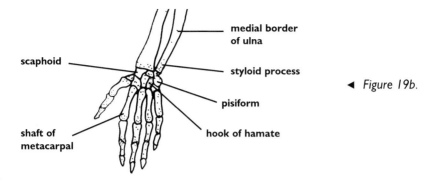

scaphoid

medial border
of ulna

styloid process

pisiform

hook of hamate

shaft of
metacarpal

◄ *Figure 19b.*

Elbow Region

1. Medial epicondyle of humerus.
2. Lateral epicondyle of humerus.
3. Olecranon process.
4. Head of radius.
5. Medial collateral ligament of elbow.
6. Lateral collateral ligament of elbow.
7. Annular ligament.

Wrist and Hand Region

1. Medial border of ulna.
2. Ulna styloid process.
3. Radial styloid process.
4. Lister's tubercle.
5. Pisiform.
6. Scaphoid and its significance in wrist injuries.
7. Shaft of metacarpal.
8. Head of metacarpal.
9. Hook of hamate.
10. Bones of the wrist and hand.
11. Ligaments of the wrist and hand are numerous and complex. However, their names and the anterior and posterior retinaculum should be known.
12. Describe and locate the anatomical snuffbox.

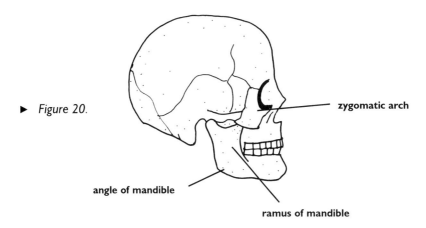

► *Figure 20.*

zygomatic arch

angle of mandible

ramus of mandible

Head, Spine and Trunk Region

1. Anterior superior iliac spine (ASIS) (*see page 42*).
2. Posterior superior iliac spine (PSIS) (*see page 42*).
3. Angle of mandible.
4. Zygomatic arch.
5. Ramus of mandible.
6. Differentiate between the spinous processes (SP's) of C2, C6, C7, T1; SP's of T4, T7, T9; SP's T12, L1; SP's L4, L5, S1 and their approximate relationship to areas of surface anatomy, e.g. iliac crest, last rib etc.

Surface Markings of Joints

Glenohumeral (G/H)

Anteriorly, the joint line is concave and lies laterally three centimetres long from the lateral border of the coracoid process. Posteriorly, it is a concave line, three centimetres long down and medially from the acromion process. The glenoid fossa faces anteriorly and laterally.

Sternoclavicular (S/C)

This is easily seen and felt at the proximal end of the clavicle. Three centimetres long, the line of this joint traces out the clavicular notch of the manubrium of the sternum.

Acromioclavicular (A/C)

Easily seen and felt at the distal end of the clavicle.

Temperomandibular (TMJ)

Anterior to the tragus of the ear.

Elbow

A three/four joint complex comprising of the humero ulnar, humero radial, proximal radial/ulnar, distal radial/ulnar joint. A two centimetres line below and joining the medial and lateral epicondyles of the humerus. It slopes downwards, lateral to medial.

Radio Carpal/Wrist (R/C)

A concave line distally between the radial and ulnar styloids.

Metacarpophalangeal Joint/Knuckle (MCP)

Easiest seen on the index finger, it lies between the head of the metacarpal and the base of the proximal phalanx.

Interphalangeal – Distal and Proximal (DIP's and PIP's)

These are the joint lines found between the phalanges.

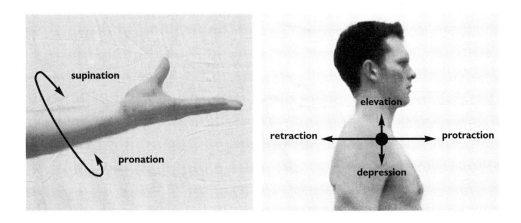

▲ Figure 21a and b. Further ranges of movement: (a) elbow; (b) shoulder girdle.

Range of Movement/Ease of Movement (Active, Passive and Resistive)

- Movements possible at the glenohumeral joint are up to 90° flexion, extension, abduction, adduction, medial and lateral rotation and circumduction.
- At the shoulder girdle they are elevation, depression, protraction and retraction.
- At the shoulder complex, movements are a combination of glenohumeral and girdle movements through elevation (above 90°).
- At the elbow they are flexion, extension, pronation and supination.
- At the wrist (radial carpal) and hand they are flexion, extension, radial deviation, ulnar deviation and flexion and extension, adduction and abduction of the fingers.
- At the thumb they are flexion, extension, abduction, adduction, circumduction and opposition.

The importance of the thumb in movements of the hand should be known.

Palpation of a Pulse

- Radial. On the palmar, radial aspect of the lower arm near to the styloid process.
- Carotid. Inside the sternocleidomastoid muscle, next to the trachea/oesophagus, in the anterior triangle of the neck.
- Brachial. Halfway down the axillary aspect of the upper arm.

Muscle Testing Lower and Upper Limb, Trunk and Spine

Sports therapists must be able to practically demonstrate safe competence in muscle testing, to identify the muscles integrity regarding strength, power etc. (*see Chapter 4, Part 2*). To assist this the therapist needs to answer the following questions before carrying out the practical tests:

- Which range would be best to test the muscles in and why?
- What would be the starting position for such tests?
- Which are the main biarticular muscles in the lower limb and what is the significance of such muscles?

Muscles/Tendons of the Foot and Ankle

1. Gastrocnemius (two heads).
2. Soleus.
3. Achilles tendon.
4. Tibialis anterior (tendon and belly).
5. Tibialis posterior.
6. Extensor hallucis longus.
7. Extensor digitorum longus.
8. Extensor digiti minimi.
9. Peroneus (longus, brevis and tertius).

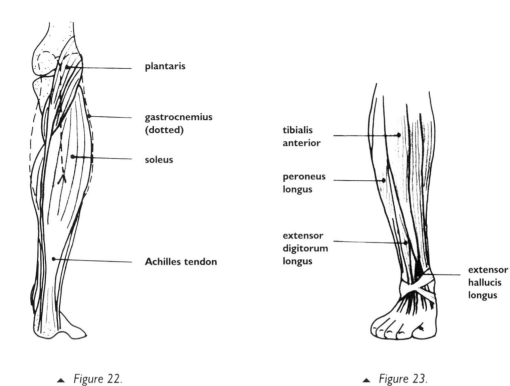

▲ *Figure 22.*

▲ *Figure 23.*

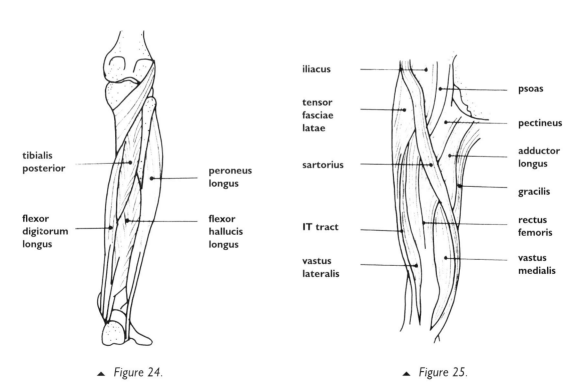

▲ *Figure 24.*

▲ *Figure 25.*

Muscles/Tendons of the Knee

1. The quadriceps as a group and individually.
2. Vastus medialis and the significance of this muscle during extension of the knee.
3. The hamstrings as a group and individually.
4. Identify the hamstring tendons at the posterior knee.
5. The hamstrings working over the hip and the knee.

Muscles/Tendons Related to the Hip

1. Psoas/iliacus.
2. Gluteus maximus.
3. Gluteus medius and minimus.
4. Quadriceps – rectus femoris.
5. Hamstrings.
6. Iliotibial tract.
7. Tensor fasciae latae.
8. Piriformis.
9. Adductors as a group: adductor brevis, adductor longus and adductor magnus.

Sports therapists should be familiar with the neurology of the lower limb relevant to the musculature, i.e. the lumbosacral plexus and the dermatomal distribution.

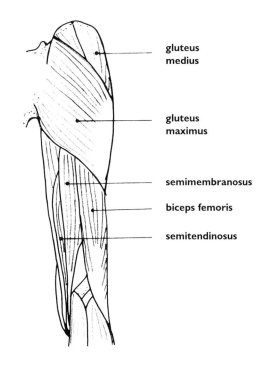

gluteus medius

gluteus maximus

semimembranosus

biceps femoris

semitendinosus

▲ Figure 26.

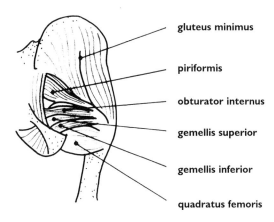

gluteus minimus

piriformis

obturator internus

gemellis superior

gemellis inferior

quadratus femoris

▲ Figure 27.

Muscles/Tendons of the Shoulder Region (G/H and Scapula)

1. Supraspinatus.
2. Deltoids (anterior/mid/ posterior aspects).
3. Biceps brachii.
4. Triceps brachii.
5. Anconeus.
6. Coracobrachialis.
7. Serratus anterior.
8. Trapezius – upper – middle – lower fibres.
9. Rhomboids.
10. Subscapularis.
11. Teres major.
12. Latissimus dorsi.
13. Pectoralis major – clavicular, sternal and all fibres.
14. Pectoralis minor.
15. Levator scapulae.
16. Infraspinatus.
17. Teres minor.

Muscles of the Spine and Trunk

1. Levator scapulae.
2. Latissimus dorsi.
3. Erector spinae – spinalis, longissimus and iliocostalis.
4. Abdominals – rectus.
5. Internal obliques.
6. External obliques.
7. Quadratus lumborum.
8. Sternocleidomastoid.
9. Trapezius – upper, middle and lower fibres.
10. Cervical neck musculature/ anterior triangle, splenius capitis, scalenus.

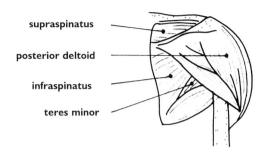

▲ *Figure 28.*

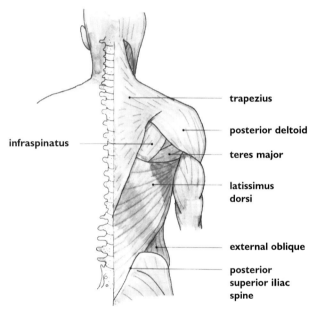

▲ *Figure 29a.*

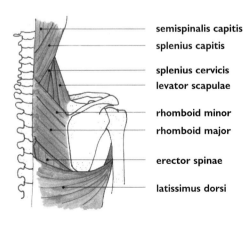

▲ *Figure 29b.*

Muscles/Tendons of the Elbow Region

1. Flexors of elbow – biceps, brachialis, brachioradialis.
2. Pronators (pronator teres/ quadratus).
3. Supinators (supinator/biceps brachii).

Muscles of the Wrist, Hand, Fingers, Thumb

1. Extensors of the wrist as a group (extensor carpi radialis, longus and brevis, extensor carpi ulnaris, extensor digiti minimi, extensor digitorum, extensor indicis).
2. Flexors of the wrist as a group – superficial, which flex the finger ends and deep/profundus, which flex the rest of the fingers (palmaris longus, flexor carpi ulnaris, flexor carpi radialis, flexor digitorum profundus and the four lumbricals, flexor digitorum superficialis).
3. Grips – power/grip, precision/pen, hook and key.
4. Thenar eminence (opponens pollicis, abductor pollicis brevis, flexor pollicis brevis, adductor pollicis).
5. Hypothenar eminence (opponens digiti minimi, abductor digiti minimi, flexor digiti minimi brevis, flexor digiti minimi).
6. Interossei – adductors and abductors of the fingers – **PADS** (3)/**DABS** (4).
7. Thumb – (extensor pollicis longus and brevis, adductor pollicis longus, flexor pollicis longus, opponens pollicis).

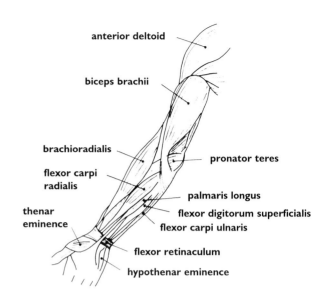

anterior deltoid
biceps brachii
brachioradialis
pronator teres
flexor carpi radialis
palmaris longus
thenar eminence
flexor digitorum superficialis
flexor carpi ulnaris
flexor retinaculum
hypothenar eminence

▲ *Figure 30.*

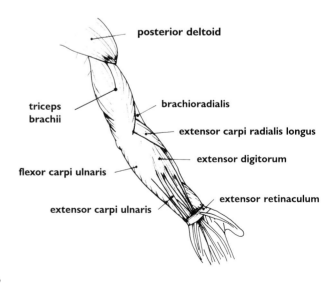

posterior deltoid
triceps brachii
brachioradialis
extensor carpi radialis longus
extensor digitorum
flexor carpi ulnaris
extensor retinaculum
extensor carpi ulnaris

▲ *Figure 31.*

8. Muscles responsible for ulnar deviation – (extensor carpi ulnaris/flexor carpi radialis).
9. Muscles responsible for radial deviation – (extensor carpi radialis, longus and brevis, flexor carpi radialis).

Sports therapists should be familiar with the neurology of the upper limb relevant to the musculature, i.e. the brachial plexus and the dermatomal distribution.

Tunnels of the Wrist and Hand

1. Carpal.
2. Guyon.
3. Extensors (6).

Part 5

Sports Injuries – Research/Epidemiology, Classification, Causes and Risk Reduction

The subject of sports injuries is a huge task and attempting to do it justice inevitably leads to aspects of the topic and specific, named injuries being omitted and information duplicated. Each injury/joint/sport can warrant a text in its own right and frequently does and so therefore the author has not attempted to discuss the multitude of specific sports-type injuries, other than to provide an overview of the common upper and lower limb injuries (*see Appendix 2*). Choosing instead, to refer the reader to the many excellent texts on each subject. **The topic will be approached from the point of view of why do injuries occur, how are they classified and how can the risks be reduced?** After all, prevention is better than cure and if it is accepted that **CURE** means complete and permanent relief of symptoms together with a return to normality, then very few injuries are ever cured to everyone's satisfaction.

Many injuries that are labelled sports injuries can so easily happen elsewhere other than in the sporting environment. The initial reaction (inflammation) and subsequent repair (healing) responses will be triggered irrespective of where and how the injury takes place. Many 'tennis elbows' can be found in people associated with the building trade, many of whom have never played tennis, squash, badminton or golf. However, there are people who think that a sprained ankle acquired whilst gardening has different characteristics, other than severity, to one obtained playing football.

There is, however, one definite, significant difference and that is the injured persons' knowledge, experience, beliefs, faith, perceptions, anticipation, needs and expectations, which, as we shall see later, are important elements in recovery. For this reason the term sports-type injuries is sometimes used. After all, the diagnosis is only a label that is based on information supplied, related to the signs and symptoms associated with a type of pain and gives no indication of the cause, other than what is obvious. The treatment of such injuries is dependent on many variables depending on which text, therapy or philosophy one subscribes to – allopathic or complementary. Both have a valid place in the total health care of the individual. However, a little knowledge/learning can be dangerous and many in sport try to increase their esteem by diagnosing injuries and passing on treatment/rehabilitation tips that for some could prove disastrous. Remember that we are dealing with individuals. At all levels in sport there appears to be conflicting 'so called' facts. What is not in dispute is that many injuries can be avoided. Let us consider pertinent issues as to why this is so.

Research and Epidemiology (Data Collection and Analysis)

In the quest for knowledge and the identification of problems, the collection and analysis of data are important aspects of the extension of such knowledge. Meaningful research is not simple but offers substantial and an existing supplement to practice. Although there are many definitions and types, research can be considered as:

> **"a formal, systematic, intensive process of carrying out a scientific method of analysis for the purpose of discovery and development of an organised body of knowledge."**
> *Professor L. Goldstone, 2001*

With scientific method involving formulation, observation, data collection, analysis and drawing of conclusions to substantiate a hypothesis related to an identified problem. Various design methods can be used ranging from the use of the classical trial v's control group type of research, through surveys to epidemiological, correlation studies. With epidemiology being considered as:

> **"The study of the distribution and determinants of varying rates of diseases, injuries or other health states in human populations for the purpose of identifying and implementing measures to prevent their development and spread."**
> *Caine and Lindner, 1996*

In simplicity, the study of causes, risks, promotion and prevention of health in populations. However, such studies should be viewed in perspective and not seen as absolute fact. According to Caine and Lindner, 1996, some of the questions that are asked relating to sports injuries are:

- Is the risk of injury greater in some sports than others?
- What types of injuries are most common in a given sport?
- What is the average time lost from injury and what is the risk of permanent impairment?
- Are some athletes more injury prone than others?
- Are particular physical or psychological characteristics associated with greater risk of injury?
- How can injury be predicted or prevented?
- How effective are the preventative measures that are implemented?

In looking at these and other questions, two types of epidemiology can be considered:

- **Descriptive, involving – How** many injuries, **Who** (person factors), **Where** (place factors), **When** (time factors) and **What** is the outcome (prognosis factors).
- **Analytical, involving – Why and How** – both causal factors.

It is also important that not only is the type of research being carried out considered but also its terms of reference. **Therefore when looking at statistics/research many variables should be considered.**

Professor Goldstone, 2001, in trying to answer the question; 'What makes for good research?' talks of **QUANTITATIVE** and **QUALITATIVE** variables and the need for **EQUIVALENT QUALITY** so that direct comparisons can be made. Such issues could be:

1. **Who** is conducting the research? i.e. governing body, doctor, physiotherapist, coach, trainer, administrator, etc. Each will have their own invested interest as to, 'the picture to be painted'.

   "95% of chronic diseases in Western Society can be treated with appropriate exercise and dietary advice."
   Rowlands, D. S., 1997

Clearly certain other interested parties involved in the treatment of injuries may want to challenge this. In February 1998 the Sports Council considered 13 sports and identified 19 million sports injuries a year with 1.4 million serious enough to be off work an average of 6 days. One quarter of these 19 million injuries were attributed to football, with skiing, running and keeping fit (aerobics, Tai Chi, etc.) the sports presenting the least injuries.

What/why is there a need and or purpose of such research? Was it to promote, to denigrate, to highlight, to expand the body of knowledge, for qualification, etc?

Evidence-based Medicine (EBM) as opposed to **anecdotal, 'unverified methods'** (*Macdonald, 2000*), is justified on the basis of proving the efficacy of a particular branch of medicine by objectivity and justified opinion, rather than subjectivity and unjustified opinion.

> **"Moving away from decisions based on opinion, past practice and precedent towards making more use of science research and evidence to guide decision-making."**
> *Walshe, K., 1995*

However,

> **"Lack of evidence doesn't necessarily equate to no evidence, it may be no evidence yet,.....evidence may be weak, or the quality of the study poor and thus no useful conclusions can be made."**
> *McLune, T., 2000*

It can also be argued that such an approach is not holistic and ignores other useful forms of evidence such as:

- Clinical experience, past and present.
- Commonsense.
- Insight and intuition of both practitioner and patient.
- Knowledge of anatomy, physiology, psychology, etc.
- Past practice and precedent.
- Life experience and philosophy (*Wickham, S., 1999*).

1. What is important – the **PROCESS** or the **OUTCOME** or both?
2. When was the research conducted – is it still relevant today?
3. Where was the research carried out – accident and emergency unit in hospital, physiotherapy department, sports clinic, private practice, club situation? This has significance for the practical relevance of such research as therapists don't generally treat people in science laboratories.
4. What are the terms of reference of such research, i.e. their definitions and designs?

"An injury is the sudden or excessive stress applied to a bodily part
which generates forces in excess of tolerable loads."
Smith, G. N., 1990

"Any impediment physical or mental that prevents peak performance."
Troop, R., 1999

An injury can sometimes be classified in simple terms because the player said it was,
or in terms of abnormal movement patterns imposed on the musculoskeletal
system. Medically it is viewed as cellular damage. All of these definitions will
provide statistically different results. Remember figures can be made to say what
they want in the hands of a good statistician.

"Even the best research if used inappropriately will not be a useful tool
in informed clinical decisions."
Green, J., 2000

This is not meant to imply people purposely distort the figures, although history
has discredited some studies and researches, but to highlight the fact that **all
evidence should be viewed in totality and not isolation**. Research data in
relation to soft tissue injury, according to the Association of Chartered
Physiotherapists in Sports Medicine (ACPSM), can be based upon:

- **Biological evidence**, providing a rationale based on an identification of a
  symptom and application of a therapy which is known to reverse that
  mechanism.
- **Empirical evidence**, relating to the valid, clinical evidence of the efficacy of
  such treatment, based on randomised, controlled trials.

Today, randomised controlled trials are the gold standard considered but an
increasingly popular and reliable form of trial is the 'meta-analysis', whereby the
results of a number of trials are pooled for communal analysis (*Isabel Walker, 2001*).

However,

"No scientific study can ever 'prove' anything; scientific research
merely provides evidence to support or reject various hypothesis."
Bledsoe, J., 1999

The above statement referred to certain claims being made about a particular
performance drink which where subsequently found to be flawed.

Convention, which relates to the argument, 'I've always done it that way', is:

> **"A socially powerful but intellectually weak dimension."**
> *Bogduk and Mercer, 1995*

Rudolph Flesch, an American author in communication skills says:

> **"Creative thinking may just be the realisation that there is no particular virtue in doing things the way they have always been done."**
> And:

> **"Unthinking clinging to tradition and precedent is inexcusable."**
> *Green, J., 2000*

It also follows that convention is not necessarily the safest and most effective way. **Certain sports are sometimes guilty of thinking that just because it has always been done that way then that is the only way.** Distinctions between **EXPERTISE** and **DUPLICATION** become blurred.

Consensus is agreement by experts in the absence of scientific evidence in the literature, based on experience and/or assumptions in such literature.

To be a safe, effective, efficient, caring, compassionate, communicating, problem-solving sports therapist who provides the best possible healthcare for any individual, at that moment in time, needs to question, review and analyse **HOW, WHAT** and **WHY** they do what they do. Continuing professional development should be about quality of experience, including reviewing, questioning, analysing and reflecting on practice and not necessarily just about quantity, by attending another course/workshop. Reflection should be an essential part of personal and professional development and all therapists, allopathic and complementary, must engage in it from time to time. This should increase their awareness of why they do what they do without causing 'paralysis from analysis' (*Dr. Simon Jenkins, 2000*). However:

> **"If people go on believing that they 'know', it makes it impossible to teach them."**
> *Alexander*

Injury Classification – Mechanism

A consideration of the Williams (1985) classification of injuries, based on the mechanism of injury, is particularly useful when considering why injuries occur and therefore how they can be avoided. There is often a difference between what sports people try to do and what they actually do which leads to injury.

INJURY	INCIDENTAL	INTRINSIC	(e.g. pulled muscle, ruptured tendon)
		INDIRECT	
	TRAUMATIC	EXTRINSIC	(e.g. bang on/blow to head, fractured wrist in a fall from some apparatus)
		INTRINSIC	(e.g. Achilles tendonitis, stress fracture of tibia)
	OVER-USE	DIRECT	
		EXTRINSIC	(e.g. blister on gymnast's hand, pressure/irritation)

Soft tissue can be loaded/damaged by the forces of:

1. **COMPRESSION**. To compact/crush, e.g. haematoma.
2. **TENSION**. To pull apart, e.g. strain/sprain.
3. **SHEARING**. To compress and tension, e.g. torn menisci.
4. **BENDING**. To overstress/stretch, e.g. strain/sprain.
5. **ROTATION**. To compress and twist beyond the 'norm' causing soft tissue spasm.

Compression and tension are the two main modes with the others being combinations of these two (*Lederman, 1997*).

Damage to hard, bony tissues can be caused by:

1. **TRAUMA** (Direct/indirect).
2. **FATIGUE**.
3. **STRESS**.
4. **PATHOLOGY**.

To reiterate by analysing the mechanism of an injury we might be able to implement measures to avoid them. This has significance not only in examination and assessment but also in planning and preparation.

Injury Classification – Physiology

Classifying injuries by looking at the body's natural response, healing and repair mechanisms, i.e. physiology, can help during treatment (*see Chapters 3 and 5*). However, time scales should be considered as a guideline.

1. **ACUTE** can be considered as the first 24–48 hours involving the inflammatory response but this period can last up to 5–6 days.
2. **SUB-ACUTE** is post-acute and lasts anything from 5–21 days until resolution, or until it becomes;
3. **CHRONIC** which is related to a non-resolved, sub-acute injury. Texts refer to this stage in terms of long duration not severity and give timings ranging from 24–48 hours, several days to weeks and beyond. The reasons for an injury not resolving and becoming chronic will be discussed during Chapters 3 and 5.

Aetiology – Causes and Considerations of Injury and Re-injury

- Personal egos and insecurities/lack of interpersonal, communication skills.
- Lack of fitness/condition – physical and mental health.
- Individual differences.
- Selection, screening and monitoring.
- Insufficient warm-up/cool down.
- Fatigue.
- U-factors.
- Changing sport/venue and training surfaces.
- Diet and nutrition.
- Ignoring the body's warning signs **PAIN – HEAT – FLUID BALANCE**.
- Going back to sport too early after injury – insufficient rehabilitation.
- Incorrect footwear, clothing, equipment, protection and proprioception.
- Over-enthusiastic, ill-advised, misguided, ineffective, ignorant adults.
- Misinterpretation/manipulation of the rules of the game.
- Inappropriate treatment/rehabilitation.
- Lack of discipline/boredom/control.
- Poor training techniques.

Personal Egos and Insecurities/Lack of Interpersonal, Communication Skills

A chain is only as strong as its weakest link. The cause and re-occurrence of injury is rarely a result of bad luck. It is more commonly the inevitable result of inefficient, ineffective medical management and an unsatisfactory relationship amongst athlete, manager, coach, trainer, 'therapist', doctor and anyone else involved in the athletes welfare. Poor communication and a reticence to 'let go' of a power base to 'allow-in' superior skills and expertise leads to 'the team' only being as strong as its weakest link. Here we are very much returning to the theme of sporting mentality. The author has personally had to treat six hamstring strains and two coccyx skin burns after an 'over-enthusiastic' training session given by several 'qualified coaches', none of whom had a current first aid qualification, but who certainly didn't think the physiotherapist had anything to offer in training.

Lack of Fitness/Condition – Physical and Mental Health

Being fit doesn't necessarily mean being healthy. Over-training can compromise the immune system (*see Chapter 2*). A person's level of fitness, which is allied to a person's aerobic and anaerobic capacity can be considered under the aspects of:

- Suppleness/flexibility/mobility – joint and muscle specific.
- Strength – agonist/concentric; antagonist/eccentric ratio.
- Speed/power – anaerobic.
- Endurance/stamina – cardiovascular/aerobic.
- Co-ordination/skill/balance/proprioception.

As well as being physiologically well, a person needs to be psychologically fit and so therefore **SPIRIT** is sometimes included in the factors of fitness. If a person is not in the right frame of mind this can lead to poor discipline and breakdown in the skill through lack of concentration. Fitness reduces injury risk in two ways:

1. By the effect it has on muscles, tendons and joints.
2. By increasing general stamina so that participants can compete for the whole duration of competition without fatigue and its risks.

The challenge is how to produce elite performance without breakdown (*Read. M., 1992*).

Anatomically and physiologically:

- The size of levers (length of limb).
- Percentage of body fat.
- Percentage type of muscle tissue and how they are energised will impose a natural limit to training no matter what is done.

Muscles can be considered as:

1. **TYPE 1.** Postural/slow twitch, which are energised via the oxidative/glycolysis, aerobic system.

2. **TYPE 2**. Phasic/fast twitch, which are energised via the **phosphagen**, anaerobic system; or via the **glycolytic**, anaerobic system.

To a large extent the human body is born with equal amounts of the type 1 and 2 muscle fibres but training can affect the length, width and characteristics of type 2, especially the glycolytic which represents approximately 20% of the total. This obviously has nutritional implications as to how the body is fuelled and the specificity of the training.

- Your level of fitness is in direct proportion to the frequency, intensity and duration of training. The re-occuring theme of **QUALITY v QUANTITY**.
- How many injuries are caused through inappropriate training procedures, where these three factors have not been adequately considered?
- Thinking that you can play yourself into shape is a good way to extend or cause injury. **Get fit for your sport and don't play your sport to get fit.**
- **You should never train with a temperature** (it is more serious than a cold, low resistance/feeling off) or with aching muscles due to fever. In these circum stances your body is far more vulnerable to injury and not in the best condition to self-repair. If you are ill or have been ill you should ensure you are fully recovered before returning to sport. An elevated body temperature can lead to myocarditis (*see Chapter 2, Part 3*).

Up to 4 days rest will not seriously affect your fitness and your cardiovascular fitness should be fine for 7–10 days.

Individual Differences

In simplicity, this is the fascination and frustration of being a sports therapist and the theme that runs throughout not only this section but also the whole of this book. That is, no two people are the same and to put them all together in one group and treat them as such is biologically inaccurate. Therefore there needs to be some logical, practical way of selecting and grouping individuals if accidents and injuries are to be minimised.

Selection, Screening and Monitoring

People working in sport will, at some stage, come across a mismatch of people to sport where the wrong people are involved in the wrong sport. This has much to do with adult and peer group pressures at too early an age without forgetting the subtle and persuasive powers of the media and advertising. At the other end of the spectrum there are some people who think they can ignore the ageing process and still play at the level and intensity they played years ago when their body is telling them they can't. Issues such as exercise addiction and habits of dedication and obsession now enter the equation (*see Chapter 2, Part 1*). Also we can return to the re-occurring theme of sporting mentality as to peoples motives, both young and old, for entering the sporting arena. Therefore, to re-iterate there needs to be some logical, practical way of selecting and grouping individuals if accidents and injuries are to be minimised.

Insufficient Warm-up/Cool Down

Athletes at all levels of sport, whilst openly extolling the virtues of this vital aspect of exercise, will practically pay scant regard to it. Some coaches even list this issue as one of the main causes of sports injuries, which seems ironic when it should be designed to reduce the incidence.

Warm-up is a systemic and comprehensive balance of physiological, psychological and neurological components that should be performed in a precise sequence that progresses from relaxed, general to highly technical skills. This development also requires a gradual progression of physical exertion.

This progression gradually narrows the athlete's focus until a deep concentration on the skill exists. Once the athlete has elevated their physical, psychological and neurological capabilities they are more likely to focus in on the training and/or competition objective in a more relaxed and physically, efficient manner. Warm-up prepares the athlete mentally and physically for performance and is most beneficial in sports requiring speed, strength, endurance and skill (*Karvonen, 1992*).

Physiologically

Muscle and blood temperature increases (*de Vries, 1986; Plowman and Smith 1997; Shellock and Prentice, 1985*). As a result of this temperature increase, metabolic rate and enzymatic activity are enhanced improving substrate utilisation (*Martin, et al., 1975*). The blood supply to/from the muscles increases. A transport system is necessary to bring nutrients to the area and waste products away from the area. Muscle contractions depend on temperature. In human beings, lowering of the muscle temperature below normal decreases muscle irritability and work capacity (*Karpovich*). Cold muscles are relatively stiff and if stretched vigorously may be injured (*Ciullo and Zarins, 1983*).

Warm-up produces more powerful muscle contraction (*Martin, et al., 1975*) as nerve impulses travel faster in warm muscle (*Karvonen, 1992*). A warm muscle is less viscous therefore contraction is easier and more efficient. A viscous muscle can cause irritation and rubbing of fibres. Passive means are helpful but to attain optimum temperature, active, dynamic work is called for. Warm-up reduces stiffness, improves range of movement and protects against unexpected movement (*Lehmann, et al., 1970*).

The stretching of connective tissue in the warm-up allows for greater range of motion and speed not to mention strength, endurance, balance and agility. Stretching as part of the warm-up is to prepare the athlete for exercise and possibly reduce injury whereas stretching to improve flexibility is to increase range of movement and ease of movement over a longer period.

The question needs to be asked **why are you doing that and what are you hoping to achieve?** Especially with the variety and multiplicity of lengthening/stretching methods/techniques that exist today, each with their claims and counter claims, it is **vital** that the sports therapist is comfortable and prepared for such a question. In itself stretching does not increase core temperature and so should not be considered in isolation but as part of the warm-up regime, following cardiovascular activity to raise heart rate and temperature. In practice slow, controlled, as opposed to ballistic stretching, in which there is a greater risk of injury especially in the young performer, is required for a minimum of 15–30 seconds (*Smith 1994; Bandy, et al., 1997*).

- A strong, pre-stretched muscle resists better than a strong, unstretched one. Pre-stretching 'takes up the slack' in a muscle. Ligaments like stretch – within limits. Stretching a muscle relaxes it and gives it greater potential and it can prevent strains and lessens the risk of injury.
- Warm-up helps proprioception and co-ordination by allowing far freer and easier movement.
- Warm-up develops body/spatial awareness – vital for young 'athletes'.
- If the body is not properly warmed-up or fatigued its defence mechanism, muscle spindles and Golgi tendon organs etc., cease to function effectively therefore running/increasing the risk of injury.
- Blood pressure and heart rate increases.
- The respiratory rate increases and oxygen uptake is enhanced (*Martin, et al., 1975*).
- There is an increase in the conversion of glycogen and its flow into the circulatory system.
- 'Working parts' are kept healthy and are less liable to disease.
- It can set off chemical reactions which prepare the body for activity, e.g. adrenaline.

Neurologically:

- The warm-up must initiate the careful laying down of neural patterns that are specific to the skills that will be utilised in training and competition.
- As a result of increased muscle temperature the central nervous system function is improved and nerve impulse transmission quickens (*Karvonen, 1992*). This is important at the beginning of exercise when athletes have to react to a variety of stimuli.

Psychologically:

- Prior to competition many players exhibit nervous tension, anxiety and sometimes aggression. For some, warm-up may provide an outlet for the build-up of such emotions/tensions and help to control arousal levels.
- Prepares the 'athlete' for competition and training by mentally focusing on the tasks. This requires a structured, well-planned warm-up routine to relax and give confidence.
- Our body is not able to give its best performance at the start. It is a unique piece of mechanical poetry but like most machines when first started it coughs and splutters into life and cannot possibly be expected to perform at high levels of efficiency. To this end a proper warm-up pattern can facilitate a shift of focus from daily events and stresses to the deep concentration required for successful competition and training. As the warm-up progresses, the specificity, intensity and difficulty of the drills should increase, goals must be set and feedback of performance must be available. The time of the day is important (diurnal rhythms). Early in the morning the body is slow to get going but gets better as the day goes on (*see Chapter 8, Part 3*).
- It also reduces tension and anxiety, via the release of endorphins, which can cause skil breakdown (*Shellock and Prentice, 1985*).

Whilst warm-up definitely appears to have physiological and psychological benefits, the scientific data regarding its effects on injury prevention and performance is inconclusive. Although there are studies that show it may help to do so (*Lehmann, et al., 1970; Shellock and Prentice, 1985; de Vries, 1986; Safran, et al., 1989; Kujala, et al., 1997*). At a more basic down to earth level its success would appear to be down to the commitment, knowledge, skills, expertise and common sense of the people involved. Those that treat it seriously will get positive results and those that 'play at it' won't.

With correct cool down, the risk of injury can be reduced by:

- The heart rate and body gradually returns to normal and recovers after exercise.

Recovery takes the form of clearing away 'blood pools' and toxic materials that are by-products of activity.

- The system is 'flushed out'. Lactic/uric acid disappears within 15–60 minutes of being deposited in the muscles/joints even in extreme cases and cool down certainly assists this removal.
- Muscle temperature is reduced and there is a reduction of muscle oedema and stiffness with athletes reporting less muscle soreness (DOMS – delayed onset muscle soreness) on the day following competition if cool down routines are practiced.
- Re-distribution of the blood is allowed and prevention of pooling.
- Athletes are relaxed emotionally and muscle relaxation is enhanced.
- Recovery time is improved with opportunity for feedback.

Fatigue

When tiredness sets in, the body's resistance level is either compromised or reduced. Fatigue is a biochemical event. When tiredness sets in, the body's resistance level is either compromised or reduced. There is a build-up of toxic waste materials in the muscle and insufficient oxygen intake to satisfy demand with the result that the muscles/tendons are not given time to recover and recharge before being called upon to perform again. This ensures they are less efficient and more prone to injury. The incidence of sports injuries increases in the last quarter of ball games. Also we must not forget the interrelationship of skill and fatigue. More tired – less skilful, therefore new skills should be taught early on in training sessions Dr. Michael Roberts says that fatigue and the sense of effort are interrelated and cannot be separated.

Due acknowledgement is given to the original authors of the following notes which has been adapted from 'Physiology And Performance' – *NCF Coaching Handbook Three, pp. 69–72 and a lecture given by Dr. M. Roberts at the SST Conference, High Wycombe F.C., May, 1999.*

When endurance fails, 'fatigue' is said to be setting in. There are a considerable number of causes of such fatigue, many of which can probably not be reduced by training.

Muscle Cell Factors

There are several potential sources of fatigue inside each muscle fibre:

- The neuromuscular junction may falter and cause 'high rate fatigue'.
- Leaks may occur in the muscle cell membrane, interfering with its vital electrical activity.

- Internal damage may result in excessive storage of calcium or the leakage of phosphate.
- If the muscle overheats, its sensitive enzymes begin to lose efficiency. When working normally, the muscle cell does actually get hotter by about 3°C. This makes its contents more fluid/less viscous, like warm syrup, and also speeds up its chemical reactions, both effects being beneficial. Heat in excess of this reduces efficiency.

On the question of lactic acid involvement as a cause of fatigue it is considered questionable because when the acid is removed fatigue still occurs.

Nutrition

Nutrition may cause fatigue via:

- Deficiency of essential nutrients, i.e. vitamin B, C and the minerals; iron, zinc, magnesium, potassium and sodium.
- Poor intake of protein which can limit muscle and immune function as well as retarded recovery from illness.
- Presence of food allergies that may cause or aggravate fatigue although there is no definitive evidence that this is so (*Dr. Alan Stewart, 1993*).

Muscle Fuel

A major cause of fatigue in longer-term endurance (i.e. events over an hour) is lack of fuel. The two main fuels are glucose (stored glycogen) and fat. Glycogen can be in two forms, Macro, which is preserved and Pro which is used in marathons. As the muscle depletes its glycogen store, a larger proportion of energy must come from fat.

The problem is that to release the same amount of energy, fat requires more oxygen than glucose. Part of 'the wall' for marathon runners may lie in this shift in the provision of energy from predominantly carbohydrate to predominantly fat (other 'bricks' in the wall are often dehydration, a rise in temperature, a steeper incline, turning into a headwind, etc., especially if several of these coincide). A further limiting factor may be the substance carnitine. This is necessary to actually get the fats into the mitochondria of the muscle cells, where they are metabolised. Carnitine itself may deplete after hours of work, and so limit the rate of fat-fuel usage. In short-term exercise the usage of creatine phosphate, especially in fast twitch fibres, can hinder fatigue.

Relaxation/Fatigue

One normally thinks of a tired muscle as being unable to make as many contractions as before, but in addition, the 'relaxation time' may almost be double. This can happen after as little as one minute of sustained strong contraction – or near the end of heavy muscle-work sessions. It rarely causes problems, except perhaps for piano players and typists, especially on colder days, but it may lead to some apparent falling off in skill level in sports requiring a delicate touch.

Elastic Component of Muscle

A very important structural feature of muscle is the elastic, connective tissue that is wrapped around bundles of muscle tissue. This is extremely important in sprinting and jumping, though its exact contribution is very difficult to measure. Fatiguing of this elastic tissue probably contributes to a reduction in muscle efficiency by limiting its 'recoil' effect.

Muscle Pain/Soreness

Non-traumatic pain in muscle (other than cramp) often slows down the rate of muscle work. It is probably caused by oedema of the muscle, i.e. too much fluid leaking out of capillaries, together with increased acidity irritating the free nerve endings in the muscle. Such pain is often worse during, or just after, 'negative' or 'eccentric' work, where the muscle has to increase its tension as it is lengthening rather than shortening. Typical simple examples are the 'down' phases of pull-ups or press-ups that are full of eccentric contractions (*See Delayed Onset Muscle Soreness, DOMS, page 72*).

Cramp is not so much a cause of fatigue as a symptom. It results from ever-increasing waves of electrical discharge down a muscle's motor nerves, but the actual cause that triggers it off is not known. Why it should occur in your feet and legs in bed has yet to be fully established. Theories range from circulatory to mineral imbalance/deficiency.

Central Nervous Fatigue

There is evidence that some cases of muscle fatigue may stem from a source deep in the brain. Experiments have shown that a muscle which has been subjected to repeated voluntary contractions until apparently exhausted may be induced to contract quite strongly by applying a stimulus to the related motor nerve. This indicates that the muscle plus the nerve/muscle junction and the attached nerve are still in a functional state, and that the lack of response is probably due to inadequate signals from the central nervous system. This form of failure may well be part of the **'psychological component'** of fatigue. Also there is an area buried deep in the brain cortex, that has some connection to a **sense of effort** which concentration can overcome. This begs the question; can the body be trained to overcome fatigue via the power of concentration?

Joint Fatigue

Muscles are not the only sites of fatigue. Joints get tired as well! Professor Basmajian, who called his book '*Muscles Alive*', discovered this. He tied various weights to people's arms in such a way that they did not need to hold them. Nevertheless, his passive weight-bearing volunteers complained of fatigue: the stretch receptors in the ligaments of the joints were complaining! Much shoulder pain in racket sports and field events may stem, at least in part, from joints as well as muscles.

Body Fat

Obesity, although not a cause of fatigue is closely linked with depression, reduced exercise and immune function (*Gershwin, N. E. et al., 1985*). Body fat should be kept to the minimum appropriate to the sex of the athlete and the sporting activity involved. It will, for example, be extremely low in Olympic gymnasts, high jumpers, squash players and most runners. Carrying an excess of body fat in such events contributes to fatigue (*see Appendix 5*).

Sleep and Rest

'Sleep deficit'/rest and sleep are important to help the body recover, re-adjust and rebalance after exercise. In fact, as has been discussed previously, many athletes today now consider sleep as 'regenerative' rest – up to four days rest will not seriously affect your fitness. Being 'macho' and 'going through the pain barrier' can have serious repercussions with the dangers of over-exertion being anything from aches, pains and cramps, to pains in the chest, severe breathlessness, dizziness, light-headedness and vomiting. This issue of fatigue and sleep deficit is important when teams travel abroad to competition. For every hour of time change, one day should be allowed for body acclimatisation with sleep patterns taking up to four days to re-establish themselves (*see Chapter 8, Part 3*).

An appreciation of the intricacy of muscle cells and the enormous complexity of homeostasis and allostasis explains why training cannot be made completely 'scientific', with exact schedules going in and precise performances coming out. These physical considerations alone ensure that there will always be differences in the way our bodies respond to training or the onset of fatigue and, of course, there are many psychological reasons.

U-Factors – Misuse, Overuse, Under-Use and Abuse

Amateur players/athletes now subject themselves to training regimes which twenty years ago were only found in professional sport. The time they spend training and the intensity of such training for some can be excessive. With the high rewards now available, professional sports men and women are pushing themselves, either voluntarily or by coercion, harder than ever before. Repeatedly pushing oneself to the limits isn't good for the body. It is estimated that running 7 miles a day or 40 miles a week will make the body more susceptible to skeletal muscle problems. Studies have also shown that a single exhaustive exercise session results in temporary immune depression lasting for a few too many hours in both trained and untrained individuals (*Berk, L. S. et al., 1985; Escola et al., 1978; Mackinon, et al., 1987; Pederson, B. K. et al., 1988; Shinka, et al., 1993*).

In such a climate, realistic goals can often become ill-defined and addiction, fanaticism, obsession and habit can become more than just an issue. Death can sometimes be the result (*Tim Noakes, 1999*). There is a thin line between the habit of dedication and the habit of obsession in the pursuit of performance enhancement. We are led to believe from the physiologists that the 'average' athlete can sustain body stress (all out) twice a week. The body needs time to recover. During exercise the body undergoes many biochemical reactions and tissue changes, with numerous micro-traumatic episodes – especially as a result of previous injury. The maximum benefit from a training session lasts approximately 48 hours. Once a week does very little and if severe can do harm. Twice a week produces slow progress. Three times a week, good progress can be made. Five times would appear to be the optimum. Everyday does not allow sufficient recovery, rest and replenishment for the body. Overuse/misuse and abuse syndromes should be recognised early with prevention being the best cure. Remember that an athlete is more susceptible to overuse injury during and after growth spurt.

Delayed Onset Muscle Soreness (DOMS)

This is muscle soreness that correlates with microscopic muscle damage, oedema and loss of strength that may persist up to a week (*Burke, E., 1997*). Causes have been attributed to actual rupture/micro-trauma of connective tissue/muscle fibres, spasm in a fatigued muscle, extensive pulling which traumatises the muscle. This causes it to swell and/or the accumulation of metabolic by products/fluid that may be the result of membrane damage or may not cause swelling, which in turn increases pressure in the area. Eccentric as opposed to concentric muscle action has also been cited (*Komi, P., and Buskirk, E., 1972*). The telltale signs and symptoms can be one to three hours' post-exercise where there is aching and sometimes cramp. One to three days' post-exercise where there is stiffness weakness and definite pain when active. One to three weeks and the athlete is still complaining of tenderness, swelling and pain on exercise (*see Chapter 2, Part 3 and Chapter 3, Part 4*).

Changing Sport/Venue and Training Surfaces

For many people, sport is as much a social event as a physical one and the thought of having to give up or change your sport is something many people choose to ignore. However, some people choose the wrong sport or have it thrust upon them at an early age, or switch to one, after a long time in another, to one which the body cannot adapt with resultant injuries. For those actually in sport, constantly changing differing environments and surfaces offers differing types of equipment, temperatures, 'give' and 'spring' underfoot that can impose extra stresses leading to injury.

Diet and Nutrition

Nutrition and diet are enormous topics. They cut across so many boundaries related to sport, exercise, training, eating disorders, body-type, performance enhancement/ hindrance, personality, psychology, energy production/utilisation, healing and repair, etc. that this section will only emphasise its importance to all aspects of sport. Further reference will be made during subsequent topics (*see Chapter 1, Part 5; Chapter 2, Part 3; Chapter 2, Part 8; Chapter 3, Part 4; Chapter 6, Part 4; Chapter 8, Parts 1 and 3*).

So much has been spoken and written on the subject that not only are we seen as a nation obsessed with eating but also we are now considered the second most obese country in the world (*BBCTV: Fat, Horizon, January, 1999*). Research in the *BMJ*, 2001, branded obesity in children as a serious public health problem. In the sporting context many issues are much the same as for non-sports people but because of the very nature of sport these issues and considerations take on much greater significance, especially for injury prevention and re-occurrence.

Nutrition is not a one-off thing but an all year round consideration. You are not only what you eat but also what you absorb and assimilate. People with intestinal/gut problems may not benefit from the healthiest of diets.

> **"Diet in itself cannot provide fitness or championship form but a poor diet can ruin both."**
> *Torrence, A., 1998*

Ignoring The Body's Warning Signs – Pain/Heat/Fluid Balance

Listen to what your body is telling you

The body is not meant to give pain. **Pain and muscle spasms** (preventing movement) are both part of the body's reaction to injury, which acts as a defence mechanism against further serious injury. Pain tells us that the pathological process is underway. Ignoring pain may impress some people but the body will not be in the least impressed. A separate section is devoted to the very important issue of pain (*see Chapter 5, Part 3*) but here are some signs and symptoms to alert the reader to the possibility of injury:

- Localising pain – usually in the joint.
- Stiffness in the joint with slight loss of movement.
- Not getting better in terms of performance even with rest.
- A change of contour of either bone, muscle or joint.
- A burning sensation, tingling or numbness in the limbs.
- Unexplained redness of the skin.
- Unexplained black or blue marks.

Heat/fluid balance is a very important consideration in sport, especially when exercising in temperature extremes.

Water is considered to be the body's most important nutrient. Sixty per cent of the body's weight is water, one third of this is considered extracellular (blood plasma, interstitial fluid, including lymph) and two thirds intracellular which is regulated by the cell itself. Much of our liquid intake is assumed to be derived from food sources (up to one litre). Water is essential to support the internal activities of the cells; to carry nutrients and oxygen around the body; to aid in the elimination of waste and to get rid of excess body heat, via the kidneys. It helps absorb essential vitamins, minerals and natural sugars as well as enabling the body to produce digestive enzymes. It helps to maintain healthy skin, hair and organs with the epidermis being made up of seventy per cent water.

Body temperature is regulated by the thermoregulatory centres in the brain (thirst and hunger both being regulated by the hypothalamus) and by the processes of evaporation, radiation and convection, i.e. breathing, sweating and going to the toilet. Even on a cool day the body uses and loses two litres of water. Any increase or decrease in the temperature/fluid balance can have psychological and physiological consequences, which can effect performance. During a dance class sweat loss may be as much as two to three litres per hour. Such sweat can only regulate body temperature if it evaporates on the skin and allows the body to cool.

So loose fitting clothing, which will absorb the sweat, will assist in the evaporation process. Heat production as a result of physical exertion with subsequent water loss by evaporation or excessive sweating leads to **DEHYDRATION**, which can lead to many problems. It is suggested that dehydration of as little as two per cent loss of body weight results in impaired physiological and performance responses (*Kleiner, 1999*).

> "Dehydration lowers blood volume and reduces flow to the muscles and brain."
> *Costain, L., 2000*

The more dehydrated one gets, the more lethargic, tired and irritable one becomes. **A dry mouth/thirst, fatigue and flushing are all late, rather than early signs, of dehydration.**

Heat gain (**HYPERTHERMIA**) can lead to:

1. **Cramps**, where the face becomes pale and the body cools and feels clammy. Calves and arms can be very painful. This can lead to;
2. **Heat exhaustion**, where the person is rarely thirsty but is sweating. Young athletes are more prone to heat exhaustion because their sweat glands are not yet fully developed, nor do they acclimatise as well as adults (*see Chapter 1, Part 6*). For every 1% loss of body fluid there will be a 10% loss of work capacity. A loss of only 3 % of the body's water content causes a 10% drop in strength and an 8% loss of speed. A 5% water loss can lead to difficulty concentrating and a 10% loss to poor balance and even delirium (*Kavounas, A., 2000*). Continued heat/fluid loss can lead to hallucinations, then circulatory collapse leading to;
3. **Heat stroke**, where there is no sweating but this is not recognised and treated incorrectly can lead to coma and possible brain damage.

HYPOTHERMIA (heat loss) is when peripheral blood vessels are dilated giving signs and symptoms of cold, shivering, slow thoughts, clumsiness leading to unconsciousness.

Going Back to Sport Too Early After Injury

> "The person who discovers a way to increase the normal speed of healing of the body will win a Nobel Prize."
> *Quigley, T. B., 1981*

As we know, as the body heals itself, sports people either assist or interfere with the processes and going through the pain barrier in the hope that it will speed up recovery is not a sensible idea. Patience, perseverance and understanding are required. Don't forget that everyone is different! **Going back to sport too early is definitely one way to extend the healing time. A sports therapist should not allow this to happen if they are following the principles of treatment and rehabilitation** (*see Chapters 5 and 6*).

Incorrect Footwear, Clothing, Equipment, Protection and Proprioception

Many foot disorders are due to the fact that people do not readily accept the importance of wearing the correct gear to suit the sport, venue surface and environment. In recent times martial arts/combat sports coaches found that the introduction of the compulsory wearing of head guards into the sport to reduce the risk of injury only 'incited' participants to try to kick each other harder, causing more not less problems!

Incorrect usage and un-serviced equipment can be the cause of sports injuries. Following the manufacturers recommendations is always advisable. Most sports recommend what should be worn as protection and those who ignore these recommendations are more prone to injury than those who do not. **Litigation for incorrect use of equipment is another issue.**

Considering that the foot is the greatest weight-bearing joint in the body, it is perhaps the most abused and misused. Many foot problems are caused by over pronation and the excessive inward rolling of the foot. One research study in the late 80's, during a Glasgow marathon by Dr. Knill Jones, Community Medical Practitioner, found rather interestingly that those wearing the most expensive running shoes were the ones most likely to have knee and other problems.

Unsuitable footwear and poor proprioception are the cause of many lower limb problems in sport. Just because a sports shoe alleges to support this, it doesn't necessarily mean it's good for you. It may be shifting your weight/balance when your weight/balance doesn't need shifting. However, running and walking shoes are now being designed tailor-made to match the vibrations of the wearer which scientists believe will reduce running times and help elderly and frail people to walk further (*New Scientist, 2000*).

Over Enthusiastic, Ill-Advised, Ineffective, Misguided, Ignorant Adults

This consideration although not new, has, as far as the author is concerned, now become one of the major issues in certain sports in the twenty-first century. Not only in relation to injury cause, its treatment, healing and repair; performance enhancement, but also child abuse and the development of young precocious talent. So much so that the author not only discusses these issues but also uses them as a re-occurring theme during this book (*see Chapter 1, Parts 2, 5, 6; Chapter 2, Part 8; Chapter 3, Part 4; Chapter 7, Part 1*).

Misinterpretation/Manipulation of the Rules of the Game – Control

With so much at stake in today's 'modern game' and the pressures and need to gain any advantage over the opposition, we are now seeing injury being caused as a direct result of 'bending the rules' which has been in sport since 'winning at all costs' became an issue. The professional foul is now common terminology in sport. What we are also now seeing are court cases for assault of – player v player; referee v player etc. with referees also being cited as the direct cause of injury for failing to 'keep control'. Managers, trainers and couches have a significant role to play in **FAIRPLAY** but sadly many are guilty of trying to justify the opposite. Lack of self-control is definitely a direct cause of injury and 'celebrations' after scoring are a constant source of concern, embarrassment and amusement (*see Chapter 1, Part 2*).

During March and May 1999, ITV screened, *Foul Play* and *When Athletes Attack 1* and in June 2000, *When Athletes Attack*. These programmes depicted a distinct lack of discipline in every sense of the word.

Inappropriate Treatment/Rehabilitation

Do we assist the body's natural healing processes or do we interfere? Chapters 5 and 6 address these very important aspects of injury prevention.

Lack of Discipline/Boredom/Control

There must be imposed discipline before self-discipline is achieved. There should be acceptable and unacceptable behaviour in treatment, fitness and rehabilitation areas/sessions otherwise the chances of re-injury will be increased. Psyching oneself up for competition is another issue that can have injurious consequences if not controlled properly.

Poor Training Techniques

In training are you achieving what you think you are achieving? Otherwise you are creating more problems than you started with. Are you using sound basic training principles to achieve your aim?

How Can the Risks be Reduced?

The answer to this question should be fairly obvious. Find out the cause and eliminate it. You neither heal a cut finger by rubbing it against a brick wall nor do you stop a headache by keep butting the garden fence. No one can play sport competitively without taking risks.

> **"Sport is an appallingly stressful business, for mind and body alike, no matter what level you do it at. Few escape without some long running, niggling, nagging ache and those who participate in it seldom do so without worry or care."**
> *Simon Barnes, Sports Columnist, The Times*

On a more practical level the risks of injury can be reduced by prevention and here are a few areas for consideration and suggested advice to be passed onto the athlete.

Education/Communication

In the list of causes and considerations of injury/re-injury one of the most challenging roles for the sports therapist is **education** and establishing lines of communication, knowing that no one can play sport competitively without taking risks and risking injury. Everyone involved has a part to play and therefore a multidisciplinary approach is advocated. In spite of what some would have you believe no one person can possibly have the knowledge, skills and expertise to totally supply the needs of the sports person. If everyone appreciates what everyone in 'the team' is supposed to be doing then the risks are considerably reduced. However, **co-ordinating, controlling and communicating** with the egos, needs a strong will if success is to be achieved (*see Chapter1, Part 7*).

Fitness

This must include all the parameters of fitness outlined previously. The message should be, **'Be fit for your sport and don't play sport to get fit'**. Training sessions should be planned, controlled and properly supervised. Off-season, pre-season, early-season and peak-season training as well as macro, meso and micro cycles of periodisation should be considered (*see Chapter 2, Part 6*). Realistic goals and targets should be set and training records and schedules maintained (*see Chapter 7, Part 3*). If training is done spasmodically, with little purpose and no records kept then injury is more likely to occur.

To avoid boredom and getting stale vary the training package. Many texts offer good practical advice on training based on sound scientific principles. Finally, train for your sport whilst accepting the fact that being good at cycling doesn't necessarily make you a good footballer, although the principles of cross-training shows that there is some benefit in 'mixing and matching' fitness regimes.

Fit to Train/Fit to Play – ARE They the Same?

The aim of any fitness test should be to try and find an athlete's weakness so they do not fail in competition (*see Chapter 2, Part 7*). During training such fitness can be assessed and controlled.

Train	**Play**
Player/coach /trainer/therapist dictates	Opposition dictates (a player can't dictate in a game or competition because there are too many factors)
Duration – can be controlled	Duration set – player can't be protected
Non/partial contact	Contact full!
Positional protection	No protection
Speed of play controlled	No speed control – type of game dictates
Pressure – none/self-imposed	Pressure to compete, win-at-all-costs, etc.
CONTROLLED ENVIRONMENT	**UNCONTROLLED ENVIRONMENT**

How can **OVERUSE** be overcome?

- Meticulous warm-up – addressing the physiological, psychological and neuro logical components.
- Mental preparation – time on their own, mental imaging.
- Physical preparation – stretching programme – individuals need own routine, such as strengthening – general, specific; mobility etc., power, sprinting, aerobic, anaerobic, endurance; skill specific and related.
- Meticulous cool down – gentle jogging, stretching etc.

Selection and Screening

"**Screening is an ideal environment in which to obtain information on fitness, medical health and talent identification.**"
Smolevski, V., 1992

During the selection, screening and monitoring process many issues need consideration if injuries are to be avoided and sporting potential is to be realised. Are they fit to train? Are they able to survive? Are their problems medically controlled (diabetes, asthma)? Also selection for the correct sport and sport specificity should be carefully monitored at the appropriate stage in the child's development. Generally speaking your tall, long-legged, ectomorph will make a far better high jumper than a short, squat muscular athlete. Jonty Skinner, 1999, highlights such issues as centre of mass, body density, physiology, anthropometry, hull length/shape, leg power and feel when assessing swimming potential. Each sport should have its own checklist. What could be included? **It is suggested the base line of any selection/screening programme is an initial personal data questionnaire that includes a medical history.** Other issues to consider are:

- **Medical factors** – the higher up the sporting ladder the more medical factors can play a part and so therefore, family history, cancer, syncope/dizziness/passing out, heart disease, pulse, blood pressure, chest expansion, peak flow, vision, urine - protein, sugar/diabetes, asthma, tetanus, etc. should be checked.
- **Experience level** – for children, training age should be considered in relation to experienced, supervised training. For adults, experience should not be confused with duplication.
- **Skill level** – tension and anxiety can break down a skill just as much as fatigue.
- **Technique** – poor technique can certainly cause injury.
- **Maturity** – there can be as much as five years developmental difference (physiological, psychological and sociological) with children of the same chronological age.
- **Heredity**, postural deformity/abnormality, body asymmetry, biomechanical malalignment and muscle imbalance – scoliosis, patella tracking, leg length discrepancy, knock knees (varus), bow legs (valgus), flat feet (pes planus) etc.
- Are we born with it or do we acquire it?

Biomechanical malalignment of the structures of the lower limb can lead to overuse or even acute injuries (*Kaufman, 1999*). There is evidence that hyperlordotic posture and reduced range of motion is linked with lower back pain (*Ohlen, 1989*). Certainly excesses or reductions of the spine's natural curve can lead to potential back problems (*see Chapter 4, Parts 4 and 5*).

Dysfunction or imbalance of the musculoskeletal system may pre-dispose or cause mechanical failure of the movement system. The imbalance may occur between the muscles providing stability becoming inhibited and weak, and the powerful mobilising muscles becoming over active and tight through poor movement patterns associated with sport, training or previous injury (*Norris, 1998*).

Tight Achilles tendons (gastrocnemius and soleus) have been implicated in ankle sprains and other overuse injuries (*Reid, 1992*).

Genetic composition – is it true that people are born to win a gold medal? **GENOTYPE** refers to:

> **"The characteristics that an individual has inherited and will transmit to his descendants, whether or not he manifests these characteristics."**
> *Hilgard and Atkinson, 1967*

PHENOTYPE is how this gene make-up expresses itself in relation to job, diet, lifestyle, posture and social environment, etc. Age and gender is an issue that crosses many other areas and this topic will be dealt with separately (*see Chapter 1, Part 6*). When talking about age, the differences between chronological (actual), developmental (physiological, social and psychological) and training (experienced structured training) should be appreciated and taken into consideration.

Temperament/Personality and Somatotype

If we consider Eysenck's (1960) scales for classifying people's personality and consider the extremes of personality types, i.e. extrovert/introvert – stable/unstable and relate these with body type and sport it can be seen how certain individuals are born to be at an advantage in certain sports.

Personality Types

Again, people's personality is not an exact science but is a combination of many factors. However, the following generalisations should prove helpful:

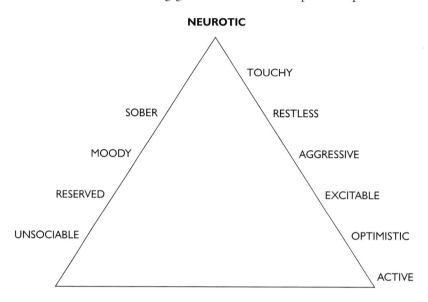

	CALM	LIVELY	
No desires to express opinions/low self-esteem			Opinionated/high self-esteem
Low levels of arousal	CALM	LIVELY	High levels of arousal
Patient	THOUGHTFUL	THOUGHTLESS	Generally impatient
Low pain tolerance	CAREFUL	CAREFREE	High pain tolerance
Works hard in training but gets tense/anxious for 'big occasion'	PEACEFUL	SOCIABLE	Poor trainer but responds to challenge
	RELIABLE	TALKATIVE	
	EVEN-TEMPERED	VOLATILE	
Attracted to sports that are predictable. Tends to be guarded apprehensive and indecisive			Attracted to sports offering unpredictability, i.e. cross-country

STABLE

In general the most successful sports people are found to be stable extroverts.

Evaluating Personal Abilities – What Makes a Sucessful Performer?

"A great performer is someone who has made his weaknesses into strengths."
Atkinson, J., 1988.

In 1988, the USSR established a fourteen point basic code of qualities necessary for top performance in gymnastics. The first four were:

1. Love of the sport and a determination in character, which will involve the following; can handle failure and success, courage/toughness, a high degree of self-discipline, a questioning and reasoning mind (why do I do it?), patience (to sustain interest, love and positive attitude), belief/faith in oneself.
2. Physical strength.
3. Co-ordination.
4. Intelligence.

It is argued that (2) can quite easily be overcome by (1).

John Atkinson, BAGA Technical Director, identified the following in assessing young gymnasts aged between eight and ten.

*   The ability, talent, physical structure. A young natural athlete with a love of exercise and activity. A child who seems to enjoy fitness for fitness' sake.
*   Someone who has a determined character and loves to work. Talent alone is not enough when it comes to achieving really high standards.
*   The right mental attitude which appears to motivate the child.
*   Someone who does not regularly show fear.
*   One who will soon co-operate with the coach/teacher and never give up the search for perfection.
*   Self-discipline – a factor of major importance in the acquisition of knowledge and approach to competitive performance.

Body shape is not gender specific but gender, exercise, diet and heredity all play a part in determining body shape and fat content.

1. **MESOMORPHY**   –   the amount of muscle mass in relation to body fat.
2. **SOMA**   –   relating to the body.
3. **SOMATOTYPING** –   body build and temperament.

W. H. Sheldon, 1940, classified bodies into three types and other research since then has identified personality traits to go with these types. Although not an exact science in selection and screening, genetic body and personality types can be useful indicators, i.e. extroverted, endomorphs – sumo wrestlers, prop forwards and shot putters; mesomorphs – scrum half; ectomorph – high jumpers; middle-distance runners could come from a mesomorphic ectomorph!

Pyknic/Endomorph

Sociable – loves comfort, easy going (adaptive), rather fat, heavily built, rounded shape. Arms and thighs usually large in relation to calves and forearms. Little muscle tone, small bones, large head, long trunk, short neck.

Mesomorph

Energetic – assertive – liking for motor activity, well-defined skeletal structure, exceptional(ly) bone/toned muscle group. Well-built, broad framed, low body fat. The most physically versatile, slender waist, wide hips, long arms and legs.

Asthenic/Ectomorph

Secretive – withdrawn – liking for mental activity, rather thin, slight, low muscle mass, low body fat. Long underdeveloped arms and legs with oversized hands and feet. Narrow hips, long and angular physique. **Schizothymes**, inflexible, suspicious or secretive.

Each individual can be categorised by a three figure classification 1 to 7 (1 low, 7 high) depending on how they relate to the above, i.e. fat to lean muscle ratio. The most common somatotypes among the general population are 3-4-4, 4-3-3 and 3-5-2. It is not possible to change these inherent characteristics, i.e. an endomorph on a severe diet will just become a hungry endomorph! With diet and training, body shape may alter but ultimately the body will return to its 'pre-determined type'. It is important to understand our own body type to adjust or modify activities. Exceeding ones' limitations can lead to injury. Also realistic goals must be set to avoid discouragement and upset.

Groupings

Groups should be relatively small to allow for adequate supervision and control. This undoubtedly will lead to higher skill levels and a greater enjoyment of the sport – not to mention reduce the risk of injury.

Skill

New skills should be taught early on in training sessions, after the warm-up, when the athlete is more amenable, in many senses of the word, to acquire the skill. Skills should also be realistically set. Asking a thirty-five year old footballer to improve his 'box splits' is asking for trouble. Research in Russia (1992) and Veritas (1995) and Germany has also identified the fact that specialization too early, i.e. pre-puberty produces the physical equivalent of a specialist but who has very little consistency outside of his/her specialism and leads to the athlete being:

- More injury prone.
- 'Burnt out' at 18.

Control

From an early age there is a need to strongly emphasise the concept of fair play and the need for and reasons to obey the rules. These concepts become increasingly more difficult to sustain once the, 'Must win-at-all-costs' concept enters the arena.

Warm-Up/Cool Down

There are many variables to consider when designing a proper warm-up/cool down routine that addresses the physiological, neurological and psychological components. The **KEY ELEMENTS/PRINCIPLES** to include and consider in a warm-up/ cool down programme to achieve the physiological, psychological and neurological aims would be:

- Initial general activities such as rubbing the skin, jogging, hopping, skipping, on the spot and/or moving etc. To raise the body temperature.
- Develop the above to actively go through a full range of movement for each upper and lower body joint, i.e. flexion, extension, abduction, adduction, medial rotation, lateral rotation and circumduction for the glenohumeral joint.
- Develop the above to concentrate on general and specific movement patterns related to the particular sport, e.g. leg/arm swings, high knees, throwing etc.
- Dynamic flexibility follows with sport specific, active stretching to prepare for the stresses of training and/or competition, i.e. from knee bent to 'kicking out' with leg swings, in an upright position to stretch the hamstrings.

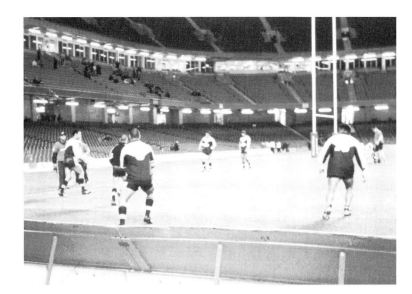

◄ *Figure 32.*
Warming-up
for the
Millennium
Rugby League
World Cup.

"The optimum time to improve static flexibility is after the workout. Muscles are already warmed-up creating an ideal window for maximum gains in flexibility. More importantly, post-workout, static stretching has a regenerative effect on muscles. This helps to calm the athlete, restore muscles to their resting length and stimulate blood flow which will reduce the muscle spasms usually experienced after workouts or competition."
Hiseman, J., 1997

- The large muscle groups can then be split into smaller units to concentrate on specific warm-up regimes in preparation for skill, drill and technique specificity.
- The element of speed, both fast and slow can be introduced in preparation for acceleration and deceleration, key components in injury prevention.

PRINCIPLES: Intensity and duration with increased skill specificity are the keys to a successful warm-up. Therefore all the above should be developed with this in mind:

- Warm-ups should be designed so that the body is fully prepared for more strenuous, sophisticated activity.
- Warm-up should do just that not tire out.
- Warm-up activities should be closely supervised.
- Warm-up should require minimal instruction.
- Warm-up should be flexible and changing to avoid boredom.
- Warm-up should be carefully planned as all other aspects of physical activity if injury is to be avoided.

Environment/Facilities/Surfaces – Hazards to Consider

These can include indoor, outdoor, grass, synthetic, all-weather, shale, clay etc., pitch, pool, track, personal, mobile, static etc., but here specifically relates to venue, clothing, footwear and protective measures. It goes without saying that **ALL POTENTIAL HAZARDS should be regularly checked and serviced according to the manufacturers guidelines/recommendations. Failure to do so can lead to litigation.**

Artificial surfaces can create problems, e.g. Osgood-Schlatter's disease and patellar tendinitis. In hockey it has been found to reduce knee and ankle injuries but the incidence of cuts, bruising and abrasions has increased. Footballers, however, claim increased stress on ankles and knees. As of yet there is no definitive evidence one way or the other. **Footwear** is essential in that it must be the right kind to do the job.

> **"The most expensive is not necessarily the best."**
> *Jones, Dr. K., 1988*

Trainers are for training, not all-round wear. Sports shoes must:

- Not be too narrow or short.
- Be cushioned yet strong enough to absorb the shock and weight bear.
- Be wide enough to allow the toes to lie flat at the widest part.
- Have a waist support that must be strong enough.
- Have a tread that must be as wide as the width and suitable for the surface on which it is going to be used to reduce torque.
- Studs if used, should be checked regularly to ensure symmetry.

Heel tabs are usually there for advertising purposes and cause more injuries than they avoid through so-called support. When out jogging try to avoid using hard surfaces, as it can cause unnecessary loading stresses to the joints. When buying shoes, go to a specialist sports shoe shop and be cautious of buying mail order. When buying new sports shoes, test gait and proprioception in and out of them and ask yourself do they alter the foot mechanics (*see Chapter 4, Part 4; Chapter 6, Part 2*). Don't just buy sports shoes because they look good. Seek advice.

Insoles/Orthotics

> **"You can correct any foot deformity with a wedge as thin as a matchbook, the trick is you have to know where to put it."**
> *Hlavac, Dr. H., 1999*

Insoles and orthotics can be used to address problems of lower extremity mechanical pathology. They can be used as a preventative as well as a supportive measure but specialist (podiatrist) help should be sought.

Clothing

The body does not perform as well in extremes of temperature, so try to keep a constant body temperature and keep warm especially during warm-up and cool down. 'Named' articles of clothing are not necessarily going to last you longer than 'unnamed' articles. Try to keep gymnasiums/sports halls at a constant temperature for your sport.

Protective Measures

Pads, guards, clothing, headgear, boxes, matting, etc., are an essential part of all sports and should be worn and used at all times, **not just during the game**. Taking off shin guards towards the end of a game when the body is tired and reactions are slower would appear to be foolish. The author has actually heard an amateur footballer saying that wearing shin pads slowed him down! The question of bandaging, strapping and taping in sport is somewhat confusing leading to widely contrasting statements and so therefore the theory and practicalities of this subject will be covered during Chapter 5, Part 6.

Diet and Nutrition/Fluid Balance

Principles, considerations and a few facts:

- Consider energy dense (fats and carbohydrates), nutrient dense (proteins) and electrolyte balance in the diet.
- Eat a **balanced diet** that is suited to you and your sport, as different sports require different energy sources. It must also be appreciated that individually tailored dietary regimes are time consuming but very necessary for the serious athlete.
- Be aware of the hazards of **slimming/over/under eating/special diets** that can seriously impair performance and result in illness and discomfort. Weight control is also an important factor in the prevention of injury. Vegan/vegetarian diets may be deficient in certain trace elements, vitamins, minerals, proteins and essential amino acids.
- Be aware of the necessity of a **sensible feeding routine**: it is not just a question of satisfying hunger but an active conscious effort to be aware of what fuel/nutrition you are putting in the engine/body.

- **WATER/ELECTROLYTE BALANCE: DEHYDRATION, HYDRATION AND REHYDRATION**. Dehydration is one of the greatest problems an athlete can have.

As stated previously, much of our liquid intake is assumed to be derived from food sources (up to one litre) and that dehydration, as little as two per cent loss of body weight, results in impaired responses (*Kleiner, 1999*).

It is suggested the best times for drinking water are when they coincide with the diurnal rhythms of high and low energy. These are first thing in the morning, to cleanse and invigorate, mid-morning and afternoon, when energy levels can be low and last thing at night, to prepare for rest. Two glasses at these times help to cut down on 'caffeine craves' and 'quick-fix' high sugar snacks. In other words eight glasses of water daily. For every cup of coffee and glass of wine one cup of water needs to be added to the daily intake. For every work out lasting 30–40 minutes, one glass of water should be added to the basic minimum. As a rough guide for every pound in weight loss during exercise it is suggested that two cups of water are drunk – not tea, coffee or alcohol. However, there is a limit as to how much water we can replace, which is dependent on the speed at which the stomach empties. This varies tremendously from individual to individual as well as the tolerance of fluid ingestion during exercise. Too much fluid during exercise can lead to intestinal discomfort and a resultant effect on performance. Up to 1 litre an hour is best taken in small frequent drinks of 150–200 mls. Every 10–15 minutes during exercise. Dancers can drink approximately a litre of water before and during dance. However, individuals must devise their own strategy of fluid intake, especially for events such as the marathon. Cold drinks empty the stomach more quickly and help reduce temperature. Concentrated drinks of glucose delay stomach emptying. Dilute solutions are best, i.e. 60% fruit juice/40% water. Ingesting large amounts of plain water or drinks with no electrolyte content over a short period of time, results in an increase of plasma volume and a decrease in sodium concentration and osmolarity of blood, making it more dilute. This dilution leads to an increase in urine leading to a loss of body fluid and a desire to drink which works against rehydration. Therefore when sweat rates and body fluid loss is high, a drink with an electrolyte solution is probably the best choice – solutions of nine per cent giving the best results. Other suggestions for maintaining water/electrolyte balance are:

- **Hypotonic drinks** are solutions with a higher carbohydrate/electrolyte concentration than body fluids and are therefore best used as energy supplementation drinks during periods of intense training.
- **Isotonic drinks** have a similar carbohydrate/electrolyte concentration to the body. They are best absorbed during recovery in the final rehydration process, i.e. *Isostar, Lucozade Sport and Liquid Power*. Salts of sodium, potassium and

magnesium are important for electrolyte/mineral balance. Tap water is regulated by various water authorities so it can be as tasty and sometimes more beneficial than the most expensive bottled mineral waters (*Health, Which Magazine, 2000*).

- **Natural mineral water** is extracted from underground sources. It is recognised by the relevant local authority, should have a constant mineral content and cannot be treated, except by a filtering process to remove grit.
- **Spring water** can have a variable mineral content, which may be above European recommended levels, but must be extracted from an underground source and can be treated. Bottled drinking water covers any product not labelled as spring or mineral and in some cases may simply be tap water that has not been treated to bring it up to bottled water standards.

"If you prefer to drink water alone after exercise, it is possible to achieve adequate rehydration if solid food, which replaces lost electrolytes is consumed at the same time. If this is not possible, some form of electrolyte solution is essential."
Carlton, I., 2001

- **Drink water, fresh fruit juice and vitamin C after competition** to help replace electrolyte depletion.
- **Avoid alcohol and coffee before competition** – it has a diuretic effect. This means that they take more than their own volume of liquid with them when they leave the body, depleting it of vital vitamins and minerals.
- **Monitor urine**. Pale yellow urine is good news but a dark colour/concentration, with infrequent urination can indicate dehydration and kidney strain.

Dieticians in Sport and Exercise Nutrition (DISEN) have produced a chart which shows a range of urine colours from those expected in a well-hydrated individual to those expected in a dehydrated and severely dehydrated individual (*Sportscare News, 2000*).

- **Carbohydrates** provide 55% of the total dietary energy. Obviously these percentages   depend on many factors, i.e. the type and amount of other nutrients present in the meals and snacks consumed. Other factors that need to be considered are the timing of carbohydrate intake and the type of carbohydrate ingested.
- **Proteins** – a body builder and provides 10% of total dietary energy. It is estimated that the body needs 1–1.5g of protein per 1kg of body weight daily.
- **Fat** slows down gastric emptying and provides 35% of total dietary energy. Fat doesn't give energy as quickly as carbohydrates but gives more. Fat is not

power-producing whereas muscle is. Remember muscle weighs 1.3 times more than fat and so therefore 'athletes' who put on weight may be changing their body fat: muscle composition. Essential fat – males – 3%; females – 13%. Stored fat – males 12%; females – 15%. Fat needs more oxygen for energy production.

- **Fibre** leaves gastrointestinal residue. In long-distance running races, take water every 15–20 minutes – not when you are thirsty. Ensure you are properly hydrated for your sport. Don't eat large meals before strenuous exercise. Wait at least 3–4 hours after a heavy meal.
- **Vitamin supplementation** is not necessary unless advised by a qualified nutritionist, dietician or practitioner. It can cause an imbalance where one might not have previously existed. The same can be said about salt tablets. However, co-operation of different vitamins, each with the other, especially A1, B1, B2, B6, C, and E may suggest multivitamin supplementation can form part of an athlete's diet.
- **Pre-match/pre-training meals** are the ones most likely to cause problems and should therefore be light but provide energy for competition.
- One week before competition could be 3–4 days of intensive work with a high protein/low carbohydrate, followed by three days involving an easy workout with high carbohydrate/low protein.

(See Chapter 1, Parts 5 and 6; Chapter 2, Part 3; Chapter 3, Part 4; Chapter 6, Part 4; Chapter 8, Part 1).

Listen to What Your Body is Telling You – Pain, Heat, Fluid Balance *(See Chapter 3, Parts 1 and 4; Chapter 5, Part 3.)*

You should not play if:

- Pain comes from a swollen joint.
- Pain intensifies when you use your body part.
- The pain is associated with infection.
- Pain continues unabated for three days.
- The pain suddenly increases the morning after injury.
- People suffering from hyperthermia need to slowly rehydrate, be cooled and be evacuated to a safer environment.
- People suffering from hypothermia need to be protected from the elements, dried, heated slowly and evacuated to a safer environment.
- In temperature extremes training should be of less intensity.

Part 6

Special Interest/Age Groups Involved in Sport

Over the years differences between sexes, age groups, able and less able bodied, has been specifically highlighted because of particular problems regarding not only musculoskeletal insult but also psychological, emotional and sexual abuse. Research and epidemiological studies emphasise the tremendous variations found within populations. It is therefore an area of concern that all working in the health care field should be aware of. You don't find 'real-people' in books and so the simple remit that you are treating, managing, rehabilitating, coaching, training, individual people will be true at all times. However, the practicalities of the situation may force people to 'lump them all together' as one group, i.e. these are all adults or these are all 10 year old children. The implications of this are that whilst they may all be adults there are many differences between males and females, other than just gender and chronological age, and whilst the children may all be chronologically 10 years old there can be as much as five years difference in terms of their developmental age. This section will look at:

1. Males and females.
2. Children in sport/child abuse in sport.
3. Veterans.
4. Less able bodied/disabled, to highlight why each can be considered a special group.

Each could provide an area of study in their own right and so the purpose of this section is to provide not only information but also food for thought and a basis for further study. **The author has a particular interest in children in sport and so that is where the emphasis of this section will concentrate.**

Skeletal, Morphological, Physiological and Performance Variations in Males and Females

The difference between men and women is not simply one of gender but the physical and physiological variations that exist which can affect performance so that it is not just a question of technical skill. The bones of a male are heavier and thicker; their muscle attachment sites more massive and distinct and their joint surfaces are relatively large compared to those of the female. Men tend to be heavier and taller than women. Characteristically males are stronger because they have a greater amount of testosterone, but possess less balance because of a higher centre of gravity. Females have a lower centre of gravity which gives greater potential for balance and stability.

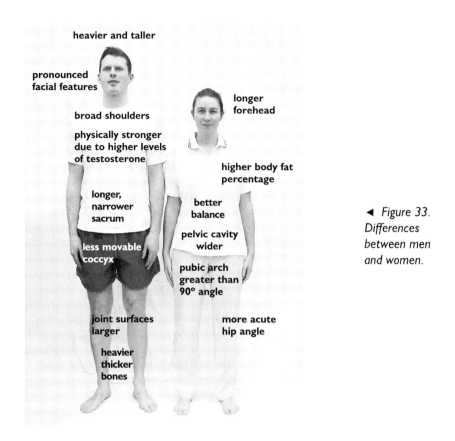

heavier and taller

pronounced facial features

broad shoulders

physically stronger due to higher levels of testosterone

longer, narrower sacrum

less movable coccyx

joint surfaces larger

heavier thicker bones

longer forehead

higher body fat percentage

better balance

pelvic cavity wider

pubic arch greater than 90° angle

more acute hip angle

◄ *Figure 33. Differences between men and women.*

The male forehead is shorter vertically, whereas the females' is more elongated vertically. A male's mandible and maxillae are relatively larger. The facial area of the male has more pronounced features, with more prominent processes, whereas the females' is rounder. The male pelvic cavity is narrower in all dimensions and deeper. The females' is wider in all dimensions, shorter and roomier. The male pelvic outlet, in comparison to the female counterpart, is relatively small. The sacrum is long, narrow, with a smooth concavity (sacral curvature); the female has a short, wide, flat concavity, which is more pronounced in a posterior direction; the sacral promontory is less pronounced.

A male coccyx is less movable, whereas the females' is more movable and follows a posterior direction of the sacral curvature The male pubic arch is less than a 90° angle whereas in the female it is greater than 90°. The symphysis pubis of the male form is relatively deep, a females' being relatively shallow.

The ischial spine, ischial tuberosity and anterior superior iliac spine are turned more inward in a male, a females' being turned more outward and further apart. The male greater sciatic notch is narrow, the females' being wide.

Females have a more acute hip angle which produces less mechanical strength advantage in executing running and jumping activities. Because of the angles of the relative position of the bones around the hips, females tend to be more varus (knock-kneed) and males tend to be more valgus (bowlegged).

Females are at a mechanical disadvantage in throwing or supporting because their shoulders are narrower and they have a greater carrying angle at the elbow than the males. Research by physiologists show that both can work equally as hard in physical activity but vigorous exercise during menstruation usually causes ill-effects. During the first days when the womb is engorged with blood, jarring or sudden torque movements should be avoided.

Another factor that can affect performance is body fat percentage and whilst fat is necessary for insulation, protection and energy, it is 'dead weight'. To re-iterate the body relies on two types of fat. The percentage of each on average is:

	STORED	ESSENTIAL
MALE	12%	3%
FEMALE	15%	13%

The average 18+ male: 15–18% in total.
The average 18+ female: 25–28% in total.
Male athletes: 10–15%.
Female athletes: 16–20%.
Elite athletes: 5–8%, e.g. an Olympic gymnast.

Obviously this is dependant on many variables, i.e. training, dietary intervention, hormones and child bearing etc. but the fact remains that women have approximately 10% more fat than men.

> **"This means male players have more active muscle tissue than females, so contributing to them being faster, stronger, more powerful and having greater endurance."**
> *Jakomy, J., Dabinett, J., and Nevill, M., 2000*

Men have larger hearts and lungs and will therefore have a greater capacity to carry oxygen in the blood, i.e. more blood volume, red blood corpuscles and haemoglobin; the greater lung power helping with a higher aerobic power. The female heart and lungs have to work harder and faster to achieve the same results. The muscle fibre tissue of a male tends to be larger in terms of hypertrophy.

Returning to the issues of 'winning-at-all-costs', some athletes will try to 'modify' these basic facts. Many female marathon runners, who have very low body fat, stop menstruation (amenorrhea), which can be a distinct advantage on the day of a major competition. Sometimes this can become obsessive when the female tries to change such gender anomalies to make themselves more one kind of gender than the other. However, the history books show that this is not a modern day phenomena.

> "Helen Stephens and Stanislawa Walasiewicz dominated women's sprinting during the 1930's. Miss Walasiewicz, born in Poland but raised in the United States, was Olympic 100 metres champion in 1932, and took the silver behind Miss Stephens in the 1936 Berlin Olympics. Miss Stephens was accused by Polish officials of being more man than woman and she took a sex test to disprove the allegation. She retired with an unbeaten sprint record, whilst her arch rival Miss Walasiewicz – who changed her name to Stella Walsh – continued her career during which she set eleven world records and won forty-one USA sprint championships. On December 4, 1980 – forty years after hanging up her spikes – Miss Walsh was out shopping at a Cleveland store when she was innocently caught in the crossfire during a robbery attempt. She was shot dead. An autopsy revealed that the athletics heroine of the thirties had male sexual organs. The Polish officials had levelled their accusations at the wrong athlete."
>
> *Giller, N., 1994*

Chidren in Sport/Child Abuse in Sport

At a time of quite dramatic social change with its impact on the whole fabric of life and social values sport inevitably has become influenced with growing concerns on all fronts.

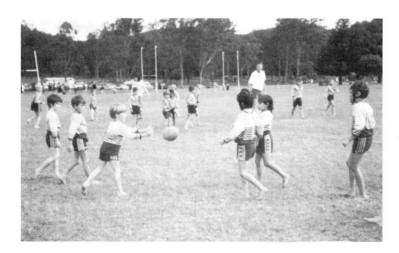

◀ *Figure 34. Children in sport.*

"There is an increasing awareness and concern on the part of parents and educationalists about the possible harmful effects on children who participate at a progressively younger age with an ever increasing intensity in sports competitions designed by and for adults."
The Child and Exercise

Yet at the other extreme:

"I feel let down because one adult came into my sporting life and ruined my childhood."
On the Line, 25.8.93

Clearly something is not quite right and there appears, as usual, to be more questions than answers, with a definite mismatch between how children perceive sport and exercise and how adults do. As previously highlighted **children participate in sport for a variety of reasons; enjoyment/pleasure, belonging/acceptance, worth/recognition, mastery/excellence, responsibility, freedom** (*NCF Coaching Children, 1999*).

Conversely there are those who don't for a variety of reasons; late development, laziness, fear of embarrassment/failure, meeting the wrong adult, lack of opportunity etc. In simplicity those that do, do so because they want to but there are those that are involved under duress. **Unfortunately the evidence of child abuse in sport for those that do participate is cause for concern.** Disuse, misuse, abuse, overuse, under-use of a growing mind and body can have serious consequences. The abuse being identified as verbal, emotional, physical, psychological and sexual. Children are generally far less fit than they were 15 – 20 years ago, and the number of obese and overweight British schoolchildren on the basis of body mass index, has increased significantly since the mid-1980's (*BMJ, 2001, see Appendix 5*). Exercise, sunshine, weight-bearing and shock absorption are integral parts of developing healthy bones. At home, many children are often allowed to spend several hours sat in a bedroom, with the curtains drawn, hunched over a computer or slouched in a chair watching TV or videos. When they do have to move from A to B, they are being transported here there and everywhere. At school, with the emphasis on league tables, PE is not seen as a high priority. As a result are we producing a potentially osteoporotic/obese adult population?

On the other hand, children are able to experience if they so wish, far more sporting activity than ever before. However, the government's latest strategy for sport, 'A Sporting Future For All', (*Hoey, 2000*) identifies not enough opportunities for children and young people to take part in sport. **Clearly there is a conflicting**

dichotomy in relation to young children and sport, those that do, which are under threat from various forms of abuse and those that don't, which are equally under threat from under-use. What is interesting is that the source is the same; adults. On the one hand from being over zealous and taking their responsibility and encouragement too far and on the other hand from abdication of responsibility of helping, guiding and being a good role model for their offsprings. The reasons for both are far from simple and obviously complex and varied. Today's society always has an excuse, by right. How has this situation arisen? Is it arrogance, ignorance or both?

We have looked in quite some detail during the text to date as to the causes and consideration of why injuries occur and in particular the human factor, (*see Chapter 1, Part 5*) and it is to this theme I wish to return.

How much are so-called responsible, experienced adults directly and indirectly responsible for encouraging 'drop-out' in sport as well as directly/indirectly causing traumatic and over-use injury in children? And could this be one of the reasons why we as a nation repeatedly fail to live up to expectation, apart from the occasional success, on the world's sporting scene, because adults disillusion so much potential talent?

One of the problems highlighted by the Government report in 2000, was that the organisation and management of sport in this country was fragmented and too often unprofessional. Research by Wright, Brown and Muir, 1999, showed that children's experiences in sport varied tremendously. For large numbers it was positive but for others it was about waiting for a go; being rejected by the team they aspired to; being subjected to unfair coaching and being belittled when they made a mistake. **It can also be argued that those children who 'make-it' in certain sports are the survivors who have made it in spite of 'the system' and/or some adults but are not necessarily the best. To gloss over this anomaly, mediocrity is then rewarded.**

Why is mediocrity hyped and rewarded in our national sport but not in others? There are now some international footballers who are worth and paid astronomical sums of money who embarrassingly favour/only kick with one foot and appear to have limited skills, in the context of the whole game. Children, and in the context of these notes are considered as 3–19 year olds, are very much influenced by what they see and hear, by and from those around them, i.e. peer group as well as adults. These people sometimes referred to as, **'a ring of influence'**, can, and most certainly do, have a positive or negative influence on how a child perceives a particular concept, situation, idea etc. Into this ring we can now most certainly include information technology, TV, video and cinema.

How much a child is actually influenced by what he/she sees, as opposed to hears, is open to conjecture but there is no disputing the fact they are certainly influenced to a degree. Negative personal rapport being a significant and positive predictor for total, somatic and cognitive anxiety and concentration disruption (*J.Sc.Med., 2000*).

There does appear to be a growing tide of hypocrisy in society today that has pervaded sport where children are concerned. Many so-called, responsible adults purport to have the best interest of children at heart but we can all be reminded of the covert and overt pressures some adults bring to bear on children.

How many are **USING** children to build themselves ivory towers or relive childhood memories/fantasies? As one national newspaper reported years ago but is still applicable today,

> **"What's the use of a mantelpiece full of medals if your child is crippled at 14?"**
> *Daily Mail, 1992*

Booth, 1986, referred to it as; *"the exploitation of young bodies."* How often do we hear on the TV or read in the press that so and so was a promising, brilliant junior but as of yet hasn't or didn't realise their potential? Why? According to Gerrard (1993):

> **"Inherent in the presentation of such musculoskeletal insult there often lurks an over-enthusiastic parent."**

The Daily Mail report (18.4.92), *'The Age of Innocence Bypasses Little Johnny'* also carried a report of how adults offer advice from the touch line and how certain 'managers' perceive their role. In these days of the sporting hooligan it is quite alarming how much interference adults, under the guise of spectator, manager, trainer are having on the sporting contest. Some schools are now having to play inter-school matches, on-the-quiet, because of interference and trouble coming from the touch/side line/bench; *"Parents battle at kids match."* (*Faye Walter, 4.10.00*). Dr. Merry, 1986, a rheumatologist with a keen interest in sporting injuries, claimed that sporting injuries were sustained by four main groups, one of which was children who were pushed too hard by their parents. But is it just parents? We've all heard or come across the alleged, sadomasochistic, adult masquerading as a teacher, coach or trainer. **Does professional sport set good examples in terms of child development, injury care and prevention?**

Again, in certain cases, I fear not, even though they might argue vehemently that they do. As with some bastions of self-regulatory bodies they close ranks if it is suggested there may be better ways to do things, in this case develop childhood talent. As Rudolph Flesch, an American author in Communication Skills says:

"Creative thinking may simply be the realisation that there is no particular virtue in doing things the way they have always been done."

As highlighted at the beginning of this book when discussing sporting mentality, certain sports do appear to have their own covert code of conduct and standard of behaviour. There is an unwritten agenda you might say, where successive moulds/clones are reproduced to carry on these traditions and where attitudes to injury care/prevention are negative, to say the least. Not that tradition and track-records-for-winning are to be pooh-poohed or changed just for the sake of change.

But this sporting mentality and condescending, hypocritical attitude, which does not allow for innovation or change, is one of the reasons why many innocent children end up injured, without developing their obvious if rather raw, precocious talent.

You can learn to ride a bicycle backwards if you are made to practise long enough but there may be other ways, with less risk and accidents! 'Prescription coaching' doesn't allow for individuality. **Abuse can be verbal, emotional, physical, psychological and sexual and many children are crucified physiologically, psychologically and, as Peterson and Renstrom (1986) put it, 'orthopaedically', long before they reach maturity.**

This is because so-called responsible adults pay lip-service to health and safety guidelines. Being injured is considered 'sissy'; foul language is acceptable at any age; twisting the rules to suit; 'fouling professionally' and conning the referee is part of the game. Wanting medical advice or a second opinion is considered heresy; needing treatment or being injured is a cop-out, and where winning is all that matters, irrespective of the outcomes as to who gets hurt in the process. All this is justified by having to accept the harsh realities of today's game and pressures. One leading sporting personality actually informed us all on TV that spitting, verbal abuse and foul play was part and parcel of the modern game involving men. This was in response to one of his players being sent off for dangerous play.

In these days of increasing litigation and compensation how long this state of affairs continues remains to be seen. Life bans are now entering the professional arena but denying someone from earning a living in the only thing they appear to be reasonable at is difficult. It must at this point be strongly emphasised that there are many adults who are doing excellent jobs, at all levels of sport and education, in developing young talent.

Injuries and problems related to children in sport are not new phenomena. Michel and Klein, 1991, reported that in recent years there had been a big increase in the number of sports-related injuries suffered by children. Scanning the literature, the problem doesn't appear to be isolated to Great Britain with articles from Australia, New Zealand and America giving the same message. In September (8.9.93) a BBC2 'On The Line' documentary looked at Chinese gymnasts in constant pain through over-training and injury. The same programme (25.8.93), *Sexual Abuse in Sport*, to repeat and quote one athlete from the script:

"I feel let down because one adult came into my life and ruined my childhood."

In this instance he was referring to his coach who had been convicted of child abuse. One national swimming coach, cited on the programme who had been convicted, was still coaching! **Most sports medicine books now devote chapters to it, governing bodies run courses about it and many commentators have raised concern in the past but the problem is still very much in evidence.**

The Arthritis and Rheumatism Council (ARC) has been highlighting evidence of arthritic-type conditions in young children, as early as seven years, approximately 1:1000 stating as yet this was not significant. How long will it be before it is? Gymnasts and dancers are notoriously early starters. The ARC has also produced literature by Dr. Wendy Dodds and others on Sports Injuries with special reference to children.

Are children just becoming status symbols to be easily disposed of when adults have finished with them and when their novelty has worn off? The author feels they are because some adults are applying adult values and criteria to evaluate young talent/performance. **"D.B. (a super league professional) wouldn't have done that,"** is one cry I hear from a rugby coach evaluating a 15 year old boy's performance during a rugby game, accompanied by a few choice swear words, before substituting the unfortunate culprit for running one way and not another.

Sometimes this abandonment, lack of encouragement and constructive criticism is disguised as; wasn't up to scratch, is injury prone, hasn't got what it takes, had the wrong attitude, wasn't mentally tough enough. We need to ask where does the attitude problem lie, with the adult or the child?

Concern and disquiet for the well-being of young children in sport, who have suffered emotional and physical trauma, long before realising their true potential, the expressions used are 'burnt-out' and 'dropped-out', is becoming more than just anecdotal. In 1989 the British Institute of Sports Coaches ran a four day conference,

'*The Growing Child in Competitive Sport*', saying that adults and in particular coaches had to change their values and philosophies in order that young children emerged from the sporting experience as responsible, autonomous, human beings.

> **"The game is not the thing – the child is."**
> *Margaret Talbot, P.E.A. Fellows Lecture, 1987*

> **"The most significant problems in children's sports are not in reducing injuries, in discovering ways to teach skills better, in finding better training methods, or in employing innovative motivational techniques. The most significant task is changing the values society has imposed upon coaches. If we want to improve children's sports, we must first change the philosophy of coaches to athletes first, winning second. Only when coaches adopt this perspective can we hope to see young people emerge from the sport experience who are responsible, autonomous human beings."**
> *Dr. Rainer Martens, B.A.N.C. Congress, 1987*

From a psychological (*Sports Psychologist, 1996*) and sociological perspective, there is no real argument in favour of early specialisation with disadvantages ranging from social isolation, bingeing, 'burn-out', drinking, drug use, vandalism, unhealthy dietary restrictions and body image problems (*Cahill and Pearl, 1993*).

The National Coaching Foundation was established to provide better coach education and many national coaching bodies are now using such courses and updating their syllabuses to include such things as child development, child protection and first aid. On 20.3.93, Gerald Sinstadt, reporting on TV on the FA's Centre of Excellence at Lilleshall stated that many young players were rejected because of too much football too early. At Lilleshall in the early 90's a significant number of the young boys at the Football School of Excellence failed a medical due to part stress fractures of the spine that they were not born with (*Hodson and Rees, 1994*). Mr. A. Hodson and Mr. D. Rees, at the FA Medical and Educational Centre have since conducted on-going research into these and subsequent findings (*Hodson, 1999*).

> **"Intensified training (for children) has no physiological or educational justification."**
> *Sports Health, 1991*

On 31.8.93, Mr. Ferguson and Mr. Wilkinson were in trouble with the FA for withdrawing children from a tournament that asked 14-year old boys to play four games in a day stating:

"England will never win the World Cup if we continue to burn out the youngsters."

Seven years later, 10.8.00, Mr. Wilkinson was still reporting to the media that in England youth development in football was still 15 years behind certain European Countries.

Early in the 90's, the FA agreed to limit the best of the country's young talent to 50 games a year. This was seen in some quarters as quite revolutionary. According to Graham Taylor, 1993, out of 650 new recruits coming into football, three quarters would be rejected because of injury or not making the grade. However, some children were playing in excess of 150 games a year and in competitive action every day. Some were being subjected to too much pressure at a younger and younger age. Whilst school, local county, English Associations, plus Saturday and Sunday teams were all creating immense conflict for youngsters, especially for the elite performers.

A damning FA report revealed in the national press, Daily Mail, 1992, highlighted the terrible toll of overuse injuries on young footballers. In response to this the FA formed an elite task force with a remit to develop young talent. Ron Noades, one of the chosen elite said that qualified coaches at clubs were the best to look after and nurture schoolboys.

The author finds this a rather sweeping assumption. After all if an insular system appears to be failing in certain areas then surely there needs to be some external input to give a more balanced diet. What is needed are coaches who understand, have the necessary knowledge, skills and expertise, can teach and develop children, as well as play and coach their sport (*see Who Should Become Involved*). Not ex-pros who are given 'jobs for the boys', who don't question and reflect on what they do and why they do it, but just duplicate and repeat the way they have been 'brought up'. The word cloning comes to mind.

Not that football is unique in this respect. At the end of the year 2000, a top English Rugby League coach quit claiming many coaches were abusing young players by a combination of too many matches and too much training (*M.E.N., 17.11.00*).

The Sunday Mail (15.8.93), reported that British Athletic bosses were to hold a series of crisis meetings to discuss, 'as absolute top priority', the injury crisis in athletics and the lack of young talent developing through to top level.

What Do We Need to Know About Children and Sport – an Overview

Many texts, publications and organisations devote time and effort to this topic. However, here are just a few key areas that must be addressed. Psychological, social, physical and skill development should all be looked at as a matter of course:

- **Children are not mini-adults**, physically, emotionally, socially, psychologically or skilfully but are growing organisms in the process of physical and psychological adaptation, adjustment and development.
- Children do not tolerate exercise as well as adults.
- Children do not adjust and adapt to travel or fatigue as well as adults.
- Children are more sensitive to heat and cold and have greater difficulty than adults in adjusting to temperature and fluid imbalance. This is because of their size, their sweat glands which although fixed in number by age three show diminished sensitivity to thermal stress up until about fourteen (*Owen Anderson, 2001*). They breathe more quickly than adults, lose water more quickly and their heart rate is higher.
- Before adolescence, children get a higher proportion of their energy from the aerobic system rather than the anaerobic. However, they do not produce it as efficiently as adults. During puberty they become more aerobically efficient with boys becoming more aerobically superior post-adolescence. Physical changes during and after adolescence increases both their aerobic and anaerobic capabilities.
- Children's tissues are significantly different than those of adults.
- A child's skeleton is a cartilaginous scaffolding that needs to ossify and calcify.
- Children's bones are more resilient, flexible and adaptable but contain growth plates or centres that are vulnerable sites if subjected to excessive stresses and strains. Injury to such areas can totally or partially stop growth, cause limb shortness, epiphyseal slip, growth to be stunted or at an angle. They can how ever, because of a better blood supply, repair quicker, if allowed to.
- The differences between Chronological Age (CA), Developmental Age (DA) and Training Age (TA) should be appreciated. CA referring to a child's actual age in years and months and DA referring to the extent to which a child's emotional, physical and social development, compares, exceeds or falls short of that of 'a typical child' of that CA. TA referring to the number of years experience a child may have gained through regular, structured learning.
- Children's growth is not uniform it is more akin to a staircase than a ramp.
- Bone growth is not consistent. Different bones grow at different rates; femur 2–2.5cm a year, radius 1–2cm a year. Upper sometimes more than lower in long bones. At the knee, growth is concentrated on the distal femur and proximal tibia.

- Children in some year groups may be up to 5 years apart in physical development. In a mixed group of 11–12 year olds there may be children whose biological maturity is in the 15–16 year old bracket.
- Girls grow outwards from the pelvis whilst boys grow longitudinally head to feet.
- Epiphyseal injuries occur because children's muscles, tendons and ligaments are relatively stronger and more elastic compared to adults. In the young elite athlete muscles will generally be that much stronger because of increased activity in these children. Ligaments can be three times stronger than the soft cartilage of the growing end plate and fracture occur (avulsion fracture).

"Tendons and ligaments are further strengthened by molecular 'cross-linking' between and within collagen fibrils. This cross-linking or molecular adhesion increases steadily with age and is one of the big differences between connective tissue in children and adults. Connective tissue becomes more robust as we pass through childhood, but it also becomes much less extensible due to cross-linking of the collagen fibrils. This, of course, is why children can increase range of mobility (flexibility) much more easily than adults...........it also partially explains why connective tissue injuries often differ between adults and children. Acute injuries that often result in torn tendons or ligaments will often result in avulsion injuries in children where the connective tissue will not rupture but instead will 'avulse' or detach a piece of adjoining bone............it has been shown in many animal studies that low intensity exercise is necessary for healthy cartilage (and bone) growth but that very high intensity exercise with compressive loads can result in diminished growth and retardation in maturation. These effects are compounded by endocrinal and nutritional factors."
Russell, K., 1999

Apophyseal injuries occur at sites where major muscle tendons apply traction to the soft bone, e.g. quadriceps at the hips and hamstrings at the ischial tuberosity. This can easily happen if children's musculature is developed rapidly due to regular training. Lachman, 1986, says that during adolescence, injury to ligaments is more likely to occur if muscular co-ordination was poor, as normal reflexes fail to cause effective agonist/antagoinist interaction to protect the joint. Salter, 1963, identified five types of epiphyseal growth plate problems caused by trauma and fracture:

1. Osgood-Schlatter's disease (patellar tendon attachment).
2. Sever's heel (Achilles tendon attachment).
3. Scheuermann's disease (thoracic spine).
4. Osteochondrosis (temporary softening of growing bone).
5. Perthe's disease (femoral head).

Osgood-Schlatter's is especially prevalent amongst 12–17 year olds, whilst 8–15 years is the danger age for avulsion fractures. **Because they are much less aware of their real limits children usually do not drive themselves to the point of injury unless unreasonable demands are placed upon them.** The incidence of stress fractures seems to be on the increase amongst children from the tender age of seven years and upwards, with long-distance running and weight-training the main culprits. Children's motor skills need systematically developing and their co-ordination, especially amongst gangly adolescents, can be poor. Children's growth and development, according to Norman Brook, can be considered in terms of:

- Infancy   0–2 years.
- Childhood   2–9 years for girls, and 2–11 years for boys.
- Growth spurt   9–10 years for girls and 11–14 years for boys.
- Puberty   11–13 years for girls and 14–16 years for boys.
- Adolescence   13–18 years for girls and 16–22 years for boys.
- Adulthood   18+ years for girls and 22+ years for boys.

We might argue they are not adults till at least 18+ with boys much later. In simplicity growth has roughly three phases:

1. Infantile conception to the end of the first year.
2. Childhood rapid growth first year to puberty. Slow steady gains.
3. Adolescence to adulthood, which is when many children experience significant growth spurts and can grow 10–13cm per annum. 75% of boys experience growth spurts between 12–16 years, girls 10–14 years.

These are periods of greatest adaptation and adjustment:

- Growth in girls tends to be complete by 16–18 years, but there can be up to 5 years of adjustment, whilst boys continue into their 20's. Post-adolescence is a period of decreasing gains – 6–12 months after growth spurt there is an increase in muscle mass.
- Growth is dependent on nutritional and hormonal balance and until the body adjusts to these the growing body is naturally stressed, becoming relatively stiff and inflexible, without further conflict by external forces! Coaching Focus, 1993, highlighted the fact that for each year of strenuous training before the menarche, delayed the event by 5 months and whilst this was attributed to low body weight and fat it also pointed out that these were in addition to physical and psychological factors.
- Children develop endurance before power that improves after puberty and subsequently declines again after 28 in men and approximately 35 in women.

- During adolescence children can become less flexible and they may lose co–ordination.
- **Children's learning passes through cognitive (reasoning) associative (relating) and autonomous (habit) phases. Don't forget they have more information to deal with, have limited experience and take longer to know what to do. So screaming numerous instructions interspersed with a volley of swear words in the hope that an immediate response will ensue may be a little optimistic!**
- Children's development passes through various stages some of which are 'critical periods', wherein events must take place or be skipped forever. Learning plateaux occur, when no apparent progress is made but consolidation is happening. These periods should not be confused with lack of effort, practise or application. It should also be appreciated that performance at one particular age in a child's development is a poor predictor of performance 2–5 years later (*Sports Med. in Primary Care, 1996*).
- Generally speaking puberty helps boys and hinders girls.

Finally, to reiterate what has been highlighted previously, research in Russia (1992) and Veritas (1995) and Germany has identified that specialisation too early has short-term gains and long-term disadvantages. Research supports the principle of early generalisation rather than specialisation.

How Can Such Knowledge Help Develop Sporting Talent and Who Should Become Involved?

> **"Talented players do not emerge automatically. If those with potential are to progress we must make sure they get the right coaching and support at every stage and are able to move on to higher levels of competition as they develop their skills............we need to ensure we have coaches of sufficient quality and quantity from the grass roots of sport to the international arena."**
> *Kate Hoey, 2000*

Adults who are going to directly influence children in a sporting sense need to have a knowledge and understanding of:

- Anatomical and physiological development of children.
- The social, psychological and emotional development of the growing body. Children of 3–19 years **DO NOT** need a constant diet of verbal abuse and threats to realise their potential.
- The irregularities in attitude, mood, behaviour and performance associated with such development especially during adolescence.

- Training theory and familiarity with the correct technical development of their chosen sport.
- How children respond and adapt to exercise.
- How children move and acquire skills.
- Nutritional knowledge and how best to fuel the growing body.
- How injuries can be caused and initially managed.
- A general understanding of the importance of what is involved in and the stages of rehabilitation after injury.

If they don't then it is suggested they either attend relevant courses to develop such skills and expertise and then practise them under the supervision of a suitably qualified adult, or let those qualified to do so get on with it. **This knowledge, skill and expertise cannot be acquired quickly** and whilst it is accepted there are 'naturals', with intuitive skills, sound theory must underpin good, pedagogical practice. If children are to benefit from their involvement with the core of experienced adults, teachers, educators and coaches that exist then it is help and support these adults want, not hindrance and interference.

Getting involved is what we would all advocate but those in charge need to keep a very tight control of who is getting involved and their motives. 'Jobs for the boys' definitely needs re-appraisal. In these days of cost cutting and value for money anyone can become involved who is prepared to put in voluntary time and effort.

In 1992, a conference at Nottingham University on After School Sports, highlighted the fact that in view of the recent changes to school management and teachers contractual obligations, anyone could fill the void unless a structured, organised body accepted responsibility for after school sport. What is the situation now as we progress through the next millennium? Such knowledge should include the following:

- The overuse/under-performance, 'overplaying syndrome' should be recognised (*see Chapter 2, Part 3*).
- Selection, screening and grouping of children for sport should take into consideration; CA, DA, TA, size, weight, physical maturity, gender, physical condition, state of excellence (skill level) aerobic and anaerobic capacity.
- Contact sports need greatest consideration in terms of height and weight, whilst running needs to consider aerobic and anaerobic development.
- Training of children should be comprehensive. It should initially be general all-round fitness with perhaps 2–3 skill sessions plus one competitive match per week. Once apophyses and epiphyses have grown (approximately 16+) and united then training can be specific if properly planned and supervised. However, Dr. Malcolm Read (1992) does point out that whilst specificity is

important it does have its dangers, even with adults. The skill is to produce elite performance without breakdown.

- Training programmes, competitive training schedules and rules applied to many sports and games are not always appropriate for the growing child. Intensive training may produce short-term improvement but the psychosocial effects may be detrimental in the long-term, i.e. many children give up sport because of too much too soon.
- not over-train fast growing children, i.e. just before their first period and breast bud development.
- Reduce training intensity during growth spurts.
- Plyometrics (dynamic stretching and contraction of muscle hopping, leaping and bounding) which require a high degree of fitness and skeletal maturity should be avoided during growth periods and in pre-adolescent children, as rapid acceleration and deceleration movements can lead to 'growth plate' problems.
- Create practise routines that meet the child's needs and abilities – training should be appropriate for bodies not to create impressions or to fit the child into the planned session. Keep instructional skills simple and meaningful.
- Remember to always include warm-up and cool down practices, encourage drinking especially in warm weather and watch for signs of distress.

As a general guide we can refer to Peterson and Renstrom (1986):

- 3–7 years – structured play, discovery and enjoyment. Develop basic movement patterns.
- 7–9 years – play, technique and all-round training. Children at this stage are receptive to learning. Co-ordination work, enjoyment and continue to develop basic movement patterns.
- 10–11 years – general basic training and all-round fitness. Playing a variety of games with simple rules. Systematic training and anaerobic fitness is considered not meaningful. Don't forget enjoyment.
- 12–14 years – general fitness training and learning techniques with some tactics. The body is in a sensitive state of development but the ability to learn is still high. Enjoyment.
- 15–16 years – preparation for specialised training. Anaerobic training. Flexibility emphasis essential to overcome stiffness. Strength training can begin but with light loads and improve with repetitions not weight. Enjoyment.
- 16 + years – specialised training. Never use heavy weights or until bone development is complete. Enjoyment.

These guidelines are not about specific fitness but are related to development and children not what to include in a PE syllabus/fitness schedule. Strength training initially is using the child's own weight because until the hormonal complement is developed in the body, things such as power training serve no useful purpose what-soever, other than to create a potential injury:

- Teach children static (isometric) stretching exercises not ballistic, bouncing ones.
- The child's needs should come first, not the coaches/teachers, winning second. Health and safety should be paramount with suitable equipment and practice procedures used at all times.
- Modification is the key word, e.g. playing area, rules, equipment etc.
- Discipline is essential. Reinforce achievement/rules/fair play.
- Rules should be introduced as a framework to build on. Adapt them and explain the reasons for, e.g. safety, avoid accidents etc.
- From an early age they should be encouraged to appreciate the need for rules and fair play and to follow them within the spirit of the game. It is important here to stress that the child needs help and guidance as to what her/his needs are, i.e. nutrition, clothing, equipment when to stop/start, when to rest etc. Explain the reasons and excesses of all things pertaining to their development, e.g. rules, sensible eating, fair play, abuse, misuse etc.
- Testing and screening children should be purposeful so that the right somatotype/personality ends up in the right sport doing the right things and not just to give an hierarchy on top/bottom, good and bad.

In essence **what children need at all stages of their development is help and guidance, an ethical and moral role model, based on sound, basic knowledge of how they develop and differ from adults not swear words, favouritism, threats, abuse, harassment, de-motivation and extra training.** Some coaches I've spoken to openly admit that it is a good idea to make children more frightened of you than the opposition. In practice this ensures temper tantrums, foul language, threats and 'childish behaviour' from the coach if he/she doesn't get his/her own way. **Why is it that some adults firmly believe that sentences must contain F, C and T words for communication to be effective?** (*see Chapter 1, Part 2*).

In working with children, adults could do no worse than read Martin Lee's 1985 article. **Although written in 1985 it is still very relevant today; in the article, words and phrases such as encouraging, friendly, helpful, quality of experience are used and encouraged as opposed to critical, demanding and dictatorial.**

In an ever increasingly, materialistic, instantly disposable, society which seems to be guided by instant gratification and an almost total lack of agreed values, is sport producing a future generation of underdeveloped, over-stressed, easily excitable, over competitive, burnt-out talent? To re-iterate the other uncomfortable scenario is that those children who are not being encouraged to exercise, preferring instead to vegetate in front of modern technology, may end up a future generation of osteoporotic, obese individuals. Balance seems to have been lost somewhere.

Man (*homosapiens*) is supposed to be the highest form of animal intelligence on the planet, but are they? In a legal sense some adults are guilty of assault and battery, and are negligent in their failure to carry out their moral and loco-parentis duty of care. Tort (*negligence*) or civil wrong doings can easily become an issue. In today's world, humans could learn a lot from the rest of the animal kingdom in terms of parental care and control.

We all have a moral responsibility and duty of care to anyone we can reasonably foresee may be affected by our actions. A growing number of adults may need reminding of this – otherwise some children may never recover from their childhood. Or is it some children may never recover from adults?

Veterans

What constitutes a veteran? Clearly as we have seen to date the question and concept of age and ageing is a pertinent issue. One that is not only open to wide interpretation but also one some people find difficult to address, especially if they have had a lifetime in sport, with varying degrees of success. When to hang up the boots, stop competing, call it a day, etc. are all issues related to age and ageing. Modification, acceptance and balance are words that become more significant as one gets older and ignoring the body's warning signs becomes more and more difficult.

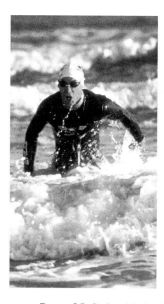 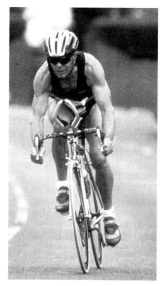 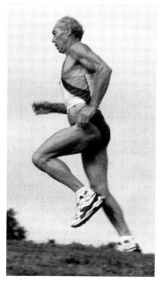

▲ *Figure 35. Richard Lake, UK International veteran age group world champion in action. Photographs courtesy of Paul Hulbert.*

Altering a lifetime of mind-set may prove to be the biggest hurdle. Certainly as we get older we can't put back what has been worn away and we don't heal and repair as well as we used to. Secondary problems, e.g. arthritis, can become more evident, unless we accept, modify and adjust. As for what age constitutes a veteran depends on who is defining the criteria, over 40, 50, 60 etc. But then the oldest competitor in the 1999 London Marathon was an American in his 80's.

Less Able Bodied/Disabled Performers

As this section of the sporting world has its own local, national and international competitions they must be given due acknowledgement in any text of this nature. The recent successes and the higher profiles of the 1996 Atlanta and 2000 Sydney Paralympic Games are testament to the enormous development and progress that has been achieved by/for such athletes. Therefore much of what is covered in this book is just as relevant to this section of the sporting community as to able bodied. Again a course of study in its own right which some sports therapists may want to become involved with/in.

Part 7

Working Relationships – P Principles

It has already been identified that one of the roles of the sports therapist is an understanding of the participants themselves and those who are directly and/or indirectly associated with these people. What role these personnel play depends on the sport, the size of the club and whether the club is amateur, semi-professional or professional. In a professional club situation, apart from the players themselves, the list could involve:

- **Administrative/ground staff.**
- **Manager.**
- **Physiotherapist.**
- **Sports therapist.**
- **Masseuse/masseur.**
- **Doctor/medical officer.**
- **Trainers.**
- **Coaches.**
- **'Kit man'.**
- **Nutritionist/dietician.**
- **Psychologist.**

Other professionals can be called upon as and when required and this list can include:

- Chiropodist/podiatrist.
- Osteopath/chiropractor.
- Dentist.
- Specialist consultant.
- Counsellor.
- Social worker.
- Sports scientist.
- Sports physiologist.

This is not to mention other agencies such as ambulance service, police, fire services and health and safety executives. What each of these roles involves, other than what is obvious, depends on many factors. Let us also not forget the role that supporters can play in creating positive and negative environments.

With so much knowledge, skill and expertise involved in one way or another, each extolling the importance of their own particular role, it is not uncommon that conflict, personality/ego clashes and disagreements can and do occur. Role definition becomes blurred and 'hierarchical pecking orders' materialise.

"It is a false premise to believe that good relationships have no conflict."
Thomas, A., 2000

By pursuing and promoting proper procedures and following established principles, peak performance may be produced without problems. However, puffed up personalities and politics may prevent and prohibit this. Alma Thomas, 2000, says that outstanding team performance occurs when:

- There is an assiduous commitment to a common target or goal.
- The team honestly believe they can achieve the goal set.
- Each individual member of the team feels that they have a significant role to play in pursuing the goal.
- The team and the individuals are treated with respect.
- There is a strong sense of purpose, co-operation and reciprocal support in pursuing the goal.

These factors being also being pertinent for individual performance that has to rely on the back-up team (*see Chapter 2, Part 8*).

It is therefore essential that all working as part of a team do so by supporting the concepts/values/ideals of responsibility, integrity, trust, competence, effectiveness, efficiency, equality of opportunity, fair play, professionalism, equity, sportsmanship, safety, encouragement, respect, effective communication, positivism, etc. For the sports therapist liasing/working directly or indirectly with such people it is vital to ensure, not only for the positive 'ethos' of the establishment but also the maintenance of a fit, healthy and happy team that:

- Good lines of communication are established, so that any problems are resolved both quickly and decisively.
- Remember a chain is only as strong as the weakest link.

- Everyone's role is clearly defined and relationships are established that are based on mutual respect, trust and a confidence in each other's knowledge, skill, expertise and professionalism. They should also be built on individual and combined experiences. Role definition requires job specifications that can be drafted by the employing institution, professional body or the individuals involved. Obviously a job description that is drafted in mutuality would appear to be the most beneficial for all concerned. However, each member of the team must be made aware of what that role involves so that potential areas of conflict can be identified. Conflict and disagreement can arise not only within an individual but also between individuals.
- Decisions are made for the benefit of the team and/or athlete and not for individual 'ego tripping'. Dr. Tim Anstiss, 1992, identified the interactive processes between doctor, coach and athlete that should take place in the decision-making process.
- Other people's viewpoints/perspectives are considered important so that modifications can be made.
- A flexible approach to the differing attitudes and expectations of all concerned is adopted.

The subject of working relationships and role definition is taken up again in Chapter 8, Part 3. In a problem-solving scenario the ability to be aware that a problem exists is a pre-requisite to solving it in a constructive way. Sometimes in sport a problem is identified but no one wants to accept responsibility for either its existence or its solution. Blaming someone else and 'passing the buck' appears to be a popular pastime. **How many games, contests and matches have been lost because it was the judges/referees fault and not the fact that one individual or team wasn't good enough to overcome the opposition.**

In sporting situations where the working ethos is based on a mutual respect of each other's role then problems are quickly identified and dealt with satisfactorily. Sport, with its different strands, is no different to health care where an ideal scenario is one where allopathic and complementary medicine is seen as a body of carers all of whom know and respect each others knowledge, skill, expertise and contribution to the whole health care picture. Whilst enormous progress has been made in the past 15 years to marry these differing perspectives, in an atmosphere of co-existence, there is still some way to go. How far has sport come?

References

1. Alter, M. J.: 1998. Sport stretch. 7, Human Kinetics.
2. Anderson, O.: 2001. Yes, children can run marathons without risk to their health. *Peak Performance*, 148: 2, April, 2001.
3. Anstiss, Dr. T.: 1992. Returning after injury – who makes the decision? *Sports Therapy*, 3:1.
4. Atkinson, J.: 1988. *Gymnast*, January/February.
5. Bandy, W. D., *et al.*: 1997. The effect of time and frequency of static stretch on the flexibility of the hamstring muscles. *Physical Therapy*, 77: 1090–1096.
6. Berk, L. S., *et al.*: 1985. The suppressive effect of stress from acute exhaustive exercise on T lymphocyte helper/suppresser ratio in athletes and non-athletes. *Medicine and Science in Sport and Exercise*, 117 (4) 492.
7. Bledsoe, J.: 1999. So what is wheat and what is the chaff about this new performance drink Endurox R4? *Peak Performance*, 123: 7–9, October.
8. BMJ. 2001. Reported in *SportEx*, 8, April 2001 as The Fat of the Land.
9. Bogduk, N., and Mercer, S.: 1995. Selection and Application of Treatment. In Refshauge, K. M., Gass, E. M. (eds): *Musculoskeletal Physiotherapy Clinical Science and Practice*.
10. Brilliant, A.: 1972. Source unknown.
11. Brook, N.: 1987. Endurance running. Chapter 6.
12. Burke, E. R.: 1997. Nutrients that accelerate healing, strength and conditioning. 19–23. *Strength and Conditioning Association*.
13. Cahill, B. R. and Pearl A. J.: 1993. Intensive participation in children's sports. 95–126, Human Kinetics.
14. Caine, D. J., Caroline, G., and Lindner, K. J.: 1996. Epidemiology of sports injuries. 1, 1–8, Human Kinetics.
15. Carlton, I.: 2001. Fluid balance: water – is it the best choice for post-exercise rehydration? *Peak Performance*, 145, February.
16. Ciullo, J. V., and Zarins, B.: 1983. Biomechanics of the musculotendinous unit: relation to athletic performance and injury. *Clinics in Sports Medicine*, 2 (1), 71–86.
17. Costain, L.: 2000. British Dietetics Association found in Water: Pure Therapy by Alice Kavounas, Kyle Cathie.
18. Denton, J.: 2000. World Class Performance – Medical Screening in Gymnastics. *NSMI News*, 18, Spring.
19. De Vries, Herbert A.: 1986. Physiology of Exercise for Physical Education and Athletics, 4th ed. 489–498, William C. Brown.
20. Dodds, Dr. G.: 1989. Body Chemistry: Effects on Soft Tissue. Northern Institute of Massage Lecture, Blackpool, 8.4.89.
21. Escola, et al.: 1978. Effects of sports stress on lymphocyte transformation and antibody formation. *Clinical and Experimental Immunology*, 32 (2), 339-345.
22. *Fit Sports Rev. Int.*: 1992, 132–133, August.
23. Fitton, P.: 2000. 'Bring on the Super Refs.' Mail on Sunday, 27.8.00.
24. Gerrard, D. F.: 1993. Overuse injury and growing bones: the young athlete at risk. *British Journal of Sports Medicine*, 27.
25. Gershwin, N. E., Beech, R. S., Hurley, L. S.: 1985. Nutrition and Immunity. Academic Press Inc.
26. Giller, N.: 1994. This sporting laugh. 2:74, Robson Books.
27. Goldstone, Professor, L.: 2001. The research agenda for massage therapists. Northern Institute of Massage, 22.03.01.
28. Green, J.: 2000. Evidence-based medicine or evidence informed osteopathy? *Osteopathy Today*, 6 (4), 21–22, April, 2000.
29. Hamer, Dr.: 2000. 'Thrill seekers'. European Cable T, 9.8.00.
30. Hilgard and Atkinson: 1967. Introduction to Psychology.
31. Hiseman, J.: 1997. Warm-up and warm down, why? *American Track and Field Magazine*.
32. Hlavac, Dr. H: 1999. Entering the foot zone. Course notes, Dr. M. Lindy, Haydock, 6.11.99.
33. Hodson, A.: 1999. Too much too soon. The risk of 'overuse' injuries in young football players. *Journal of Bodywork and Movement Therapies, 3* (2) 35–91.
34. Hoey, K.: 2000. A sporting future for all. *Faster Higher and Stronger*, 13–15, Summer, 2000.
35. Jenkins, Dr. S.: 2000. Demystifying the penalty-kick. Found in *Sportscare*, 20, Autumn, 2000.
36. Journal Science and Medicine and Sport 2000, 3 (2) 110–9, June 2000.

37. Karvonen, J.: 1992. Importance of warm-up and cool down on exercise performance. *Medicine and Sports Training and Coaching*.

38. Kaufman, K. R., Brodine, S. K., Shaffer, R. A., Johnson, C.W., Cullinson, T. R.: 1999. The effect of foot structure and range of motion on musculo-skeletal overuse injuries. *American Journal of Sports Medicine*, 27 (5): 585–593.

39. Kleiner, S. M.: 1999. Water an essential but overlooked nutrient. *J. Am. Diet Association, 99*(2): 200–206, February.

40. Knill, Dr. J: 1988/99. How much do we know? BASM Conference, Manchester.

41. Komi, P., and Buskirk, E.: 1972.The effects of eccentric and concentric muscle activity on tension and electrical activity of human muscle. *Ergonomics*, 15: 417–434.

42. Kujala, U.M., Orava, and Jarvinnen, M.: 1997. Hamstring injuries: current trends in treatment and prevention. *Sports Medicine*, 23 (6), 397–404.

43. Lachmann, S.: 1986. Soft Tissue Injuries in Sport.

44. Lakomy, J., Dabinett, J., and Nevill, M.: 2000. Physiological differences between elite male and female games players. *Faster Higher and Stronger*, 9, October, 2000.

45. Lederman, Dr. E.: 1997. Fundamentals of Manual Therapy, Churchill Livingstone.

46. Leese, L.: 2000. 'British humour is so peculiar,' Mail on Sunday, 23.1.00.

47. Lehmann, J., F., Massock, A. J., Warren, C. G., and Koblanski, N. J.: 1970. Effects of therapeutic temperatures on tendon extensibility. Archives of *Physical Medicine and Rehabilitation*, 41, 481–487.

48. Macdonald. R.: 2000. Research. *Osteopathy Today*, 6.02, 6.

49. Mackinon, et al.: 1987. The effects of exercise on secretory and natural immunity. *Advances in Experimental Medicine and Experimental Biology*, 216A, 869–876.

50. Martens, Dr. R.: 1987. BANC Congress.

51. Martin, B. J., Johnson, W. R., and Kramer, G.F.: 1975. Effects of warm-up on metabolic responses to strenuous exercise. *Medicine and Science in Sport and Exercise*.

52. Martin, L.: 1985. The importance of positive relationships. *Coaching Focus*, 2, Autumn, 1985.

53. McClune, T.: 2000. The evidence base of osteopathy. *Osteopathy Today*, May, 2000.

54. Michel, L. J., and Klein, J. B.: 1991. 'Sports injuries in children and adolescents.' *British Journal of Sports Medicine (GB)*, 25:1, 6–9, March, 1991.

55. *New Scientist*, 2000. No. 2251, 12.8.00.

56. Nicholls, A. H.: 1972. Developing a curriculum. 32–47.

57. Nigg, B., Wakeling, J.: 2000. High tech. shoe design. Human Performance Laboratory, University of Calgary, reported in *Sportscare News*, 20, Autumn.

58. Noakes, T.: 1999. Sudden death and exercise. *Sports Science News Journal* (Internet Site), 1–11.

59. Norris, C.M.: 1995. Spinal stabilisation: muscle imbalance and the low back. *Physiotherapy*, 81(3): 127–138.

60. Norris, C. M.: 1998. Sports injuries: diagnosis and management, 2nd. ed.

61. Northern Institute of Massage Sports Therapy Course, Seminar II: pre-2000. Young sports people and injury.

62. Ohlen, G., Wredmark, T., and Spangfort, E.: 1989. Spinal saggital configuration and mobility related to low back pain in female gymnasts. *Spine,* 14 (8): 847–850.

63. Pederson, B. K., et al.: 1988. Modulation of natural killer cell activity in peripheral blood by physical exercise. *Scandinavian Journal of Immunology*, 27: 673.

64. Peterson, Dr. L., and Renstrom, Dr. P.: 1986. Sports injuries: their prevention and treatment. Chapter 9. Risks to children and adolescents.

65. Plowman, S. A. and Smith, D. L.: 1997. Exercise physiology for health, fitness and performance. 498–507, Boston, USA: Allyn and Bacon.

66. Quigley, T. B.: 1981. Sports health. Southmayd and Hoffman.

67. Read, Dr. M.: 1992. The Achilles Tendon. SST Annual Conference, Solihull.

68. Reid, D. C.: 1992. Sports injury assessment and rehabilitation. Churchill Livingstone.

69. Rowlands, D. S.: 1997. Biochemistry of Exercise. *Sportscience News*, September/October, 1997.

70. Russell, K.: 1999. Connective tissue: children are not small adults. *Coaches Report* (CAN) 5:4, 28–29.

71. Safran, M. R., Seaber, A. V., and Garrett, W. E.: 1989. Warm-up and muscular activity prevention – an update. *Sports Medicine*, 8, 239–249.

72. Sapega, A., et al.: 1981. Biophysical factors in range of motion exercise. *Physician and Sports Medicine*, 12(9), 57–65.

73. Shellock, F. G., and Prentice: 1985. Warming-up and stretching for improved physical performance and prevention of sports-related injuries. *Sports Medicine, 2*, 267–278.

74. Sims, G.: 1999. Eyes wide shut, *Inside Sport (Aus)*, 21–22, 24–29, June, 1999.

75. Skinner, J.: 1999. All swimmers are not created equal. *Swimming Technique*, April–June, 1999.

76. Smith, G. N.: 1990. Sports Therapy Diploma, Course Notes, STES Ltd.

77. Smith, C. A.: 1994. The warm-up procedure: to stretch or not to stretch. A brief review. *The Journal of Orthopaedic and Sports Physical Therapy*, 19 (1), 12–17.

78. Smolevski, V., and Suchilin, N.: 1992. BAGA Coaches Conference Papers; the Soviet plan for technical preparation in gymnastics.

79. Sport Psychologist. 1996: 10, 341–366.

80. Sports Health. 1991: 9, 23–24.

81. Sports Medicine in Primary Care. 1996: 2 (12), 87–89.

82. Stewart, Dr. A.: 1993. Fatigue and nutrition. An article taken from, 'Tired all the Time.'

83. Taylor, G.: Manchester Evening News, April 20th, 1993.

84. The Child and Exercise: An Overview. *Journal of Sports Science*, 4. 3–20, 3.

85. Thomas, A.: 2000. Managing conflict. *Faster Higher Stronger*, 9, October, 2000.

86. Torrence, A.: 1988. Sports nutrition. Society of Community Medicine Conference, Manchester.

87. Troop, R.: 1999. Sports injuries. *Peak Performance*, 117.

88. Veritas: 1995. From childhood to champion athlete.

89. Walker, I.: 2001. A single scientific study proves nothing. *Peak Performance*, 148, April.

90. Walshe, K.: 1995. Given in evidence. *Health Service Journal*, 29.06.95.

91. Walter, F.: 2000. 'Parents battle at kids match,' Manchester Evening News, 4.10.

92. Webborn, Dr. N.: 2000. Continuing professional development in sport and exercise medicine – a discussion paper. *Sportscare News*, 20, Autumn, 2000.

93. Wickham, S.: 1999. Evidence informed midwifery – what is evidence informed midwifery? *Today*, 51, 42–43. Autumn, 2000.

94. Wright, J., Brown, R., and Muir, P.: 1999. 'Children's participation in sport.'

95. Zneimer, J.: 1999. Pitch rage – a worrying trend. A football playing psychologist's view. Premier Sports Medicine Millennium Newsletter.

Bibliography

1. Babkes, M. L., Weiss, M. R.: 1999. Parental influence on children's cognitive and affective responses to competitive soccer participation.

2. BASM Conference, Manchester: 1986. 'Prevention of sports injuries.'

3. Bohner, W.: Key factors in coaching: developing female gymnasts.'

4. Caine and Lindner: 1996. Epidemiology of sports injuries.

5. Coaching children and young performers/people. 1999.

6. Coaching Focus No.2, 'Competitive sport and young children.' Autumn, 1985.

7. Coaching Focus, No.22, Eating disorders in sport. Spring, 1993.

8. Coaching Focus No.27, The development of young people and the role sport has to play.

9. Crouch, M.: 1998. Protecting children: a guide for sports people.

10. Daily Mail: 1992. 'England will pay for too much play, the age of innocencemby-passes little Johnny,' 18.4.92.

11. De Pauw, K., and Gavron, S.: 1995. Disability and sport.

12. Drinkwater, B.: 2000. The encyclopaedia of sports medicine, 8. Women in sports.

13. Encyclopaedia of sports medicine, 6, The child and adolescent athlete. Blackwell, 1996.

14. Exercise and the immune system. Source unknown.

15. Fentem, P. H., Bassey, E. J., and Turnbull, N. B.: 1988. The new case for exercise.

16. Gleeson, G.: 1986. The growing child in competitive sport. Hodder and Stoughton.

17. Griffin, J.: Diet problems in sport. Coaching Focus No.10, Nutrition and Sport.

18. Hamill, B.: 1993. Coaching Focus No.27, Weight training and weightlifting for children.

19. Hugger, M.: 1999. Coaching young performers.

20. Hungerford, M.: 1998. Beyond sports medicine. Sports Massage Training Institute.

21. Karpovitch: Physiology of muscular activity. Saunders and Saunders.

22. Kingsley, K.: Inappropriate training: its significance and ill-effects.

23. Lee, M.: 1985. The importance of positive relationships. Coaching Focus, No. 2, Autumn.

24. Maffulli, N.: 1995. Colour atlas and text of sports medicine in childhood and adolescence. Mosby.

25. Maffulli, N., and Pintore, E.: 1990. Intensive training in young athletes. *BJSM*, 24:4.

26. Mager, R. G.: 1962. Preparing instructional objectives.

27. Manchester Evening News, 17.11.00, Bernard quits as coach.
28. Morrisey, D.: Injuries in young people and their prevention.
29. NCF Introductory Study Pack 7, Working with children, 1, Coaching Children.
30. Northern Institute of Massage, Sports Therapy Course, Seminar 2: 1990. 'Young sports people and injury.'
31. *Peak Performance*, Kids and sport. Issue No.148, April 2001.
32. Rowley, S.: 1986/1990. The effects of intensive training on young athletes.
33. Russel, B.: 1998. The growth of physical characteristics in male and female children. *Research in Action*.
34. Russel, K.: 1998. The growing athlete: connective tissue. Coaches Report, 29.
35. Russel, K.: 1998. The growing athlete: a look at skeletal differences. Coaches Report, 27.
36. Saunders, J.: 1994. Schoolchildren and sport. *Sports Care Journal*, 1.
37. Sharp, C.: Aspects of anatomy and physiology of the sports woman.
38. Sharp, C.: 1994. Aspects of training and sport for children. *Sports Care Journal*, 1:2.
39. *SportsCare News*, 2000. New 'Pee Chart' available, Dieticians in Sport and Exercise Nutrition (DISEN), 21: Winter 2000. DISEN P O Box 22360, London, W13 9FL.
40. Sterling, P. and Eyer, J.: 1988. Allostasis: a new paradigm to explain arousal pathology. Ed. Fisher, S. and Pearson, *J. Handbook of life stress cognition and health*, 629–649, John Wiley and Sons, New York.
41. Taba, H.: 1962. Curriculum development: theory and practice.
42. TOYA and Sports Injuries – Sports Council Publication. 1990. *Coaching Focus*, No.14, Summer.

Chapter 2
Exercise, Training, Fitness and Performance

Quitters never win and winners never quit!

True strength is a measure not of the body but of the soul.

Part 1

What is Exercise?

> "Any activity resulting in physical exertion that is intended to maintain physical fitness, to condition the body or correct any physical deformity."
>
> *Oxford Concise Medical Dictionary, 4th edition*

But is it good or bad for you? The answer to this will, to a certain extent, depend on whose opinion you seek. Was it Mark Twain who said that the only exercise he got was visiting the graves of his friends who used to take exercise? People will always think of reasons for and against taking exercise.

> "The only reason I would take up jogging is so that I could hear heavy breathing.....again."
>
> *Erma Bombeck*

"Exercise is bunk. If you are healthy, you don't need it: if you are sick, you shouldn't take it."
Henry Ford

"I have always said that exercise is a short cut to the cemetery."
John Mortimer

"I like long walks, especially when they are taken by people who annoy me."
Fred Allen

"Too much health is unhealthy."
Leo Rosten

"There is no human activity, eating, sleeping, drinking or sex, which some doctor somewhere won't discover leads directly to cardiac arrest."
John Mortimer

These views, however, are purely subjective and any serious consideration of the subject requires a more objective approach.

Part 2

The Case For and Against Exercise

For

The benefits of exercise for individuals, when of suitable intensity, which is regular and carried out sensibly, far out weigh the risks (*Fenton, Bassey and Turnbull, 1988*). Exercise is of general benefit at all ages because it is necessary for the preservation of optimum function and structure of muscles, bones, joints and the cardiovascular system. According to Dr. Peter Sperryn:

"Physical activity is beneficial to health in a general way and, whilst not necessarily guaranteeing the individual longer life can improve the quality of his daily life and delay deterioration in fitness due to age and inactivity."

This ensures that even when one individual is constrained through ageing or disease, work capacity and fatigue can be maintained and avoided.

AGE IS A STATE OF MIND – AGEING IS A FACT OF LIFE

But if exercise is so beneficial for the body, why is it the cause of so many referrals and visits to the Accident and Emergency (A & E) units at the local hospitals? (*Nicholls, J., 1986*). The following may help us to answer that question.

The benefits of exercise can be considered as **PSYCHOLOGICAL AND PHYSIOLOGICAL**.

Psychologically, exercise:

- Improves attitude to longevity and outlook.
- Helps reduce tension, anxiety and stress.
- Is more effective than drugs in treating long-term serious depression.
- Enhances mood by altering brain chemistry
  (*Sharp, 1994; Murray and Pizzomo, 1998*).
- Improves confidence, memory, concentration and decisional efficiency.
- May reduce handicap and help avoid or delay the necessity for institutional care.

Physiologically, exercise:

- Can induce physical fitness (*Murray and Pizzomo, 1998*).
- Delays physical decline in the over 60's.
- Reduces the likelihood of developing coronary heart disease by the reduction of arterial blood pressure, improving the transport of blood lipids with less likelihood of these being deposited in the artery walls. There is also a reduction of blood clotting factors and of sympathetic activity and adrenaline release. There is also the added benefit in that cardiac muscular activity improves its strength and efficiency.
- Attenuates (reduces) blood pressure associated with hypertension. Training causes hypertrophy of the heart and skeletal muscle (*Lakomy, et al.*, 2000).
- Improves oxygen uptake and cardiovascular functions.
- Contributes to the prevention and treatment of chronic conditions.
- Assists weight reduction.
- Can thicken hyaline cartilage, so that greater forces can be tolerated by the joint – this process exists 10–30 minutes after activity cessation.
- Increases tissue sensitivity to insulin.
- Maintains or increases bone density even after menopause. To slow the rate of osteoporosis the vital factor is that the exercise has to be weight bearing (*Sharp, 1994*).
- Can improve pregnancy (unfit mothers usually have a 'hard time').

In simplicity exercise contributes to a reduction in mortality and morbidity and adds to enjoyment of life; people feel better and they function better. A person's quality of life young or old can be greatly enhanced. Exercise is now available on prescription from certain GPs in certain areas, for example rehabilitation after heart attack.

"Physical activity must be one of the most undervalued interventions to improve public health."
SportEX, 2001

Against

Exercise can:

- Cause **INJURY** via U factors, i.e. overuse, abuse, misuse.
- Become **ADDICTIVE** as a result of the release of the body's own opiate-like substances.
- Cause **SYNCOPE** (dizziness).
- Compromise the immune system, which can lead to a multitude of problems and eventually cause **DEATH**.

Noakes, T., 1999, discusses predisposing, triggering factors and screening for risk factors, i.e. Marfan's Syndrome and various arrhythmias, in sudden death and exercise. In Issue 3 of the NCF publication, *FHS*, April 1999, John Bryant, the Deputy Editor of the Times, touches on all of these issues when he considers the most dangerous performance enhancer of all to be obsession, related to the addictive aspects of exercise. An obsession that begins with a habit but a habit that has both positive and negative aspects. The positive allows the athlete to fully relax after they have indulged their habit and completed their planned training session. The negative is that when things start to go wrong the athlete will not or cannot break the habit. There is, he says, a thin line between the habit of dedication/ commitment and the habit of obsession. One giving positive results whilst the other can become destructive.

Another area where this issue comes to the fore is in relation to diet and body form. Gill Horgan, 1994, asks the question: *"Is the motivation behind exercise the pursuit of sporting excellence or the pursuit of slimness?"*

She goes on to say: *"There are those people who use diet as a means of improving performance and those who use diet as a means of controlling their weight. What are the consequences of both? The image of the modern day female athlete – healthy, slim and brimming with vitality is one to which many women aspire. But are those athletes healthy? Do they have enough energy to enjoy life outside their sport? Are they controlling their weight or is their obsession with the weight controlling them? Weight control and disordered eating issues have become heavily associated in the public mind with the female sector of the population, and especially female athletes.*

Although it is recognised that males, including male athletes can be susceptible to eating disorders, predominantly at risk are females in the 15–25 year age range. They are told that in order to improve their performance they have to train hard and eat the right diet. But are they eating the right diet for the right reason and indeed are they eating the right diet? There are many athletes who are so serious about their performance that they will manipulate their diet in order to achieve success. It is well known that gymnasts and skaters are judged highly on their aesthetic quality and many an endomorph has attempted to diet into becoming an ectomorph and has ended up being a hungry endomorph with an eating disorder. They forget that, not only is natural ability, training and mental preparation necessary for success, but also that overall good nutrition is essential for training and recovery and must never be skipped in favour of weight loss. Athletes who have to attain a set weight in order to compete in certain weight categories often compromise this overall good nutrition in favour of quick weight loss without any thought for the future. In both cases there is a coupling of excessive exercise with dieting, binge eating and food obsession, leading to disordered eating, guilt and a negative attitude towards food. In extreme cases this disordered eating leads to anorexia and bulimia nervosa."

Eating disorders, such as anorexia and bulimia nervosa and weight management issues are not solely found in sport but there are issues related to such that all working in sport should be aware of.

> **"At any one time, 60,000 people in the UK are known to be suffering from anorexia or bulimia, although the real figure is thought to be closer to 150,000–200,000. Around 10% of sufferers are male."**
> *Jasmine Challis, 1992*

Exercise Induced Syncope

Syncope (dizziness), can be defined as:

> **"A brief, sudden loss of consciousness and muscle tone secondary to cerebral ischaemia, inadequate oxygen or glucose delivery to the brain, is common following exercise, especially long duration and static exercise."**
> *John Davis, 2000*

Affecting 3% of the population, some of the causes can be considered as; neurally mediated (vasovagal), orthostatic and vascular, cardiac arrhythmias, structural cardiac disease, neuralgic and non-cardiovascular. John Davis cites vasovagal reactions as the primary cause of syncope in athletes following exercise with other contributing factors such as; volume depletion – coma, hypoglycaemia, anxiety attack – hyperventilation and in extreme cases, cardiac arrythmias or structural cardiac disease. During history taking/consultation the issue of syncope should be addressed (*see Chapter 4*).

Some people also play sport/indulge in exercise to get fit without due consideration to the risks. These factors whilst significant in themselves can be attributed at times to such issues as sporting mentality and/or at other times to predisposing factors, i.e. heredity, genetics, etc. with exercise not being the direct causal factor (*Tim Noakes, 1999*). One such problem that cuts across the injury/addiction scenario relates to Part 3, Exercise and the Immune System.

Part 3

Exercise and the Immune System – the Overuse/Overtraining/ Under-performance Syndrome

During Chapter 1 when looking at the causes of injury/re-injury, the issues of U–factors, fatigue and associated problems were raised. Here we further consider the issue of doing too much. The prime task of the immune system is to discriminate between the body's own substances, **SELF**, and foreign substances, **NON-SELF**.

> **"It is a well known fact that exercise is good for the immune system but the demanding training programmes of many athletes may damage the immune system, leaving them open to infection and illness."**
> *Dr. Lynn Fitzgerald, 1994*

Such damage, as a result of physical and mental stress, can result in the action of the body's natural cells, molecules, chemical and hormones being suppressed or controlled so that the individual becomes more susceptible to infection by the 'non-self', i.e. viruses, bacteria, fungi and small parasites. Stress can be from examinations, training intensity/monotony (*Kreider, 1998*), competition, diet, pre-existing medical conditions, environmental, psychosocial (*Urhausen, et al., 1998*), travel (*O'Conner, 1991*), psychological and emotional. Anxiety and depression are psychological states that can manifest themselves physically as tension. Anyone can be affected and research has identified that the effects can last from a few to many hours in trained and untrained individuals (*Berk, L. S., Tan, S. A., Nieman, D. C., and Eby, W. C., 1985; Escola, J., et al., 1978; Mackinnon, L.T., et al., 1987; Pederson, B. K., 1988; Shinkai, S., 1993*). Even a single exhaustive exercise session results in temporary immune depression lasting a few hours. With regards diet, the general findings are that an inadequate supply of carbohydrates in the diet during and after strenuous exercise is associated with a bigger stress hormone response to exercise (*Sport and Exercise Nutrition Conference, 2000*). There also appears to be cumulative, long-term effects of regular hard training. Training or competing in such a state can further exacerbate the problem and in extreme circumstances may lead to death (*Wesslen, I., Pahlson, C., Frimon, G., Fohlman, J., et al., 1992*).

> **"Extra training as a result of poor performance can lead to further problems."**
> *Rachel Wheeler, 1995*

However, reaction to poor performance is usually just that rather than rest (*Smith, C., Kirby, P., and Noakes, T. D., 1997*). Therefore, returning to the re-occurring theme of sporting mentality, temper tantrums by managers, coaches and trainers **after a bad result and demanding extra training may not be the best solution to addressing the issue of poor performance.**

With children and young performers this knee jerk reaction is even more questionable (*see Chapter 1, Part 6*). **The mechanisms by which exercise and the immune system are interrelated is not yet fully understood but psychological, endocrinological, physiological and immunological factors play a role in the failure to recover from exercise.** Many articles and research data can be referred to that will increase our knowledge and awareness (B*udgett, R., 1990, 1994, 2000; Collins, D., 2000; Sharp, C., 1995*). Such awareness and knowledge has lead to management advice and certain guidelines being formulated involving a positive, holistic approach of rest and regeneration strategies. These can involve rest, relaxation, counselling, psychotherapy, massage, hydrotherapy, nutritional advice, tapering training loads and avoiding monotonous training regimes. Planning, monitoring and communication are keys to preventing the over-training syndrome.

The Overuse/Overtraining/Under-performance Syndrome

Many factors have contributed to the development of sport in recent times – improved training, coaching, methodology, equipment etc. but as with all things there is a price to pay for such advances and improvements. Overtraining, staleness, overwork, overreaching, burn-out, chronic fatigue and sports fatigue syndrome are just some of the terms, states and conditions associated with not only exercise and recovery but also doing too much exercise. As with most conditions of the body, there isn't universal agreement as to what each actually is. Neither are the terms and conditions new (*John Byant, 2000*). Overtraining is no different in this respect as some coaches and trainers would argue that no such condition actually exists as it's purely a subjective opinion (*O'Conner, 1997*). Overtraining can be defined as:

"Excessive training characterised by long lasting fatigue and worsening of competitive performance with further attempts to improve physical condition."
Michael Gleeson, 1997

Overreaching (short-term reaction) can be defined as:

"A planned, excessive overload with inadequate rest. Poor performance is observed in training and competition. Successful recovery should result from short-term (that is a few days up to one or two weeks) interventions."
Sports Coach, 1999

Overreaching therefore causes physiological changes that if recovery occurs within two weeks is a vital part of training for improved performance (*Budgett, R., 1990*). Overtraining Syndrome (long-term reaction) is a complex condition and in the absence of illness, injury, anaemia, poor nutrition and disease can be defined as:

"Untreated, overreaching that results in chronic decreases in performance and impaired ability. Other problems may result and may require medical attention."
Sports Coach, 1999

This condition is considered secondary to the stress of training and is often associated with frequent infections and bouts of depression. In recent times the Unexplained, Under-performance Syndrome (UPS) has been defined as:

"A persistent, unexplained performance deficit (recognised and agreed by the coach and performer) despite two weeks of relative rest."
Budgett, Dr. R., 2000

Dr. Budgett has also identified that UPS is not a new piece of terminology, but can result from a variety of related circumstances. For example, staleness, excessive long-term stress or short-term, additional challenges and is not the same in all performers, with a difference in reported symptoms between sprint and endurance athletes. Factors to spot the overuse/training syndrome:

- Poor/under-performance ('performance incompetence') in training, practise and competition, not attributed to illness or injury, is usually the main complaint and a good indicator of overtraining.
- Loss of appetite.
- Loss of energy.

- Loss of libido.
- Depressive loss of drive/enthusiasm.
- Disturbed sleep, vivid dreams, nightmares and waking unrefreshed can occur in 90% of cases (*Koutedakis, Y., Budgett, R., Faulmann, L., 1990*).
- Increased infections especially respiratory.
- Reduced healing – cuts and abrasions.
- Muscle pain/soreness/stiffness/heaviness and weakness.
- Fatigue and an expected sense of effort (*see Chapter 1, Part 5*).
- Prolonged Chronic Fatigue Syndrome. But in this condition the symptoms must last 6 months (*see Chapter 2, Part 6*).
- Hormonal and haematological changes.
- Increased resting pulse.
- Excessive sweating.
- Mood swings, anger, anxiety and irritability.
- Psychological depression.
- Nutritional problems such as loss of appetite and diarrhoea.
- Repeated bouts of colds, sore throats, flu-like illnesses mimicking post-viral fatigue syndrome.

As a result of this the athlete may miss weeks of training, be out of action for years, or worse still, may never return to competitive sport. Sometimes the syndrome can be graded 1–4 based on problems experienced before, during and after exercise.

Part 4

Exercise – Some of its Uses in Treatment, Training and Rehabilitation

The subject of treatment and rehabilitation will be dealt with more specifically in Chapters 5 and 6 but the following will serve as an introduction. The physiologists inform us that movement/exercise can effect tissues in various ways:

- **MECHANICALLY** it stresses tissues and affects collagen alignment.
- **HORMONALLY** anabolic stimulation is increased with exercise and endorphins and enkephalins effect pain reduction (*see Chapter 5, Part 3*). It can stimulate testosterone and the growth hormone.
- **HISTOLOGICALLY** there is an increase in collagen fibres and fibre diameter.
- **BIOMECHANICALLY** there is an increase in collagen turnover.
- **ANATOMICALLY** there can be reabsorption of bony attachment sites with inactivity and resultant changes in the mucopolysaccharide, ground matrix.

In terms of training response the aim is to:

"Cause biological adaptation to improve performance on specific tasks."
Norris, C., 1997

These responses/changes can be considered as:

- Cardiopulmonary for stamina.
- Muscular for strength.
- Joint tissue to affect stretch, increases in size, range/ease of movement.
- Anabolic and catabolic.
- Enzymatic muscle cell activity.

As sports therapists we need to be aware that **exercise is like medicine, when applied to the right condition, in the right dosage and the right time can be beneficial but to the wrong condition, in the wrong dosage at the wrong time, it can prove harmful.** Athletes need to be advised as to the benefits of active exercise and be given some as part of their treatment regime. This is home management **NOT** home treatment. Lederman, 1997, informs us that to affect the motor system, movement needs to be centrally initiated and therefore active, as opposed to passive. This can have various effects. By involving the person in their own recovery it can have a greater placebo effect (*see Chapter 5, Part 2*).

It also re-enforces the fact that the problem belongs to the athlete. Most athletes usually only want to 'perform', expecting someone else to 'put their problems right'. Subconsciously it also informs them that by helping in their own recovery/rehabilitation there are benefits, i.e. they may return to full, functional, fitness faster and this can have financial benefits.

Having said that, exercise induced injuries may form a large percentage of those people who seek treatment. In a more sports-related sense exercise places a tremendous stress on the body. **Physically any stresses placed upon any mechanism will result in that mechanism** (i.e. the body) **absorbing such stress up to a point until there's breakdown** (The Stress Factor).

Intense training brings about progressive fatigue and a decrease in effectiveness in the athlete's activity. The athlete can become injury prone. Exercise can place tremendous stress on the tendons – remember they exert the pull, and the ligaments, which, amongst other things, determine the range of movement. Stretching them to excess can lead to strains and sprains. Fluid can accumulate, creating soreness and stiffness (*DOMS – Delayed Onset Muscle Soreness – see Chapter 1, Part 5*). Massage is in fact passive exercise for the body but massage techniques can stimulate the circulation and loosen fibres that have been bound together. This enhances lymph circulation, lubricating the muscles, decreasing friction and help to remove toxins and acids. Lung ventilation and circulation can be improved because massage can help peripheral circulation, increasing the number of capillaries and their lumina (central cavity size), as well as oxygen availability and absorption. It can also assist the body in aligning torn myofibrils in a parallel fibrillary network helping to create soft pliable scar tissue (*see Chapter 5, Part 4*). In simplicity exercise can be used to:

- Increase range of movement/ease of movement – actively, passively and resistively.
- Increase strength – high loads/low repetition.
- Increase endurance/stamina – low loads/high repetition.
- Increase general fitness – cardiovascular.
- Improve morale/motivation.

Part 5

Some Factors to Consider When Developing an Exercise

- The aim of the exercise. Is it to strengthen, increase flexibility etc.? Remember if you aim at nothing you hit it every time and think you are successful!
- Its relevance. Is this exercise beneficial for my sport?
- Environment. Is the environment suitable?
- Which structures are being targeted? e.g. muscles, neuromuscular mechanisms.
- Timing. Is this the best time to introduce this exercise into the training programme in terms of warm-up, fatigue, developmental and skill factors?
- Starting position/length/leverage/isolation. Is this the best starting position for mechanical advantage, i.e. will it limit trick movements?
  Will it work the relevant structures in the best way?
- Repetitions. How many will achieve your aim? Repetition is necessary to achieve skilled performance. Lederman, E. 1997, reminds us: *"A single motor event will be lost very rapidly if it is not repeated over and over again."*
- Speed of execution. How fast or slow?
- Type of muscle contraction and contraction time. Isometric, isotonic or isokinetic? How long to hold the contracted position?
- Compensatory/trick movements. e.g. use of momentum/inertia in strengthening exercises.
- Teaching ability. Has the exercise been taught, coached and progressed correctly?
- Resistance/gravity. Muscles need an overload (or resistance) to hypertrophy.

- Muscle imbalance. If the exercise is symmetrical is this the way it is being performed?
- Fitness component imbalance. Getting the balance is the secret. Is cross training beneficial?

Obviously specialist knowledge, skill and expertise is required to address these issues/factors but the sports therapist must be aware of such issues even if they do not possess the necessary knowledge, skills and expertise to implement themselves.

Part 6

Training and Training Principles

Why Train?

"To condition the body and mind to resist fatigue and to develop the maximum potential of muscle strength, heart, lungs and muscle endurance, motor skills and co-ordination and in the general physical and mental experience and judgement necessary for success."
Dr. Peter Sperryn, 1983

Because of the intricacy of muscle cells and the enormous complexity of body homeostasis and allostasis, training cannot be completely scientific with exact schedules going in and precise, predictable performances coming out. If it were we would all win a gold medal. Also the ability to tolerate and recover from exercise is highly individualised (*see Chapter 2, Part 8*). However, long-term planning and development of athletes has become highly sophisticated with the **TRAINING YEAR** being split into:

1. **PHASES**. i.e. training to compete, training to win, etc.
2. **PERIODS**. Pre-season, pre-competition, post-competition. **PERIODISATION** can use;
3. **CYCLES** which can be phased into **macro**, which are lengthy periods planned with a particular goal in mind and consisting of preparation, competition and recovery. **Meso**, which consist of two to six weeks focusing on different components of fitness, and **micro** cycles, which are daily routines that make up the meso cycles.

By being aware of these regimes and the latest thinking and development of such, and following guiding principles, coaches and trainers decide on the most effective training for any physical activity and try to maximise the effect that training has on an individual. Sports therapists need to be familiar with these regimes and aware of how the coach/trainer works in order to complement this activity with their own knowledge, skills and expertise. The factors to consider when developing an exercise can be used in conjunction with these principles.

The Principle of Overload

"A planned, systematic and progressive increase in training with the goal of improving performance."
Sports Coach, 1999

To improve the fitness of the various body systems we need to overload them. This means we need to make them work harder than normal. We call the extra demand on the system 'stress'. We can improve our aerobic ability, muscular strength and endurance as well as our flexibility by gradually increasing the amount of stress that we place upon them.

Stress can be increased in four ways. By increasing the:

1. Intensity of exercise. This means that we actually work harder, lift heavier weights or fun faster.
2. Frequency of exercise. We train more often and allow less time for recovery between training sessions.
3. Duration of exercise. We train for longer periods of time and so prolong the stress situation.
4. Quantity of exercise. Quality in terms of specificity is considered superior to quantity just for the sake of it. **LESS FOR MORE CAN BE THE MOTTO HERE**.

Super/Overcompensation

Initial intense training causes under-performance but if the athlete is allowed to recover as a result of periodisation, supercompensation occurs and there is an improvement in performance (*Morton, R. H., 1997*). These transient signs and symptoms and changes can include reduced vitality, increased tension, depression, anger, fatigue and confusion (*Morgan, W. P., et al., 1988*). Hard training causes microscopic, muscle fibre damage (*Costill, D. L., et al., 1988*), as well as producing a shortage of glycogen and potassium in the muscles. These changes, known as 'overreaching', are physiological and normal if recovery occurs within two weeks. Time is needed to allow the muscle fibres to heal as well as to replace fuel supplies in the muscles. It has been found that tissue healing is aided by light training. This is one reason why many athletes do hard and easy training on alternate days.

The Principle of Progression

The effects of training can be seen most easily in the early stages. Almost any increased amount of regular stress will produce improvement in the body parts being stressed. As the body adapts, the intensity of the training will have to be gradually increased if improvement is to be continued. The fitter a person becomes and the nearer they get to their potential limit, then the harder it is to increase fitness.

It is most important that the overload is increased progressively. **Too much stress too soon can cause breakdown and injury. This is never more so than with children** (*see Chapter 1, Part 6*). Too little stress can lead to staleness and boredom. Planning is vital. Variations on the theme and cross training can overcome this.

The Principle of Specificity

Fit for what? The effects of training are very specific. This means that if you wish to build-up the strength of your upper arm muscles you need to perform physical exercises that put stress on the particular muscles concerned.

Heart – lung endurance can only be improved through activity that puts prolonged stress on the heart! In the same way the balance needed for sea surfing will only be improved by training sessions which are similar to the actual event. It must not be assumed that an exercise designed to improve flexibility will also improve strength or endurance.

Training effects are so specific that it is perfectly possible for a 110-metre hurdler to have a very flexible trunk and yet be unable to do a back bend. If you want to improve a particular part of your body in a particular way, then you must find a way of stressing it that closely resembles the actual movement you wish to perform. A sprinter must include a large amount of speed work in his training. This will ensure that the fast twitch muscle fibres are fully developed. The slow twitch muscle fibres essential for endurance-type activities can be developed by training which puts prolonged steady stress on the body. Sportsmen and sportswomen who need both speed and endurance must include both types of activity in their training.

The Principle of Reversibility

If you don't use it you lose it. The body will also adapt to less stress. It takes only 3–4 weeks for your body to get out of condition but general fitness is fine for 3–4 days, i.e. cardiovascular. Deterioration can be seen most readily in aerobic activity as the muscles quickly lose much of their ability to use oxygen. Anaerobic activities are less readily affected by lack of training. This is because the use of oxygen is not as crucial. Strength gains are lost at about one third of their rate of gain. If muscles are not used they atrophy and waste away. Both speed and strength is gradually lost 5–6 days after training. As muscles become weaker and smaller they become more prone to injury. Weak muscles also take longer to heal following injury.

The Principle of Variation

If training programmes are repetitive and lack imagination and thought then athletes can soon become bored, lose their motivation and discipline, which can lead to injury.

The Principle of Adaptation

This is related to the way the body adapts to the training programme.

The Principle of Recovery

This is one that can be overlooked in the pursuit of excellence. It is during the recovery periods that the adaptations to training take place. Rest 24–48 hours after vigorous exercise; 72 hours after exhaustive vigorous exercise although top athletes consider rest as 'less strenuous periods'. Sleep is now considered as 'regenerative rest'.

The Principle of Individuality

Different athletes respond differently to the same training session. Many exercise training regimes and schemes, involving progressive resistive exercise, can be found, i.e. De Lorme and Watkins (strength), MacQueen (power) and Zinovieff or Oxford (endurance) (*see Appendix 3*).

Communication with exercise/fitness trainers and reference to the many excellent texts on the subject of exercise and fitness training will increase the sports therapists' knowledge in the area.

Part 7

Fitness Testing

During Chapter 1 the parameters of fitness in relation to causes and avoidance of injury were considered but fitness testing, according to Lynn Booth (1997), is not about testing fitness but is about:

"Making decisions regarding resuming, continuing or increasing intensity of activity following injury."

At various stages in the treatment (*Chapter 5*), training (*Chapter 2*) and rehabilitation (*Chapter 6*), the fitness of the patient will have to be tested. This is usually done at various levels depending on which authority is consulted. **But it must be remembered that no man has ever been declared fit on a bed.** The following are guidelines and not intended as definitive prescriptions.

Early Training

In order to commence early training, the injured limb or joint should fulfil the following criteria that relates to the early to intermediate stages of rehabilitation, (*see Chapter 6*):

- It should have about 50% of normal power.
- It should have about 80% of its range of active movement.
- Ease of movement should be improving and not hinder progress.
- Swelling should be down to about 20%.
- The joint or limb should be almost stable even though it may be supported by strapping at this stage.
- There should be no pain at rest.
- There should be no gradual increase in pain as workload increases.
- Slight discomfort and stiffness during or immediately after exercise is acceptable.
- Treatments continue during this phase of early training at least.
- There is a need for the trainer, coach and therapist to know what each other is trying to achieve with the athlete.

Pre-discharge Stage of Rehabilitation

This stage may last for between 3–5 days. During this stage the athlete will be expected to do everything that might be asked of them upon their return to full unrestricted training. In addition they must show themselves capable of reproducing such work over a number of days. This type of 'fitness test' is principally used after an injury of some severity that has meant a player has been out of full training for a number of months. In a clinic/club situation this test has still to be very demanding, otherwise the player will be vulnerable to further injury. Any weakness **MUST** be found:

- There should be an absence of pain.
- There should be no swelling.

- There should be full strength/power.
- There should be full range of joint movement.
- There should be full ease of movement.
- There should be full extensibility of muscles, especially bi-articular, e.g. rectus femoris.
- Endurance should be tested, e.g. 20 minutes jogging, 'multistage, fitness, bleep test'.
- Speed should be tested, e.g. 100m sprint and shuttle runs.
- Plus specific functional tests depending on the types of skills and the demands of the sport, e.g. block tackles in soccer, scrummaging in rugby, lunging in badminton etc.

Full Fitness Testing Session

All elements of fitness and sports specific function will be included in this session. This is a full, 'to the limit' session lasting for 2–2½ hours depending on the sport in question. In football for example this is a session which could take place on a Thursday prior to a game on the Saturday. Reaction to such a session may be checked on the Friday during which time a light session is done.

The aim of this type of fitness test is to assess fitness to play on a Saturday after an injury which has been carefully treated and rehabilitated over 5–14 days.

Pre-match Fitness Test

This is a fitness test done on the morning of a game and is only done if the injury has only been very mild and has occurred in the last few days or even the day before. Such a session might last between 15–30 minutes and just gives an extra check that there hasn't been any adverse reaction from the injury that might prevent the player from participating in the event or game. Consideration needs to be given to the level of participation, i.e. child, recreational, amateur, professional. An amateur footballer might ask; 'can I play' and you, as a sports therapist, have to make that decision. What criteria can be adopted? The player is pain free; there is no swelling; he/she has full power/strength; he/she has full extensibility; he/she has full range of movement/ease of movement; he/she can sprint. As for sports specificity with regards football the following could be considered:

- The player can, skip, hop, side-skip, back-peddle and sprint flat out and stop dead.
- The player can twist and turn.
- The player can jump and land safely from various heights.
- The player can block tackle and kick a ball that is right up against an obstacle.
- The player can trap and pass a stationary ball over varying distances.

- The player can volley a ball.
- The player can head a ball.
- Can the player respond to any physical activity asked of him/her without hesitation?

If all of the above can be done with no adverse reaction/reticence then the player could be considered for selection. Key factors to consider in fitness testing:

- Clinical – has sufficient time elapsed and has the injury healed?
- Anaerobic fitness.
- Aerobic fitness.
- Skills.
- Psychological.
- Can the athlete do all they are expected to do upon their return to full training and reproduce it?

Part 8

Factors Affecting and Improvement of Performance

Outstanding team performance occurs when:

- There is an assiduous commitment to a common target or goal.
- The team honestly believe they can achieve the goal set.
- Each individual member of the team feels that they have a significant role to play in pursuing the goal.
- The team and the individuals are treated with respect.
- There is a strong sense of purpose, co-operation and reciprocal support in pursuing the goal (*Thomas A, 2000*).

Although sports science and medicine have contributed greatly to our knowledge in recent times much is still unpredictable. **The multifaceted nature of sport, and in particular the human factor, means that being able to predict, with absolute certainty, outcomes by following prescriptive processes instantly projects one into the realms of millionaire/guru.** In fact just trying to quantify the factors never mind trying to qualify their significance is enough to send some people into shock! Something is surely going to be omitted.

- What constitutes great performance/perfection?
- How can one prepare for elite performance?
- How can one produce peak performance without breakdown?

These and similar questions are ones that all involved in sport are seeking the definitive answers to. Subjective value judgements have to be viewed alongside objective criteria. A great performer could be considered as one who has made his/her weaknesses into his/her strengths. Whilst the athlete that has made the fewest mistakes in preparation is usually the most successful.

Many of the factors that can affect fitness and performance have either been considered and discussed, or will be considered and discussed in this chapter and so therefore their inclusion here serves to re-emphasise their importance. Also, although the following are put into neat little compartments for convenience, as with everything related to the body, there is considerable overlap and integration. The following lists are by no means exhaustive and are included to emphasise the complexity of trying to devise a winning formula to gaining that extra 1–2% advantage over the opposition (*see Chapter 8, Part 1*).

The Human Factor

Each athlete possesses individual strengths, weaknesses, needs, demands, beliefs, perceptions, expectations and knowledge which can/will have an effect on out-comes and the improvement of performance. Allied to this is the fact that all the personnel involved in the health and welfare of the athlete, i.e. the coach, trainer, therapist etc. will also have such personal qualities.

The key to success lies in marrying the differing perspectives to avoid conflict (*see Chapter 1, Part 7*). Failure occurs because such individuality and issues are not appreciated and/or addressed which will/can have a negative effect on both individual and team morale/improvement/performance.

What is important – the outcome or the process? When aiming to produce peak performance without breakdown, it is both. The re-occurring theme of sporting mentality plays a significant part here as the knowledge, skill, expertise and common sense of the personnel involved allied to **INTENSITY AND DURATION** will always play a significant part in improving performance. In fact the issues of how long – **DURATION** and how severe – **INTENSITY** appear to govern most issues in sport. Also the ability to tolerate and recover from frequent hard training is one of the most important qualities in elite performance (*Budgett, R., 2000*).

A negative approach when dealing with people can reduce energy levels and reduce performance. Encouraging facial expressions with smiles as opposed to scowls and verbal praise, when earned, are far more akin to improving performance than foul language and 'dirty looks' (*Uyens, H., 1996*). This obviously is food for thought regarding the half-time team talk when the team is losing. Empathy and positive communication is vital (*see Chapter 1, Part 6*).

Failure, or lack of success, can be viewed in relative terms either materialistically or as a relative value judgement. It depends on who is defining the criteria. Also coming under the heading of the human factor, previously discussed issues such as addiction, fanaticism, obsession, dedication, commitment, habit and motivation can all have a positive or negative effect on performance (*see Chapter 2, Part 2*). Closely akin to the human factors, in fact the psychologists may argue that the human factor should be put there, are the psychological considerations.

Psychological Factors

- An individuals' psychological profile (genotype, phenotype, temperament, personality introvert/extrovert, stable/unstable, etc.) How well they cope under pressure and/or cope, perform under stress. How they deal/cope with stress, success, failure and recover from training are issues that differentiate the winners from the also-rans. These can then be matched to their physical profile (*see Chapter 1, Part 5*).
- Anxiety/depression are psychological states that can physically manifest themselves as tension, which can lead to skill breakdown.
- Stress – mental, physical, financial etc. Whilst stress is necessary and natural and not a bad thing too much can have catastrophic effects on the mind/body. The key is how a person deals with it.
- Sleep deprivation. The importance of not only sleep but also the quality of sleep and its significance on performance has long been accepted (*see Chapter 8, Part 3*).
- Arousal and motivation. Here we return to the issues of intensity and duration. Too much can take the competitor, 'over the edge', whilst not enough doesn't get them there.
- Morale – individual and team being vital for success.
- Placebo. Everything appears to have a placebo (*Hammond, Dr. P., 2000*), and can be a very powerful tool in the mind – body connection (*see Chapter 5, Part 2*).
- Seasonal Affective Disorder (SAD). The amount of sunlight and its effect on people is very much related to the mind – body connection. The fact that emotional states influence our physical health has been recognised, even by allopathic medicine for over a century (*Wood, Dr. C., 1990*).

Anatomical and Physiological Factors
(*see also Chapter 1, Part 6*)

The following can all have an effect on an athlete's performance:

- Heart function/blood quality.
- Lung function and inspirational muscle training (*McConnell, A., 1999*).
- Muscle fibre type.
- Limb length and its relevance to the leverage system.
- Muscle fat ratio.
- Enzyme efficiency.
- Somatotype – endomorph, ectomorph and mesomorph (*see Chapter 1, Part 5*).
- Warm-up/cool down (*see Chapter 1, Part 5*).
- The ability to tolerate and recover from frequent hard training.
- Overtraining/overreaching (*see Chapter 2, Part 3*).
- Fatigue and the sense of effort (*see Chapter 1, Part 5*).
- An individual's genotype (inherent potential) and phenotype (how such potential is expressed and influenced by 'a ring of influence') (*see Chapter 1, Part 5*).
- Skills, talents and experience.
- Chronotypes – is the athlete a morning lark or a night owl?
- 'Biological body clocks' can be affected by internal/endogenous or external/exogenous factors (*see Chapter 8, Part 3*).
- The body core temperature governs the body's physiological systems. External cues can be rest, exercise, daylight, darkness, meals, diet and social influences.
- Jet lag or circadian dysrhythmia (*see Chapter 8, Part 3*).
- Direction and length of travel (*see Chapter 8, Part 3*).

Environmental Factors

- Nature versus nurture.
- Altitude. The affect of altitude training on physiology and performance, although individualised, suggests that competing and training at altitude can be beneficial. Competing at sea level and training at altitude can be beneficial but the research is mixed. Training at a moderate height is best i.e. 8–10,000 feet, and living high and training low gives the best of both worlds (*Gundersen, 1997*). It is suggested that if the athlete is training at altitude then they should arrive at least 1–2 weeks before competition and stay there as long as possible before competing, i.e. less than 1 hours' drive away. The effects of altitude are lost after about 1–2 weeks, unless the athlete lives there but this again is very individual (*Davis, J., 2000*).
- Temperature.

Technical/Innovative Factors

- Equipment design.
- Inappropriate training. Not setting standards ensures failure.

Nutritional Factors

- Mineral deficiency.
- Chemical components.
- Diet.
- Supplementation, ergonomic aids etc.
- Alcohol.
- Smoking.
- Caffeine.

(*See also Chapter 1, Part 4; Chapter 2, Part 3; Chapter 3, Part 4; Chapter 6, Part 4; Chapter 8, Part 1*).

Medical Factors

Sports therapists should be aware of some of the common ailments that can affect 'athletes'. The effects can be detrimental to preparation, performance, their ability to repair and recover as well as having a psychological effect on their mental state and attitude. As previously stated, the role of the sports therapist crosses many boundaries and in order to refer 'athletes' to the relevant specialisms a little knowledge can prove useful as well as being a dangerous thing in the wrong hands!

Suspicion of medical ailments should always be referred to the medical practitioner/club doctor. Some supplements now being taken by athletes, i.e. *Echinacea*, are thought to reduce the duration of the common cold (*see also Chapter 8, Part 1*). Elite athletes should always seek advice as to the effect of such drugs on their performance before taking over the counter medication for any condition. **DRUG TESTING** is now an integral part of sport and relevant personnel should be informed. However, medical conditions are not a barrier to sporting excellence, as Steve Redgrave, Olympic Rowing Gold Medallist, and Gary Mabbutt, former professional footballer and all the contestants at the Sydney 2000 Paralympic Games will testify.

The following information, which has been dealt with on a systems classification, is given in good faith as a starting point for further study and in no way suggests/infers sports therapists are medically, or should be medically, qualified. They should, however, be aware of certain medical conditions.

Respiratory System

Asthma is a condition in which breathing becomes distressingly difficult. The muscles in the air passages go into spasm, causing narrowing so that it is difficult for air to flow from the air spaces in the lungs. The spasm can be caused by allergy (e.g. dust, animals, pollution), chest infection, nervous stress or exercise. Approximately 5% of the population are asthma sufferers and with the present increased amounts of environmental pollutants in the atmosphere, the number of sufferers is increasing.

'Exercise-induced asthma' is understood to be due to the cooling and drying of the airways that can occur 6–8 minutes after exercise in certain conditions. Cooling is the cause in 50–60% of cases. Post-exercise airway constriction is perhaps a better name for the condition since the effects are not fully evident until about fifteen minutes after exercise. Symptoms and signs are coughing followed by an audible wheeze and difficulty in taking a deep breath or exhalation.

The treatment of asthma comes in two forms (preventative and symptom relief). Treatment with certain drugs prior to exposure to an irritant can lead to reduced sensitivity and a reduction in airway constriction. Other drugs (e.g. *Ventolin*) taken after exposure to an irritant can help to reverse the airway constriction. In some cases exercise may serve to alleviate some of the asthmatic symptoms since the hormonal responses to exercise and the temperature changes may serve to dilate the breathing passages.

Most asthma sufferers use an inhaler with medication (e.g. *Ventolin, Intal, Becotide*) to reverse the constriction. If the sufferer has no medication, does not respond to medication, or if the attack is prolonged and the breathing is severely distressed, an ambulance should be sent for. Encourage the person to contact a doctor. Chest infections shouldn't be ignored and treatment and rest are important.

Cardiovascular System

'Athlete's heart'. Training, particularly for endurance events over several years, increases the heart size and reduces the resting pulse.

Myocarditis (inflammation of the heart muscle) may occur in people who exercise with an active viral infection. 'Post-viral Fatigue Syndrome' after viral infection. Personal Bests (PB's) are hard to achieve and often this lasts for 4–6 weeks after recovery. Reducing training or even complete rest gets better results than trying to 'train through it'.

Central Nervous System

Headache/migraines associated with nausea, visual disturbance, allergic reaction or vascular disturbance can be triggered by exercise, cold winds, hunger, excitement or overtraining.

Many people suffer from **stress, tension, anxiety and depression** and quite simply the cause should be found. Depression can be exogenous – due to outside circumstances (no medication will help). You must find the cause and correct. It could be endogenous where intrinsic factors are to blame. Medication can help. Note that the arousal curve, i.e. 'psyching oneself up' can cause a breakdown in skill if overdone.

Genitourinary System (Excretory)

Haematuria (blood in the urine) can be a normal occurrence in an endurance runner due to the continual buffeting of the bladder. However, it can be the start of kidney disease or stones in the urinary tract. Small traces of blood and protein can be found in sports people after exercise but on waking should be clear of either of these. If not a medical practitioner should be contacted.

The colour and content of the urine is a good and reliable indication of **dehydration. THIRST IS NOT**. If the urine is dark yellow and in small amounts, extra fluids (water) should be taken until frequent amounts of clear urine are passed (*see Chapter 1, Part 5*). Passing of blood should always be investigated.

Digestive System

Digestion and eating. When food is taken, blood is directed away from the muscles to the gastrointestinal tract in order to aid absorption of the nutrients. Exercise hinders this process and may cause indigestion/stomach cramps. Food is better absorbed at night (early evening) when exercise has ceased.

There are several causes of **constipation** but in athletes it may be through lack of sufficient fluid which helps the utilisation of carbohydrates as the energy source. The use of certain drugs can cause it. Four types of **diarrhoea** leading to dehydration due to fluid loss are:

1. **Viruses**. Rest and take plenty of fluids with electrolyte supplementation, *Dioralyte* or *Rehydrate*.
2. **Food poisoning**. Keep off milk/fatty foods and protein (they stimulate acid secretion).
3. **Travel**. Usually changing climate can cause it.
4. **Anxiety**. Relaxation and reassurance needed.

Skin Conditions

These can be bacterial, viral or fungal and personal hygiene is very important.

Scrum pox is an affliction well-known among rugby forwards and is the generic term for a variety of complaints, of which the most common is '*herpes simplex gladiatorum*'. Symptoms are facial lesions, particularly in the beard area, cold sores and blisters. It can also manifest itself as *herpes genitalis*. The Rugby Football Union advises afflicted clubs that anyone with any skin rash should not play until given medical clearance, and that players should shower after games, rather than wallow in communal baths. Players are also advised to wear swimming trunks under shorts, rather than a jockstrap.

Acne and boils can be promoted by unwashed skin and unwashed sports wear. A course of tetracyline lasting up to 6 weeks may help acne.

Tinea (fungal infections) for example, athlete's foot, occurs especially in warm, moist parts of the body. *Daktarin* and *Canestan* cream and improved hygiene may help.

Insect bites are not easily treated. Some sprays may deter. Antihistamines, such as *Triludan* or *Hismanol* may relieve if taken thirty minutes after being bitten. **DO NOT** squeeze the poison sac as this will force the poison into the skin.

The Immune and Lymphatic Systems

As a general guide the signs and symptoms of illness related to the lymphatic and immune systems that should raise suspicion as opposed to a common cold are a history of chronic fatigue and recurrent physical illness, especially the skin (dryness and scaly), gastrointestinal and respiratory.

Myalgic Encephalopathy (ME), Chronic Fatigue Syndrome (CFS) and Post- viral/infection Fatigue Syndromes (PVFS/PIFS) are characterised, if by nothing else, a disagreement by the medical profession as to its nomenclature, causation and management (*Dr. Charles Shepherd, 2000*). Chronic Fatigue Syndrome (CFS), which has been referred to previously (*see Chapter 2, Part 3*) is characterised by "severe, disabling fatigue as the principle symptom." (*Sharp, et al., 1991*). The fatigue:

- Should be of definite onset that is not lifelong.
- Must have been present for a minimum of 6 months and for more than 50% of the time.
- Must affect physical and mental functioning.

Other symptoms such as myalgia, mood and sleep disturbance (but not a clinical sleep disorder) may be present. Patients excluded from the definition are those with:

- Food intolerance.
- Weight fluctuations.
- Rashes of unknown origin, and enlarged, tender nodes.
- Swellings, lumps and bumps of unknown origin (*see Chapter 3, Part 6*).
- Established medical conditions known to cause fatigue.
- A diagnosed schizophrenia, a proven organic brain disease, substance abuse, manic depressive illness or an eating disorder. Other psychiatric disorders, such as anxiety or depressive illness need not necessarily be excluded.

The Post-infectious Fatigue Syndrome (PIFS) is characterised by the same symptoms as CFS but in addition there must be definite evidence of an infection at onset or presentation, and the syndrome must be present after the onset of infection (*Futuda, K., et al, 1994*).

Specific Conditions/Considerations

Menstruation

(Amenorrhea – the absence or stopping of).
(Dysmenorrhea – painful discharge).

Period irregularities occur in endurance athletes and the menstrual cycle may cease altogether if the person is lean with low body fat. Not having a period on the morning of a major sporting event can, I am told, be 'a blessing'. A recent study in the Journal of Sports Medicine, 1998, suggests that exercising during menstruation results in an increased risk of ACL injury. This is thought to be due to an increase in oestrogen production that results in a decrease in connective tissue strength.

Appendicitis

In acute appendicitis the aching pain usually begins in the pit of the stomach and migrates to the lower right quadrant, referred to as the 7 o'clock position. However, the pain could be the result of 'a psoas spasm' as well as other conditions.

Chronic Glycogen Depletion

This condition may occur due to insufficient dietary intake. It is important that performers have a balanced diet both in terms of quality and quantity. The importance of this balance is clarified by relating the human body to a car. Would you put treacle and tar into your petrol tank and expect it to perform to a high standard? Increased training volumes means an increase in mileage – food intake can be related to the petrol in the tank. To drive the car further without adjusting the petrol intake has the simple effect of causing the car to splutter, stall and eventually come to a grinding halt.

Equally important is the quality of the food intake; for most performers a well balanced diet is sufficient. However, in some sports due to their specialist form of training, the balance of nutrients may need to be adjusted. This should only be achieved with appropriate input from both medical and nutritional experts. It is important that not only are training volumes monitored but also training effects to ensure that the performer is responding positively to training levels.

Diabetes

This is a condition in which insulin production (in the pancreas) either ceases or becomes ineffective, and which affects 2% of the population. Insulin is a hormone necessary for carrying glucose into the working cell and its absence causes blood glucose levels to rise (hyperglycaemia) which then becomes noticeable in the urine. The liver throws out more glucose in an attempt to supply the needs of the working cells, but without insulin this glucose is unable to cross into the cells and blood sugar levels rise even higher. If the condition remains untreated, the individual will lapse into a coma and eventually die. There are two forms of diabetes.

Type 1 insulin dependent/diabetes mellitus, is a condition in which insulin ceases to be produced due to damage to the pancreas. This type usually affects children and young people and may often result in anxiety and depression. This medical condition can be controlled by regular injections of insulin and attention to carbohydrate intake. Diabetics can suffer from hypoglycaemia (too low blood sugar levels) if too much insulin is injected/produced, sufficient carbohydrate is not eaten or as a result of prolonged and/or strenuous exercise without adjusting diet and insulin. The reaction results in nausea, dizziness, sweating, confusion and blurred vision that eventually results in coma and will lead to death if untreated. It can be readily remedied by giving quickly digested glucose (e.g. sugary drink). If there is no improvement, medical help should be sought directly.

Type 2 usually affects older people (especially those who are overweight). In this condition, insulin is produced but the system has become insensitive to it. However, it can be controlled either by orally administered tablets or a carefully controlled diet. Exercise can help the body to become more insulin sensitive and can improve this condition.

Exercise places the body under stress and can make diabetic control difficult if insufficient carbohydrate is ingested or if insulin amounts are not reduced prior to the exercise. Therefore exercise can worsen a hyperglycaemic condition. However, exercise can help to alleviate anxiety and depression and diabetics will often be encouraged to engage in physical activity and learn to juggle the insulin levels, carbohydrate intake and energy output to keep everything under control. If working with a diabetic, therapists should:

- Discuss the condition with the performer and establish the treatment, e.g. number of injections per day and;
- How this is adjusted to accommodate exercise.
- Encourage blood glucose testing before and after exercise.
- Be aware of the symptoms of exercise-induced hypoglycaemia (i.e. clammy skin, trembling, dizziness, nausea, blurred vision, staggering, bad temper, tingling of lips and mouth, hunger).
- Always have a supply of glucose on hand.
- Treat the performer normally.

Sports Anaemia

This has been recognised as a major problem within the female sporting population, brought about by low iron levels. For many medical practitioners, this has been seen to result from over-training, but is now recognised as a distinct condition. The extent and nature of anaemia within the performer is difficult to assess, as a wide range of haemoglobin levels are exhibited. This may result in an increase in blood volume rather than in haemoglobin concentration.

This condition may affect the ability of the immune system to protect the body against viral infection and results in flu-like symptoms with accompanying mood changes such as depression. The practice of compensating with excessive iron supplements can have equally adverse effects characterised by diarrhoea, abdominal pain and constipation with an increased risk of infection.

Overtraining and Illness

Returning to the re-occurring theme of overuse, sports therapists should recognise the fine dividing line between normal healthy function, breakdown and ill-health. The process leading to ill-health may occur as a result of a mismatch in training volume and a performer's failure to adapt to the effects of training (*see also Chapter 2, Part 3*). This is manifested by fatigue. The principle of overload as a means of developing fitness, means that whilst it is normal to experience fatigue and training effects, in some cases these training effects linger for a longer period of time and the performer may drop deeper into the fatigue zones.

The use of training diaries, a common practice with elite performers, is a good way to identify problems before they arise or modify training periods if they don't appear to be as effective as they should. For further conditions reference can also be made to Chapter 3, Part 5 and Chapter 5, Part 4.

References

1. Berk, L. S., Tan, S. A., Nierman, D. C., and Eby, W. C.: 1985. The suppressive effect of stress from acute exhaustive exercise on T lymphocyte helper/suppresser ratio in athletes and non-athletes. *Medicine and Science in Sports and Exercise*, 17(4): 492.
2. Booth, L.: 1997. When is fit, fit? OCPPP Seminar, Manchester, November, 1997.
3. Bryant, J.: 2000. Editorial. *Faster Higher Stronger*, 8, 5, July, 2000.
4. Budgett, R.: 1990. The overtraining syndrome. *British Journal of Sports Medicine*, 24: 231–236.
5. Budgett, R.: 1994. The overtraining syndrome. *British Medical Journal*, 309: 4465–8.
6. Budgett, R.: 2000. The unexplained under-performance syndrome (UPS), under-recovery and overtraining. *Faster Higher Stronger*, 8, 5–9, July, 2000.
7. Challis, J.: 1993. Eating disorders. Found in *Coaching Focus*, Eating Disorders in Sport.
8. Collins, Professor, D.: 2000. The Zulu Principle, helping to avoid under-performance. *Faster Higher Stronger*, 10–11, July, 2000.
9. Costill, D. L., Flynn, M. G., Kirway, J. P., Houmand, J. A., Mitchell, J. B., Thomas, R., Park, S. H.: Effects of repeated days on intensive training on muscle glycogen and swimming performance. *Medicine and Science in Sport and Exercise*, 20; 249–54.
10. Davis, J.: 2000.Exercise induced syncope: a case study analysis. Society Sports Therapy Annual Conference, Luton, 21.5.2000.
11. Davis, J.: 2000. Altitude training, live high, train low. SST Annual Conference, Luton, 21.5.2000.
12. Eskola, J., Ruuskanen, O., Soppi, E., Vilijanen, M. K., and Jarvinen, M.: 1978. Effects of sports stress on lymphocyte transformation and antibody formation. *Clinical and Experimental Immunology*, 32(2): 339–345.
13. Fenten, P. H., Bassey, E. J., and Turnbull, N. B.: 1988. The new case for exercise. Health Education Authority.
14. Fitzgerald, L.: 1994. Immune system profiling and the dangers of overtraining. *Sports Care Journal*, 1:1.
15. Foster, C., Lehmann, M.: 1999. Overtraining syndrome. *Insider*, 7:1 Isostar Sports Nutrition.
16. Fukada, K., Straus, S. E., Hickie, I., Sharpe, M. C., Dobbins, J., Komaroff, A.: 1994. The chronic fatigue syndrome: a comprehensive approach to its definition. *Am. Int. Med.*, 121: 953, 59.
17. Fulcher, Dr. K.: 2000. Physical activity and chronic fatigue syndrome. *SportEX*, 5, June, 2000.
18. Gleeson, M.: 1994. Overtraining muscle damage and immune function. *Frontline Feature*, NCE.
19. Gleeson, M.: 2000. Maximising your immune system and preventing infection. *Faster Higher Stronger*, 8, 21–23, July, 2000.
20. Hammond, Dr. P.: 2000. 'Mind Over Matter'. TV, February, 2000.
21. Horgan, G.: 1994. 'Is the motivation behind exercise the pursuit of sporting excellence or the pursuit of slimness?' *SportsCare Journal*, 1:2.
22. Koutedakis, Y., Budgett, R., Foulman, L.: 1990. Rest in underperforming elite competitors. *British Journal Sports Medicine*, 24: 248–252.
23. Kreiders, R. B., et al.: 1998. Overtraining in sport. Human Kinetics.
24. Kuipers, H.: Training and overtraining: an introduction. 1998. *Medicine and Science in Sport and Exercise*, 30, 1137–1139.
25. Kurashova: 1990. Sports Massage Congress/Canada. Sports Massage Therapy Institute.
26. Lakomy, J., Dabinett, J., and Nevill, M.: 2000. Physiological differences between elite male and female games players. *Faster Higher Stronger*, 9, October, 2000.
27. Lederman, E.: 1997. Fundamentals of manual therapy: Section 2, 108.
28. Mackinnon, L. T., Chick, T. W., van As, A., and Tomasi, T. B.: 1987. The effect of exercise on secretory and natural immunity. *Advances in Experimental Medicine and Biology*, 216A: 869–876.

29. McConnell, Dr. A.: 1999. 'Gaining that extra 1 or 2 % in performance legally.' *SportEx*, 2, October, 1999.
30. Menstruation and the increased risk of ACL injury. 1998. *Journal of Sports Medicine*, 26 (5): 612–618.
31. Morgan, W. P., Costill, D. C., Flynn, M. G., Raglin, D. S., O'Conner, P. J.: 1998. Mood disturbance following increased training in swimmers. *Medicine and Science in Sport and Exercise*, 20: 408–414.
32. Morton, R. H.: 1997. Modelling, training and overtraining. *Journal of Sports Science*, 15: 335–340.
33. Murray, M., and Pizzomo, J.: 1998. The encyclopaedia of natural medicine. Churchill Livingstone,
34. Nichols, J.: 1988/9. Epidemiology of injury. Prevention of Sports Injury Conference, Manchester.
35. Noakes, T.: 1999. Sudden death and exercise. *Sports Science News Journal*, Internet Site, 1–11.
36. Norris, C.: 1997. Exercise progression for the promotion of full function. Dynamic Tissue Healing and The Effects of Physiotherapy. OCPPP Seminar, Manchester, 15.11.97.
37. O'Conner, P. J.: 1997. Overtraining and staleness. In: Morgan, W. P.: (ed), Physical activity and mental health, 145–160, Taylor and Francis.
38. Oxford concise medical dictionary, 4th ed., 1996.
39. Pederson, B., Tvede, N., Hansen, F. R., et al.: 1988. Modulation of natural killer cell activity in peripheral blood by physical exercise. *Scandinavian Journal of Immunology*, 27:673.
40. Sharpe, M. C., et al.: 1991. A report – chronic fatigue syndrome: guidelines for research. *Journal of the Royal Society of Medicine*, 84:118–121.
41. Sharp, Professor, C.: 1994. Exercise, weight loss, health and fitness. *SportsCare Journal*, 1: 5.
42. Sharp, Professor, C.: 1995. Overtraining syndrome. *SportsCare Journal*, 2:1.
43. Shepherd, Dr. C.: 2000. Careful exercise in the management of chronic fatigue syndrome. *SportEX*, 5, June, 2000.
44. Shinkai, S., Kurokawa, Y., Hino, S., Hirose, M., Torrii, J., Watanabe, S., Shiraishi, S., Oka, K., and Watanabe, T.: 1993. Triathlon competition induced a transient immunosuppressive change in the peripheral blood of athletes. *Journal of Sports Medicine and Physical Fitness*, 33(1): 70–78.
45. Smith, C., Kirby, P., and Noakes, T.: 1997. The worn out athlete: a clinical approach to chronic fatigue in athletes. *Journal Sports Science*, 15, 341–351.
46. Sperryn, P. N.: 1983. *Sport and medicine*. 1:1, 15.
47. SportEX, 2001, Health Promotion News, Page 5, Issue 8, April 2001.
48. Sports Coach (AUS): 1999. Overtraining syndrome in athletes: the challenge of prevention. 22:1, 16–18, Autumn, 1999.
49. Sport and Exercise Nutrition Conference, Loughborough University, 2000. Reported in *SportsCare Journal*, 19, Summer, 2000.
50. Thomas, A.: 2000. Managing Conflict. *Faster Higher Stronger*, 9, October, 2000.
51. Urhausen, et al.: 1998. Ergometric and psychological findings during overtraining: a long-term follow-up study in endurance athletes. *International Journal of Sports Medicine*, 19, 114–120.
52. Uyens, H.: 1996. Society of Sports Therapy Conference, London, 28.4.
53. Wheeler, R.: 1995. Overtraining – the physiotherapist's view. *SportsCare Journal*, 2:1.
54. Wesslen, I., Pahlson, C., Friman, G., Fohlman, T., et al.: 1992. Myocarditis caused by chlamydia pneumonia and sudden death in a Swedish elite orienteer. Lancett, 340: 427.
55. Wood, C.: 1990. Sad cells. *Journal of Alternative and Complementary Medicine*, October, 1990.

Bibliography

1. Eriksson, B. O., Mellstrand, P., Peterson, Renstrom, P., and Svedmyr, N.: 1990. Sports medicine, health and medication: a complete self-help guide.
2. Macauley, D. (ed.): 1999. Benefits and hazards of exercise.

Chapter 3
Injury, Inflammation, Healing and Repair

Man cannot discover new oceans until he has the courage to lose sight of the shore.

Death is nature's way of telling you that you were seriously ill.

A basic understanding of fluid exchange and how this can be affected, the response of the body to injury and the processes/mechanisms involved in healing and repair will ensure that intervention when treating helps **such** processes. It also ensures that it **doesn't interfere** negatively with them therefore delaying repair, recovery and return to sport.

Part 1

Tissue Fluid Dynamics

Sixty per cent of the body's weight is water. One third of this is considered extracellular (blood plasma, interstitial fluid, including lymph) and two thirds intracellular which is regulated by the cell itself. Synovial fluid is a viscous putrification of blood plasma containing some proteins.

The transport systems of the body are designed, amongst other reasons, to affect protein transportation. Normal fluid balance exchange occurs as a result of various opposing forces/pressures, concentration gradients, factors and mechanisms and in simplicity can be considered as follows.

Hydrokinetic requires energy or a mechanical force to move fluid along osmotic and hydrostatic pressure gradients. This is important for tissue growth, nutrition and healing which may be impaired in the absence of mechanical stress in immobilised areas. **Blood pressure is the lateral, outward pressure exerted by the blood to vessel walls as a result of ventricular contraction (systole and diastole)**. At the arterial end of the capillary loop/bed the force is greater than at the venous end. One reason for this being the frictional effect of the fluid on the vessel walls as it is forced through the system. Blood travels around the body at three feet per second.

Oncotic or colloid, osmotic pressure, is an attractive force resulting from the existence of the plasma proteins (prothrombin, fibrinogen, albumin, globulin etc.). The plasma proteins provide the pressure/concentration constancy to the system.

Hydrostatic is fluid tension within the tissue that affects protein transport. **Interstitial pressure** is the minor pressure exerted by fluid that has 'seeped out' into the interstitial, cellular spaces and which will eventually be taken up by the lymphatics.

Diffusion is movement not requiring mechanical force or external pressure, i.e. concentration gradients which affect small solutes such as oxygen and sugars. Finally there is the **membrane permeability**, which is considered, amongst other things, as a 'gating mechanism' to allow the passage of certain molecules (solutes and gases) through its channels whilst opposing the passage of larger molecules (plasma protein, red blood corpuscles etc.). Dodds, 1989, highlighted the fact that diet can metabolically change the membrane, via fatty acid composition, over a three-month period.

The net result of these forces, where nutrients and oxygen are forced out of the vessels to bathe the tissues, and waste products, such as carbon dioxide, are re-absorbed to be expelled from the system, should be that tissues have neither gained nor lost fluid (**equalisation**). In a 24-hour period the whole system is cleansed and filtered, with a small percentage taken up through the lymphatics.

Part 2

Structural Changes and Affection to Flow

It has been shown (*Lederman, 1997*) that this can be disturbed/affected both intrinsically where the tissue structure itself is effected, i.e. the muscle tissue may swell, and extrinsically where there is nothing wrong with the tissue but there is pressure on it, e.g. Carpal Tunnel Syndrome. Both lead to structural changes, leading to oedema, leading to pain. Some of these factors can be:

- Alteration to normal blood pressure.
- Cardiac failure. The strength of the heartbeat is regulated by mechanical, neural and chemical factors.
- Gravitational problems.
- A reduction in the lumen diameter in the blood vessels; a 10% reduction can lead to a 3% reduction in blood flow *(Lederman, 1997)*.
- A decrease in the plasma/osmotic pressure as a result of dietary deficiency, disturbed protein synthesis (liver disease) and/or loss of plasma proteins (kidney disease).
- A disturbance to lymphatic drainage.
- An increase in the permeability of the capillary walls to proteins can be as a result of **TRAUMA**, which can lead to a reduction in osmotic pressure and reduced re-absorption. This trauma can be viewed as **'a disturbance of the semi-permeable membrane,'** *(G. N. Smith, 1997)*. This creates a free interchange of fluid because the membrane has now become freely permeable, which creates more potential for pitted oedema. As a result of which is an increase in blood, leading to increased fibroblastic activity, increased formation of elastic and collagen fibres, thickening of tissue, thus creating the potential for more scar tissue. This leads to pain and/or congestion leading to hypoxia, increased metabolic waste and a change in the cellular environment, leading to further pain.

Part 3

Soft and Bony Tissues – Injury, Repair and Treatment Implications

INJURY is:

> "Any impediment, physical or mental, that prevents peak performance."
> *Troop, R., 1999*

> "The sudden or excessive stress applied to a bodily part which generates forces in excess of tolerable loads."
> *Sports Therapy Education Services Ltd., 1990*

Lederman, 1997, informs us that injury is the result of abnormal movement patterns imposed on the musculoskeletal system because the afferent discharge, signalling input is not totally synchronised with the efferent discharge response. In other words our responses and reactions in certain situations are not fast enough.

Living tissues will absorb stresses until such time as overload causes breakdown. Soft tissue is unique in its ability to absorb such stresses (*Greene, E., 1987*). In fact, periodic, moderate stress is essential for tissue nutrition and healing. Soft tissue can be stressed by; tension, compression, rotation, bending and shearing forces (*see Chapter 1, Part 3*). The injury itself causes, in medical terminology, cellular damage, with the resultant release of enzymes and chemicals that affect other cells and triggers the inflammatory response.

Soft Tissue

The standard texts tell us that mild, moderate and severe muscle injuries can take up to seven days, three weeks and three months to recover whilst a ligament takes two weeks, six weeks and six months respectively. However, this is dependent on many variables. Soft tissue injury and repair consists of three phases:

1. **INFLAMMATORY/LAG PHASE**, involving a vascular, cellular, chemical response.
2. **PROLIFERATION/RESOLUTION/REGENERATION/ REPLACEMENT PHASE**, involving the laying down of collagen.
3. **MATURATION/REMODELLING PHASE**, which re-orientates the tissue.

These stages are carefully orchestrated, mutually dependent, overlapping processes, which are not totally discrete but where each step stimulates the next response. This can be known as **THE CASCADE EFFECT**. The whole process is designed to progress and return towards the restoration of *status quo* or homeostasis. A goal in the healing process is to promote re-generation, with minimal scar tissue and keep replacement, with excessive scar tissue, to a minimum.

If sports therapists are going to assist the body in this process, they need to be aware of what the body is trying to achieve. Don't forget that the body heals itself – therapists just assist it. However, by adopting unsuitable methods *ad hoc*, we can interfere with natural processes and actually delay, if not stop, good repair. The duration of the phases as previously mentioned is dependent on many variables not least the knowledge, skill, expertise and common sense of the practitioner. The above phases can also be considered in terms of:

- **ACUTE**, involving the inflammatory response.
- **SUB-ACUTE**, post acute and lasting until resolution, or until it becomes;
- **CHRONIC**, which is related to a non-resolved, sub-acute injury. Texts refer to this stage in terms of long duration not severity but later physiological considerations for why an injury can become chronic will be discussed.

The Inflammatory/Lag Phase – 'The Vulnerable Phase' (4–6 Days)

INFLAMMATION, which can last from 4–6 days, is the body's response/reaction to injury irrespective of the cause and precedes specific repair. Inflammation is natural, normal and necessary for repair and has two aspects:

1. **IMMUNOLOGICAL**, to clear debris.
2. **MECHANICAL/REPARATIVE**, by putting in and taking out the correct fibres and ground matrix. In simplicity it is the body's warning system designed to protect, localise and rid the body of harmful microorganisms and foreign matter, i.e. dead cells, toxic waste products, therefore preventing infection. It is also designed to stop further aggravation of the injury site. This reactive phase consists of a mainly vascular, cellular and chemical response, resulting in the textbook signs of:

1. Heat (calor).
2. Redness (rubor).
3. Pain (dolor).
4. Swelling (tumor).
5. Sometimes fever.

All of which brings about **LIMITATION OF MOVEMENT**.

Haemostasis (blood clotting) is complementary to and a very important part of the inflammatory process and as it is part of the reaction, healing and repair mechanism all sports therapists should possess a knowledge of it. The following is a simplified overview.

Haemostasis consists of physical and cellular responses, i.e. **vascular spasm**, which occurs immediately after trauma, via various reflexes and muscle spasm, causing the blood vessels to contract, therefore reducing blood flow.

A platelet plug is formed **via agglutination** (sticking together) of platelets that fill holes in the blood vessel walls so as to avoid further blood loss but inhibiting blood flow. **Blood clot**, which in severe trauma can take 15–20 seconds, whilst in minor trauma can take 1–2 minutes. There are over 30 different substances effecting blood coagulation, some pro some anti, in what is known as the 'classical theory of coagulation'. **Clot retraction**, which occurs several minutes after clotting, is where the edges of the damaged blood vessels are drawn together.

How Are The Cardinal Signs of Inflammation Initiated?

Heat and Redness

Initially the **PHYSICAL/VASCULAR RESPONSE** with short vasoconstriction (5–10 minutes), leads to a reduction in cell permeability and a reduction in blood flow (stasis). Combined with the initial injury and cell damage, this leads to a reduction in oxygen and nutrients, resulting in **HYPOXIA** leading to further cell damage.

Then there is **ACTIVE VASODILATION** by the opening up of thousands of capillaries, increasing blood flow, with bradykinins being potent vasodilators. Increased cell permeability is helped by serotonin and histamine released from mast cells. The heat and redness takes a few hours to develop with the resultant increase in local temperature increasing the metabolic demands, which in turn results in increased vasodilation.

Swelling

Increased cell permeability is also caused by disruption of the semi-permeable membrane from the initial injury. This allows inflammatory, plasma exudate (plasma proteins) to seep through the vessel linings into interstitial spaces. This together with leakage from damaged blood vessels creates inflammatory exudate/oedema which will be high in proteins and inflammatory cells giving a high suction force/osmotic pressure, drawing out more fluid into the tissue. This is facilitated by axial flow in the blood vessels changing to marginal flow. Inflammatory swelling starts to develop approximately two hours after the injury and may continue for up to four days. This swelling increases tissue pressure causing pain, pain causing neuromuscular inhibition, movement is reduced, muscle strength decreases, normal walking patterns are lost and the patient will say the joint does not feel normal and will remain so until all of the swelling is reabsorbed. Immediate swelling is indicative of bleeding into the joint – **HAEMARTHROSIS** (which is clinically significant!). This exudate contains fibrinogen that forms fibrin that is a necessary part of the body's defence mechanism against infection. However, too much inflammatory exudate leads to excessive fibrin formation leading to scar tissue.

COMPLEMENT is a component of blood plasma consisting of approximately 20 protein compounds. These are inactive enzymes that become activated in sequence (**THE CASCADE EFFECT**) to catalyse a series of reactions involving:

1. Killing foreign cells by cytolysis:

    'The breakdown of cells particularly by destruction of their outer membranes'. (*Oxford Concise Medical Dictionary, 4th ed.*).

2. Causing vasodilation by increasing the size of the lumen in the blood vessels.
3. Enhancing **phagocytosis**:

    'The engulfment and digestion of bacteria and other foreign particles by a phagocyte, i.e. leucocyte, macrophage'.
    Oxford Concise Medical Dictionary, 4th ed.

The cellular response consists of the cellular activity outlined above plus the migration of white blood cells through the vessel walls, known as **DIAPEDESIS**, i.e. monocytes, neutrophils and macrophages, which happens within a four hour period, which peaks, then disappears within a few days. These are brought to the area as a result of the increased blood flow. The red blood corpuscles are manufactured in certain bones, femur, humerus, sternum and are stored in the red and yellow marrow.

White blood corpuscles although produced in the lymphatic tissue are also stored in the marrow. **Chemotaxis/Chemotropism** is a response where there is movement that is positive (toward) or negative (away from) to a chemical stimulus.

Pain

Pain results from pressure or irritation on the nociceptors (pain receptors) as a result of the swelling and release of chemicals and dying cells. This tells the body something is wrong and limits movement by making it hurt. 36–42 hours post injury is a vulnerable, risk time as relatively little is happening, the inflammatory stage is receding and the sub-acute, healing, response/repair has not yet got under way. Macrophages clear the area of debris by phagocytosis and signal the end of the acute, inflammatory stage.

Resolution/Replacement/Regeneration/Proliferative Phase – 'The Tension Phase' (5–21 Days)

Tissue repair is the replacement of dead cells with living cells. There are a number of ways in which the inflammation can terminate and repair and healing continues.

Regeneration/resolution is where the exudate is absorbed and debris removed; tissue is replaced like for like and the irritant is removed. **Fibrosis replacement** is where fibrous tissue is formed as a result of the reaction. In other words new cells are formed from connective tissue which are slightly different from those they replace (the fibres and ground matrix have differing ratios), resulting in scar tissue. Sometimes this phase is referred to as **proliferation or granulation (new tissue)** when fibroblasts and endothelial cells form new, granulation tissue to control contracture. Granulation can be considered 10–16 days post injury. The new tissue will have no tensile strength and can tear quite easily.

Granulocytes, leukotrienes and prostaglandins assist protein turnover. Protein helps build tissue as well as affecting fluid dynamics. Collagen/protein turnover can be considered five days post injury, with tensile tissue strength being only 20% of normal. This process may take up to three weeks to complete.

The Maturation/Remodelling Phase

This is the stage of cross-linking and re-orientation following the regeneration phase. **Three to four weeks post injury is a critical time because unless the tissue has strength and proprioception it is liable to re-injure.** It is a continuous process and may last a few weeks or up to six months depending on the damage and interference with the tissues. During this phase the collagen contracts.

Scar Tissue

During the re-modelling phase of tissue repair our aim is for good quality repair, via regeneration/resolution, as opposed to poor quality repair, via replacement.

This can occur because during haemostasis, the clot is invaded by fibroblasts and forms connective tissue (scar) all through the clot. Conversely this extra tissue can dissolve and resolve.

> **"Contrary to early thinking, voluntary, skeletal muscle has tremendous powers of regeneration and will completely repair if treated and rehabilitated properly."**
> *Lederman, E., 1998*

The belly of the muscle possesses a better blood supply than the tendons, which don't heal as well. Ligaments heal slowly but because they do not possess any specialised cells, such as osteoblasts in bone formation, healing is by fibrous scar tissue. Scar tissue has only 70% of the tensile strength of the tissue it is replacing and is less pliable. A possible mechanism for the formation of scar tissue in muscles is the creation of an imbalance between the muscle and connective tissue components during the deposition of collagen, thus rendering the tissue more passive with the resultant loss of certain mechanical properties, e.g. elasticity.

Chronicity is related to a non-resolved, sub-acute injury. The suggested reasons for this are stress/overuse; the introduction of a new injury on an existing one; and/or inappropriate treatment/rehabilitation that interfered with rather than supported the natural physiological process.

Chronic inflammation is when there has been minor repetitive trauma to a non-resolved inflammatory response. To combat this the body lays down extra tissue, i.e. collagen to protect the area, which causes stiffness. **Stiffness after rest is a classic, chronic response**. However, according to Dr. Lederman, this fibrotic build up can be reversed quite quickly via active techniques that can increase blood flow 30 fold! During the sub-acute phase the priority should be one of restoring movement within the limits of pain, i.e. strength and stretch.

Suppuration is where pus is formed. This consists of dead leukocytes and bacteria and if this discharges, **an ulcer** occurs. **Necrosis** is where the tissue cells die; and this will depend on the cause of the inflammation, the defence system of the body and the particular tissues affected. **Gangrene** results when the whole area becomes a mass of dead cells.

Treatment Implications

Clearly for the sports therapist how the body is overloaded, injured, reacts to intervention and repairs has many implications in treatment, the aims, objectives, principles and practicalities of which will be discussed in Chapter 5. Repair is usually a combination of regeneration and replacement.

In essence what a sports therapist should be trying to do is change the environment in which repair takes place so that the tissues are capable of meeting the functional demands placed upon them as they slowly return to sport. By looking at the phases of tissue repair and treating the primary site correctly this can be achieved. Brukner and Kahn, 2001, identified six principles in the overall management of most sports injuries:

1. Minimising the extent of the initial damage.
2. Reducing associated pain and inflammation.
3. Promoting healing of the damaged tissue.
4. Maintaining or restoring flexibility, strength, proprioception and overall fitness during the healing phase.
5. Functionally rehabilitating the injured athlete to return to sport.
6. Assessing and correcting any predisposing factors in order to reduce the likelihood of re-occurrence.

A good practitioner therefore visualises and adopts techniques to assist physiology not bend the physiological fact to assist the technique (*Lederman, 1997*). He/she is always aware that modalities designed to assist repair can also re-injure and appreciates that success is dependant on many variables, not least intensity and duration. Therapeutic discomfort is acceptable, knowingly causing pain is not.

Tension and Compressional Loading

Soft tissue can be injured by tension, compressional, bending and rotational forces and so therefore in treatment/rehabilitation the need is to progressively and safely load the tissues so they will subsequently be able to deal with future loading. However, in treatment, **Lederman's work (1998), shows that tensional loading is not good for fluid exchange and results in thick dense tissue with an increase in stiffness and strength. Whereas compressional loading is good for fluid exchange but leads to thin, mechanically low quality tissue.** Therefore it is vital that the **WHY** and **INTENTION** of treatment are clear in the planning of treatment and rehabilitation programmes. Most practitioners/therapists when asked how to treat an acute injury respond with:

> "The universally accepted procedure of RICE, i.e. rest, ice, compression and elevation for the immediate care of acute sports injuries."
> *Knight, 1995*

Therefore by looking at some of the conventional, consensual, empirical and biological evidence (ACPSM, 1998), the priority of treatment for an acute condition would appear to be as follows.

PROTECT the injury in the early stages of the healing process for at least up to three days, depending on the severity (*Karlsson, 1996; Levin, 1993; Reider, et al., 1993*). **The mode of protection must be capable of accommodating oedema** and can be crutches, slings, braces, Plaster of Paris and taping.

COMPRESSION should be applied via a pressure/compression bandage. This would be to reduce the amount of space the oedema could go into, giving the capillary chance to repair. In terms of oedema reduction the evidence suggests (*Rucinski, 1991*) that **compression should not be combined with elevation if the limb can be elevated above the heart. However, compression is necessary in the dependency position when elevation cannot be maintained.** Remember that compressional forces are good for fluid exchange.

REST should be applied to the injured part immediately following injury as mobilisation could disrupt the healing process (*Jarvinen and Lehto, 1993; Burrough and Dahners, 1990*). The part should not be moved outside the pain barrier. Active rest and isometric contractions at this stage will assist fluid dynamics, whilst stimulating the nerve and blood supply.

COOL the area by applying crushed ice in a damp cloth. This can affect metabolism, if applied long enough, but the cold must be cold enough to avoid reflex vasodilatation and kept that way, i.e. a minimum of 8–10 hours will affect metabolism, keep vasoconstriction and reduce the inflammatory response. As cold is transferred through conduction the **most effective duration of the application appears to be 20–30 minutes applied every two hours** (*Taba, 1992; Ho, 1990; McMaster, 1978; Knight, 1989*). The first 24 hours should involve this regime.

ELEVATE the part to alter the pressure gradients and assist lymphatic/venous return and removal of oedema. However in terms of oedema removal, evidence suggests (*Rucinski, 1991*) that when elevation can be maintained above the heart level, compression **should not** be applied simultaneously. The reasons for this are that it compromises lymphatic and venous return and causes a possible 'rebound phenomena', caused by a sudden shift of vascular or lymphatic fluid. This phenomenon only occurs when compression and elevation are done together and not when elevation is carried out alone.

This suggested clinical approach to acute injuries is considered safe and effective but **what is still not clear to the author is exactly in what order these steps are to be taken to be most effective in assisting the inflammatory process?** There is no disputing that the acronyms **RICE, PRICEM, RICEM,** etc. help to give a guideline and a protocol to deal with an acute injury but looking physiologically at all the evidence to date, perhaps **COMPRESSION, COLD, ELEVATION, REST/PROTECTION** would be the most effective.

Research has shown that to control and minimise the swelling, treatment as soon as possible after injury to the knee prevents secondary damage; dramatically reduces pain and disability; reduces movement loss; allows movement without excessive limitations and allows comprehensive assessment after 72 hours. This means that early and appropriate rehabilitation is possible which may prevent common complications, i.e. arthrofibrosis (symptomatic loss of knee flexion and extension) and is cost effective as it reduces the time lost at work and sport (*Noyes, et al., 2000; Shelbourne and Rask, 1998; Macdonald, 1995*).

By applying cold, the physiological and therapeutic benefits will be felt and whilst cooling has little effect on haemorrhaging, it does limit the amount of secondary hypoxic injury and oedema. It decreases the metabolic needs of the cells by reducing the oxygen consumption, as long as the cold is cold enough and continuously applied. Cooling also results in less tissue damage and less oedema. The cold will also affect some pain relief (*Arnheim and Prentice, 2000; Peterson and Renstrom, 2000; Knight, 1995; Low and Reed, 1994*).

Compression and cooling effectively applied by 'cryocuff' for the first 24 hours after injury has been shown to be safe and effective in minimising and controlling swelling and indicates less pain when compared with other methods of applying compression and cooling. A Robert Jones compression needs to be kept on even during sleep and elastoplast and tubigrip can lead to complications (*Shelbourne and Rask, 1998; Zaffagnini, et al., 1998; Whitelaw, et al., 1995; Scheffler, et al., 1992*). Cryocuff can be used for up to five days and can be changed and monitored every hour so that in the case of post anterior cruciate ligament reconstruction surgery, passive extension can be checked.

Elevation can alter the pressure gradient to assist venous and lymphatic drainage. It eliminates the effect of pooling in the extremities by increasing the venous and lymphatic drainage of blood from the injured area to the central circulatory system. The greater the degree of elevation, the more effective the control of swelling (*Peterson and Renstrom, 2000; Arnheim and Prentice, 2000; Whitelaw, et al., 1995*).

Resting the injured part, not the whole body, gives the body time to respond, repair and heal. These measures combined with the patient being advised on active, controlled rhythmic pumping methods, e.g. isometrics, would appear to assist the body's natural healing.

Applying pressure/compression as priority one, would immediately reduce/minimise the amount of available space into which the inflammatory exudate could flow by increasing the extracellular pressure and this will reduce the amount of plasma proteins collecting into the interstitial space. This will assist capillary repair (*Arnheim and Prentice, 2000; Prentice, 1999; Zuluaga, et al., 1995*). **By applying cold, the physiological and therapeutic benefits will be felt**.

To recap, the **LAG PHASE** involves this vascular, chemical, cellular bodily response and is the first 4–6 days following injury when a 'fibrin scaffold' is being laid down. There is no increase in tensile strength during this time. If you break down the 'fibrin scaffold' too early by mechanical means you will elongate this lag phase, delaying repair and increasing the healing time. If connective tissue is stretched then interfacing tissues, involving the nerves and blood vessels must also be affected. However, after 36 hours, controlled movement must be initiated otherwise there is increased likelihood of chronicity. During the first 4–6 days don't put the soft tissue under too much stress. Remember at five days there is collagen/protein turnover.

Work around the injury and the rest of the body. Work with what you are presented with, i.e. possible restricted range of movement, ease of movement, stiffness, discomfort and pain. **Pain being a red flag/barrier not to be passed as opposed to a red rag to a bull to be charged at** (*see Chapter 1, Part 2*). During this inflammatory stage when macrophages will eventually clear debris there should be **no stretch** to injured tissue. Remember tensional forces are not good to assist fluid exchange. Work by Dr. E. Lederman in the late 1990's suggests **the aim of the manual therapist in the early stages of repair should be to improve tissue nutrition and drainage, reduce inflammatory exudate and pain via early mobilisation, involving rhythmical, non-painful techniques. This will avoid undue stress on the tissues, will affect fluid dynamics (blood and lymph flow) and support metabolic needs**. Therefore, during the early stages of repair:

1. **NO STRETCH**.
2. **NO STATIC**.
3. **LOW LOADS** – the load must not be greater than the tensile strength.
4. **EARLY MOBILISATION** with passive motion within the pain-free range.
5. **SLOW, RYTHMIC PUMPING**.
6. **DYNAMIC COMPRESSION** which must be deep enough to deform the tissues therefore affecting the lymphatics. The protocol of compress/decompress/compress/decompress is suggested. The direction can be considered as proximal first, to create a reservoir, then periphery to the centre and finally distal.
7. **OSCILLATIONS** involving active, pain-free movement of the limb between two points determined by the therapist. The therapist can use their limbs to act as boundaries. To develop this the therapist can provide low level resistance as the patient moves.

For Muscles

CONTRACT – RELAX, with 50% effort and a two second time interval for six minutes will create a two and a half minute hyperaemia, which can then be effleuraged immediately after cessation. Dr. Lederman considers this a powerful tool to assist fluid dynamics, and it has been shown to improve flow 30 fold! However, a force beyond 50% is considered not as effective. Combining this with **MID TO INNER, not stretched position, CONCENTRIC MUSCLE WORK** will also assist blood flow.

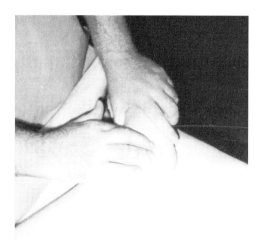

◀ *Figure 36.*
Transverse friction
to ATF ligament on
stretch.

For Joints

Controlled, gentle, passive movement is better than active to assist synovial fluid pumping. This can take the form of 10 cycles a minute for 20–30 minutes. A cycle consisting of full flexion to full extension, etc. Again movement as opposed to stretching.

Massage

Massage is contra-indicative directly onto the site of an acute injury or to an inflamed organ but by understanding the pathophysiology, the experienced practitioner can use common sense because it has been claimed that:

- Massage can stimulate the release of the body's own anti-inflammatory, pain relieving agents.
- Certain types of massage actually increase the inflammatory response triggering the body to complete the job. Sometimes it is necessary to 'go back to the beginning' by imitating the inflammatory response, i.e. the use of friction techniques and deep pressure mobilisations. Such techniques can also help to ensure the development of an orderly fibrillary network and 'spin' the fibres that are present approximately 48 hours after injury (*Cyriax, J., 1984*).
- Massage helps the dilution and removal of the irritants via the lymphatic system.
- By increasing blood flow into and out of the area the process may be assisted.

As a general guide, massage above and below the site of an acute injury would appear to assist the body's natural healing, with more specific techniques being introduced depending on the stage of healing and repair.

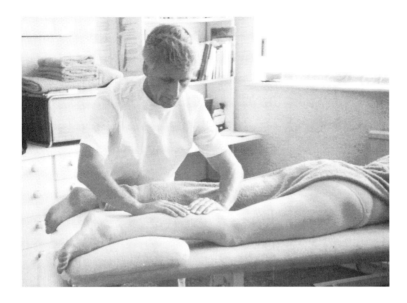

◀ *Figure 37. Massage to the legs.*

However, reference to Chapter 5, Part 4, will give a more objective insight as to the efficacy of massage. **Also the acronym HARM, which stands for heat, alcohol, running and massage, helps to remind sports therapists of the activities that could possibly undermine the effectiveness of any protocol** (*Zuluaga, et al., 1995*).

REGENERATION PHASE is considered 5–21 days post injury when there is a greater increase in tensile strength. Fibroblastic activity increases. Fibroblasts are the precursor to collagen synthesis.

Fibroblasts are 'blind' because they do not know either what type of tissue is being worked on or the direction of the fibres. Fibrous scar tissue is laid down in 'kinks and curls'. This will cause anatomical shortening as the scar organises and consolidates unless appropriate manual therapy techniques are applied, i.e. cyclical stretching, movement leading to functional tasks. Note that steroids plummet tensile strength and increase collagen activity. **All tissues that can't stretch are the slowest to heal, i.e. ligaments and cartilage**.

Following the lag phase the aim should be to direct the repair and remodelling process towards increasing the tissues' tensile strength by promoting the normal laying down of collagen; reducing excessive cross-linkage and promoting the normal development of mechanical behaviour, i.e. flexibility. One way is with specific stretching that loads and tensions the tissue. This stretching needs to be slowly controlled. Specificity is vital to scar tissue. Therefore just stretching is not good enough (*Hunter, G., 1997*). Scar tissue has plastic properties. It is not elastic but can be stretched and moulded to give a position of length. Cross-fibre, lateral rolling, lateral, twig-snap style and slowly, controlled linear or longitudinal stretch are examples of what may be required.

Remodelling

Regular, continuous stretching is still important during this stage to assist healing, prevent excessive contracture and prevent re-injury.

Neural Tissue

The nervous system consists of dynamic, pain sensitive structures. On a continuum it has:

- Mechanical.
- Electrical.
- Thermal.
- Chemical aspects which need consideration during injury.

Mechanically, nerves can be injured by:

1. **Compression** that will cause neural tensioning and pressure changes within its cellular components and ultimately will interfere with nerve physiology. The critical variables are force and time sustained which leads to vascular impairment and ischaemia.
2. **Stretching**. There is a lower limit of approximately 8%, which will affect venous return and an upper limit of 15% which causes vascular standstill.
3. **Distension**. Swelling occurs as a result of the pressure.

According to Dr. Lederman, 1998, the way to affect the nervous system is to mimic/imitate natural processes via cognition and volition. These are vital if the injured athlete is to know what they are doing; and **repetition**, which is vital to allow for adaptation.

> **"A single motor event will be lost very rapidly if not repeated over and over again."**
> *Schmidt, R. A., 1982/91*

Bony Tissue

Long bone is formed from a cartilaginous framework which hardens/ossifies/calcifies by the deposition of certain salts, mainly calcium, magnesium and potassium. Flat bones are similarly formed from membranes. These two types of bone formation are known as **ENDOCHONDRAL** and **INTRAMEMBRANOUS** respectively. Growth originates from ossification centres in the cartilage models that are found in the centre and ends. These two areas are separated by an epiphyseal cartilage or growth plate. Eventually the growth centres join up. In children the growth points of the bone are at the epiphysis of the long bones and the periphery of the flat bones. At about 20 years of age the main length of the bone is achieved and then growth continues by an increase in bone diameter. This is achieved by the combined action of:

Osteoblasts, the bone-forming cells, are small cells that originate in the periosteum, synthesise and secrete a ground matrix called **osteoid** which helps build new bone around the outside of the bone. **Osteocytes** are mature non-dividing osteoblasts that have become surrounded by extra cellular material. **Osteoclasts**, the bone re-absorbing cells, are giant multi-nucleate cells that erode the bony walls of the medullary cavities, thus increasing its diameter.

This process of ossification and sculpting of the bone is known as **osteogenesis** and ensures that bone gain outstrips bone loss. The process of osteogenesis is approximately in balance from early childhood to middle age. Up to approximately 20 years of age ossification exceeds re-absorption and between 20–35 years osteogenesis is in balance.

Between 35–40 years of age the process reverses and bone gain at the periosteal surfaces loses its impetus whilst bone loss at the inner, endosteal surfaces, increases in rate. Thus the thickness of compact bone diminishes and the diameter of the medullary cavity increases. The result being that in old age bones become more hollow and are less able to resist compression and bending.

Osteoporosis is known as the 'the silent epidemic', and is when the osteoblastic and osteoclastic balance is disturbed. It is one of the most common and serious of all bone diseases. It is a condition of abnormal thinning of bone because there is a loss of matrix and minerals, i.e. calcium, magnesium, boron etc. This renders the bone brittle and fragile and susceptible to 'spontaneous fractures'. Therefore manipulative treatment would be contra-indicative. The 'growing child' needs exercise (weight bearing/shock absorption), sunshine and a varied healthy diet to assist the healthy development of the cartilaginous framework. In fact, in the treatment of osteoporosis, diet and weight bearing exercises are recommended (*see Chapter 1, Part 6 and Chapter 2*).

Sports therapists should also be able to recognise the signs and symptoms of a fracture and be able to administer first aid before transfer to hospital. Therefore it is important that sports therapists should have some knowledge of how bones become injured and subsequently repair. It should also be appreciated that different texts have different classifications.

Continuing the overview from Chapter 1, **a fracture can be considered as a break in the bone, resulting in the loss of continuity, with or without displacement**.

Aetiology of Fractures (#)

Fractures can be caused by '**U-FACTORS**' – **OVERUSE, MISUSE, ABUSE, DISUSE**, in other words:

- **TRAUMA**. A sudden injury, which can be direct or indirect violence to the bone, i.e. **DIRECT** – a blow, kick, (transverse, crush, compressed, impacted, angulated, double comminuted).
- **INDIRECT**. Twisting or falling with non-contact (avulsion/stress/spiral/oblique). Muscular action where the bone detaches at the tendon (avulsions) is uncommon but does happen.
- **FATIGUE**. Overuse which overloads an already vulnerable area.
- **STRESS**. i.e. abnormal loading – (see stress fracture below).
- **PATHOLOGICAL**. **DISEASE** i.e. tumours (benign or malignant) hormonal disorder, etc.

'**STRESS FRACTURES**' are caused by overload or fatigue and are found in the lower $1/3$ tibia, lower $1/3$ fibula and metatarsals, especially the 3rd.

Categories of Fractures

1. **CLOSED FRACTURE** (**UNDISPLACED**). There are no breaks in the skin and the fracture is contained in local tissue.
2. **AN OPEN FRACTURE** (**COMPOUND**). There is a break in the skin as well as the bone. These are prone to infection and set up a '**WOUND TOILET**'.
3. **COMPLICATED FRACTURE** (**DISPLACED**). The surrounding structures and organs are injured. These can involve a joint or a dislocation, i.e. the end of one bone breaks off and goes into the joint.
4. **COMPLETE/INCOMPLETE FRACTURE**. These terms are sometimes used to refer to whether or not the break has extended through the bone.

These can be divided into **TYPES OF PATTERNS OR FRACTURES**, which relate to the shape adapted by the fracture surfaces and are distinguished on X-ray.

These can be:

1. **GREENSTICK**. An incomplete fracture of the diaphysis of a long bone. Usually found in children.
2. **TRANSVERSE**. The break is straight through at right angles to the diaphysis. This fracture is a poor healer.
3. **ANGULATED**. When one end of the bone is at an angle to another.
4. **OBLIQUE**. The bone is fractured at an oblique angle.
5. **SPIRAL**. The bone is fractured creating a spiral pattern.
6. **DOUBLE**. More than one break.
7. **COMMINUTED**. A bone is broken in more than two parts.
8. **IMPACTED**. A fragment of bone has impacted into another.
9. **AVULSION**. The bone is detached at the tendon attachment, usually at the epiphyseal growth plate.
10. **CRUSHED/COMPRESSION**. This usually relates to the spine or calcaneus.

Fractures/dislocations are sometimes named after the person who 'discovered' them i.e.:

1. **COLLE'S**. Radius resulting in a 'dinner fork deformity'.
2. **POTTS'**. Ankle/tibia and fibula. Originally classified by Percival Potts, it has since been expanded to include fourteen variations.
3. **SMITH'S**. Ulnar.
4. **BENNETT'S**. Thumb/1st metacarpal.

Fracture Sites

Almost any bone in the body can be fractured and therefore the sports therapist should familiarise themselves with the most common and the most serious, e.g. the ankle and the cervical respectively. **Compact bone healing and repair** is not constant and two stages may occur at the same time.

The Injury Itself

'The fracture (#) site' involves four components involving cellular damage. The fracture damages:

1. The periosteum and endosteum.
2. Blood vessels are damaged, which leads to hypoxia, cell death and necrosis. This is initiated because lysomes release enzymes that affect other cells/blood vessels. In a fracture the parts nearest to the fracture become ischemic and die.

3. Extracellular substances, fascia, adipose tissue etc. whose function is affected and disrupted.
4. Extravasated blood leads into extra cellular spaces.

Inflammation/haematoma/blood clot – coagulation, as discussed previously creates a 'wound toilet'.

Phagocytosis of Clot and Clot Debris

Non-granular (cytoplasm with a few granules), histiocytes, monocytes and macrophages (natures vacuum cleaners), clear the area of different, noxious agents i.e. inflammatory exudate, small fragments of bone without a blood supply. All of the above stages take about five days.

Cellular Proliferation/Granulation Tissue (New Capillary Tissue) Leading To Callus Formation

Within eight hours of the break, cells rush to the site. Early osteoblast cells grow sub periosteal (from under the periosteum) and endosteally (inside the **MEDULLARY CAVITY**) towards each other forming a '**BRIDGE OVER BREAK**'.

Callus Formation – 'Clinical Union'

This occurs when **CHONDROBLASTS** and **OSTEOBLASTS** lay down **HYALINE CARTILAGE, COLLAGEN FIBRES AND BONE** respectively. The osteoblasts secrete non-lamellar osteoid – lamellae being thin bands of calcified matrix arranged concentrically around an haversian canal. This becomes impregnated with calcium salts (calcified) to form **IMMATURE, WOVEN BONE**. This is the first sign of 'clinical union' after about three weeks for an upper body spiral/oblique fracture. This is recognisable on X-ray as a big white blob/bulbous collar and is dependent on:

1. Periosteal stripping.
2. The size of the haematoma etc.

Consolidation

New bone (woven/non-lamellar) is made into mature bone by **OSTEOBLAST** activity and **CALCIFICATION**. As bone is made stronger, it is laid down along lines of stress. This is approximately double the time of callus 'clinical union', i.e. 6 weeks.

Remodelling

This is constant but inconspicuous. This is when the repair process removes excess callus and opens up the medullary cavity. **OSTEOGENESIS** and may take weeks, months and even years. **METABOLIC BONE DISEASE** can occur during the remodelling phase.

Cancellous Bone (Intra-membranous) Healing and Repair

Compared to compact bone, it possesses a quicker healing time and union because it possesses:

- A uniform spongy matrix.
- No medullary cavity therefore there is a broader area for healing.
- An open mesh framework.
- Union doesn't have to occur endosteally sub periostally.

Treatment and Management Implications

The role of the sports therapist in the treatment and management of fractures and dislocations is during the initial first aid and later during the rehabilitation as an exercise therapist.

Signs and Symptoms

For this a little acronym may help:

- P̲ay – pain, usually deep.
- T̲om – tenderness.
- L̲oss of function/mobility.
- S̲welling. There may be some discolouration/bruising.
- D̲ – Deformity – unnatural contours when compared.
- I̲f – irregularity of natural contours/immobility.
- U̲ – unnatural movement.
- C̲an – crepitus.

Beware of Shock!

Rib fractures are not uncommon in contact sports and should be suspected if:

1. There is pain over the area especially during deep breathing, coughing and sneezing.

2. There is tenderness and swelling over the fracture site.
3. Compression of the thoracic cage is locally painful. To test, one hand is put on the sternum and the other is put on the thoracic spine and the hands are brought together. There should be a pain free springy feel. An alternative, with the hands in the same position is to resist the inspiration of the patient.
4. X-ray confirmation and exclusion of lung damage.

First Aid Treatment
(*see Chapter 4, Part 1*)

These are basic guidelines and are not intended as definitive treatment:

1. **DO NOT** move the casualty unless he/she is in danger or give them anything to eat or drink.
2. **SECURE AND SUPPORT** the injured part with a sling or bandaging either to the trunk or the other limb. If the bone is protruding through the skin do not put pressure over it but build up pads around it to bandage over.
3. **SEND** for an ambulance. The person needs to be X-rayed for confirmation of a fracture.
4. **TREAT** the person for shock.
5. **STAY** with the person until they have been transferred to medically qualified personnel.

NOTE: Treat severe sprains as fractures and if in doubt, always refer to the hospital.

The hospital management will consist of:

1. Reduction.
2. Immobilisation.
3. Preservation of function/rehabilitation.
(1) and (2) may not be necessary but (3) most definitely is to:

*   Preserve function.
*   Rapidly restore function once there is union.
*   Maintain levels of general and local fitness.

Rehabilitation can begin after 24–48 hours and can consist of either the whole body and/or self help, home exercise regimes. Massage and mobilisation to joints above and below the fracture site, once the medical people have dealt with it, can prove beneficial. Subsequent soft tissue work, i.e. when the plaster has been removed and surgeon has stated that the fracture has knitted and there is a good callus formation can:

- Promote healing by stimulating the nerve and blood supply, which in turn will increase the supply of nutrients to the area and remove toxic waste debris (i.e. dead cells, etc.) The nerve and blood supply is vital to the body in healing itself.
- Help prevent/reduce swelling/oedema, adhesions and muscular atrophy and weakness.
- Help the absorption of lymph, effused blood and damaged tissue.

However, as stated before, a basic understanding of the stages involved in such healing will help to assist the repair as will an appreciation of the efficacy of any treatment modality.

Part 4

Factors Affecting, Influencing and Delaying Healing and Repair

The texts inform us that without complications muscle can take 7 days, 3 weeks–3 months to repair depending on the severity, whilst ligaments can take 2 weeks, 6 weeks–6 months. With bones, consolidation times can vary from 6–24 weeks depending on the type of bone and the type of fracture. However, healing and repair are not constant and can be affected by:

1. **THE KNOWLEDGE, SKILL, EXPERTISE AND COMMONSENSE OF THE THERAPIST/PRACTITIONER** (*see Chapter 1, Parts 1–3*).
2. **INTENSITY AND DURATION, REST/PROTECTION**, e.g. strappings and coverings (*see Chapter 5, Part 6*).
3. **VASCULARITY**, (blood supply), which is essential for healing, e.g. the scaphoid bone is a poor healer because only its proximal $1/3$ has a blood supply. Upper limb fractures heal better than lower limb.
4. **TEMPERATURE** excesses may retard or damage tissues (*see Chapter 5, Part 7*).
5. **IRRITATION** if persistent will slow healing. The irritant needs to be removed. One type of muscle tear that is very slow to heal is when muscle fibres tear at the insertion of the tendon into the periosteum (i.e. tennis elbow) because scar tissue is under stress all the time and gets very little rest.
6. **TYPE AND DEGREE OF VIOLENCE.**
7. **TYPE OF INJURY**. Is it soft tissue or bony tissue? (*see Chapter 3, Part 3*).
8. **REST** is needed for the body to re-adjust, rebalance and recover from the shock/stress fatigue of both the injury and the treatment. With bone, weight bearing, immobility and movement are significant factors.
9. **INFECTION** delays healing and may cause further damage. This must be overcome.

10. **NUTRITION**. Good nutritional status is essential for repair (*Davidson, et al., 1979*) and the studies that have been done on nutrients known to promote health and healing show promising results (*Bucci, L., 1997*). Also bringing essential nutrients directly to the injury site appears to markedly enhance healing (*Acta Chir. Scan., 1977*).

- **Free radicals** are at least partly to blame for muscle damage soreness and reduced endurance (*Burke, E. R., 1997*).
- **Vitamin C**, enhances iron absorption, is required for collagen biosynthesis, assists wound healing and stimulates the immune system. As a water-soluble antioxidant it specialises in scavenging oxidants and free radicals in the water regions of cells and blood (*Burke, E. R., 1997*). **Zinc and certain amino acids** are also related to collagen synthesis.
- **Arganine** may stimulate insulin production, enhance the production of critical protein structures, improve immune functions and also increase the synthesis of nitric and nitrous oxide, which dilate blood vessels and promote the delivery of oxygen to damaged tissues (*Am. J. Surgery, 1991*). **Arganine hydrochloride** supplementation can boost collagen deposition whilst, **Arganine aspartate**, can improve protein synthesis (*Surgery, 1990*).
- **Vitamin E** may help muscle soreness and damage (*Dekkers, J. C., 1996*). **Pycnogenol**, a water-soluble bioflavonoid, which is extracted from the bark of a French pine tree. A natural anti-inflammatory, there are no known side effects. As an antioxidant it is 50 times more effective than vitamin E and 1,000 times more effective than vitamin C. Binding to collagen it claims to improve the strength of arteries, veins, capillaries and the skin (*Passwater, R. A., 1985*).
- **Proteolytic enzymes** assist the elimination of inflammatory debris and initiate regeneration. This means that damage control, repair and new tissue generation is carried out more forcefully and precisely. Clinical trials in the supplemental use for healing and repair of such enzymes are encouraging (*Dietrich, R., 1965 and Donaho, C., 1962*). Found in living cells two of the most common sources come from fruit papin from papayas and bromelain from pineapples. **Combination supplementation, that are 'enteric coated'** to help resist breakdown by stomach **enzymes, of bromelain, papin, trypsin and chemotrypsin are best** (*Bucci, L., 1995*).
- **Glucosamine, an amino acid**, has many functions in the body ranging from water transportation, promotion of post exercise rehydration, the main source of energy for immune system cells, regulation of body pH and the stimulation of protein and glycogen synthesis. It is the major precursor of glucosaminoglycans (GAGs), which are the tissue framework onto which collagen models attach. Synthesised from glutamin and glucose it is the body's rate limiting step in GAG production and consequently the rate limiting step

in re-modelling of the connective tissues. Following soft tissue injury this limit does not allow the body to make sufficient glucosamine for optimal healing. Also as we get older the body's ability to synthesise glucosamine declines because of the reduction in the level of the converting enzyme glucosamine synthetase. The combined effects of these is that connective tissue repair declines. Man made glucosamine bypasses the rate limit in the GAG production system, increases GAG levels and increases connective tissue synthesis (*see Chapter 8, Part 1*).

"Evidence at present is not strong enough to warrant recommending an athlete to use this supplement, but there are some suggestions of a possible role in stimulating the anabolic process."
Professor R. Maughan, 2000

With regards to bone mineral balance, e.g. calcium, magnesium and boron are also vital. NSAIDS assist cell permeability and reduce pain. Steroids toughen cell membrane.

11. **ALCOHOL/SMOKING** can cause vasodilation (*see Chapter 8, Part 1*).
12. **AGE/GENDER**. The young heal better than the old and in approximately half the time. Again we come back to the question of age and the ageing process.
13. **MOVEMENT/IMMOBILITY/EXERCISE**. Exercise is like medicine – it is beneficial in the correct dosage and to the right condition, but it can do harm in the wrong dosage and to the wrong condition. What we do know is that it is essential for good bone formation (*see Chapter 2*).
14. **THE INTERACTION BETWEEN THE THERAPIST/ PRACTITIONER AND THE ATHLETE/PATIENT** (*see Chapter 5, Part 2*).
15. **PERSONALITY TYPES AND HYPOCHONDRIACS, POSITIVES, NEGATIVES, PLACEBOS AND NOCEBOS** (*see Chapter 1, Part 5; Chapter 5, Part 2*).
16. **SOMATOTYPES**, i.e. endomorph, mesomorph, ectomorph (*see Chapter 1, Part 5*).
17. **SECONDARY/ILLNESS GAIN** – 'the compensation culture' (*see Chapter 5, Part 2*).
18. **TYPE/SIZE OF TISSUE/FRACTURE/BONE**, the more specialised the tissue the less the power of regeneration.

There are those that:

• Will regenerate in most circumstances bone, epithelial and connective tissue.

As we know bone regenerates by the formation of callus; different types of bone (cancellous and hard) and fracture (transverse/spiral) and the site of fracture (upper body/lower body) will affect healing.

- Will regenerate in favourable conditions, i.e. liver, thyroid and kidney.
- Cannot regenerate, i.e. nervous tissue. Nerve tissue is poor and only 80% successful if it does, although research has shown that some white fibres in the spinal cord will regenerate in favourable conditions. Skeletal muscle was once thought to have little power for regeneration and the healing was by fibrosis or scar tissue, which takes the place of normal tissue or forms adhesions between normal tissues and so affects function. However, Dr. Eyal Lederman, 1998, now refutes this (*see Chapter 3, Part 3*). The belly of a muscle has a better blood supply than the tendon, which doesn't heal as well. Ligaments heal slowly but because they possess no specialised cells, healing is by fibrous tissue. Fascia is usually the first to show signs of change in postural problems. Obviously the size of the area affected will affect the rate of healing. With particular reference to bone we have:

19. The degree of **PERIOSTEAL STRIPPING**. This will affect osteoblastic activity.
20. **THE THICKNESS OF THE BONE**. The femur and fibula will have different healing/repair times, e.g. fibula 3 weeks to union, femur 14 weeks.
21. **THE CLOSENESS OF THE FRACTURED ENDS AND TISSUE FRAGMENTS BETWEEN THE BONE ENDS** (sequestra). This is when splinters and dead bone are not removed by phagocytosis and fibrosis occurs causing a fibrous union.
22. **INTERNAL FIXATION**. Screws, nuts and bolts after surgery.
23. **FAT EMBOLISM**. This is not common but serious and can occur within a few days of a lower limb fracture.

NOTE: 1, 14, 15, 16 and 17 are related to factors that are not easily quantifiable but are a constant source of discussion throughout the whole of this book.

Part 5

Complications of Injury

These complications can be considered as slight, severe or catastrophic.

Bones

- **INTRINSIC**. Related to the fracture itself.
- **EXTRINSIC**. Attributable to associated injuries.

- **IMMEDIATE**. Relate to arteries, nerves, viscera (internal organs), joints and skin.
- **DELAYED**. i.e. infection.
- **LATE**. Considered 'life or career threatening', e.g. an impacted fracture can cause shortness with <1cm being tolerable but >1cm requiring a heel lift, with possible osteoarthritis occurring later.

Intrinsic/Delayed

- **INFECTION**. In a compound/open fracture a 'wound toilet' is created which can lead to hypoxia, ischaemia and pus formation.
- **DELAYED UNION**. Here the intervening fascia hasn't clinically united and after 3–4 months the fracture site is still mobile.
- **NON-UNION**. This is worse than delayed union as there is no callus formation which could be because of infection, blood supply, movement between fracture ends, soft tissue imposition, traction distortion, synovial fluid dissolution, corroding metal in the fracture site, tumour and/or pathological reason.
- **AVASCULAR NECROSIS**. The common sites of which are the head of the femur, the proximal half of the scaphoid bone and the body of the talus.
- **MAL-UNION**. Through malalignment the fracture site will lack strength.
- **SHORTENING**. This could be because of mal-union, crushing, loss of bone and epiphyseal interference. Crush injuries to the hand can result in oedema retention with nerve disturbance.

Extrinsic/Immediate

- **INJURY TO MAJOR BLOOD VESSELS**.
- **INJURY TO NERVES**. This is when there is a transient physiological block, e.g. neuropraxia (nerve compression) but recovery is spontaneous. Axonotmesis is when there is an interruption of the axon.
- **INJURY TO THE VISCERA**. e.g. lung puncture.
- **INJURY TO TENDONS**.
- **FAT EMBOLISM**. Creating non-union/delayed union.
- **INJURY TO JOINT**. This causes stiffness and can include **SUDECK'S ATROPHY** (Reflex Sympathetic Dystrophy Syndrome) where there are neurovascular and vasomotor changes. The limb becomes cyanotic and cold and there is swelling, loss of power and sensation in the fingers. It occurs a couple of weeks post injury and sometimes follows a Colle's or Pott's fracture. **VOLKMANN'S ISCHEMIC CONTRACTURE** is where there is persistent spasm of the brachial artery following supracondylar fracture of the humerus.

Joints

1. **DEFORMITY**. There are three occasions when this may occur:

- Ligament tears, which result in an altered relationship between joint surfaces.
- Fractures are always potential sources of deformity when the bones are not perfectly aligned.
- Adaptive muscle shortening, muscles not being in 'natural resting position', can produce deformity as a result of insufficient extensibility in the muscles over a joint to produce full joint extension.

2. **GAIT**. Because of stiffness the athlete will have an antalgic gait with a possible limp.
3. **LIGAMENTS**. If ligaments are allowed to heal in a lengthened position they can lose their proprioceptive and controlling ability on the related joint. This can lead to instability, resulting in the joint being less able to protect itself at its end range. Irritation of the periosteal attachments can lead to calcification of the ligaments that further reduce its ability to function correctly.
4. **SECONDARY ARTHRITIC CHANGES**. Any disruption of the hyaline joint surfaces initiates a degenerative, 'wear and tear' cycle with damage which increases with further stress and strain. The effect on the joint is cumulative and leads to further structural changes, such as 'pitting' and 'osteophytic lipping', which affect function. Consideration should also be given to the effects of intra-articular fractures and meniscal lesions.
5. **SOFT TISSUE ADAPTATION**. Soft tissue contracture as a result of poor repair, leads to a loss of correct function.

Muscle

1. **CYST FORMATION**. Poor haematoma re-absorption results in a small sac of fluid being left within the muscle fibres which steadily degenerates. This sac develops a lining because of the pressure from the surrounding tissues and a cyst is formed. A soft fluctuant area can be felt early on in the centre of the bruise.
2. **INFECTION**. This is less common than in skin injury. Injections, proteolytic enzymes, steroids and local anaesthetics into muscle may predispose it to infection.
3. **MYOSITIS OSSIFICANS**. Also known as heterotopic bone formation, charley horse and cork, depending on from which part of the world you originate, and is when direct violence to a muscle results in bleeding either intra or inter muscularly. The haematoma may become invaded by osteoblasts, calcium is deposited and calcifies. The degree of osteoblastic activity will determine the severity of the disability and resultant tethering. The risk factors

for further injury are increased. Initial x-rays may not detect the calcification for 5–12 days.

4. **MUSCLE SHORTENING ADAPTATION**. This can be the result of scarring and/or poor rehabilitation post trauma.

5. **SCARRING**. This can be a major problem, e.g. hamstrings. Haematomas are invaded by repair cells from the surrounding tissues to replace damaged fibres with collagenous scar tissue. The scar tissue contracts and the tissue heals in an 'unnatural resting position'. There is obvious loss of flexibility and mobility with resultant discomfort and pain. This situation can become permanent if ignored and frequently leads to re-occurrence, as scar tissue possesses less tensile strength than the tissue it has replaced.

Tendons

Most complications of tendon injuries are the result of inappropriate treatment, e.g. injections into the tendon (*Smith, G. N., 1997*). We can also add to this inappropriate manual frictions. If the inflammatory response fails to resolve the healing/repair of the tendon follows a degenerative continuum. Inflammatory changes produce fibrosis, thickening and scarring, causing a thickening of the paratenon and fibrous sheaths. If this state is not addressed and is further aggravated by additional stresses then a tiny lesion can develop in the tendon resulting in microscopic loss of continuity of the collagen fibres (focal degeneration).

This can lead to avascular necrosis, partial and total rupture of the tendon. Malcolm Read, 1992, informs us that the Achilles tendon has a natural rupture rate of 3% in tendon pathology. Another complication can be soft tissue adaptation where, as previously discussed, the damaged tissue ends up in a shortened position with the resultant loss of normal function. An **AVULSION FRACTURE** is the result of a strong tendon pulling on its anchorage/attachment causing the bone to give.

Skin

1. **EXCESSIVE GRANULATION TISSUE**. Healing grazes, especially if infected, become covered by bright pink, protruding flesh known as 'proud flesh'.

2. **INFECTION**. Invasion via bacterial, viral, fungal or parasitic sources can cause local irritation leading to cellulitis and generalised septicaemia.

3. **HYPERTROPHIC SCAR TISSUE**. Some people are prone to very thick scars, commonly post infection.

4. **SCAR TETHERING**. Tethering is the adherence of scar tissue to the underlying tissue resulting in loss of mobility and suppleness for such tissues.

Part 6

Swellings, Lumps and Bumps

This subject is one that requires the therapist to have a knowledge of, an awareness of and a familiarity with:

- The difference between a hard and soft tissue lump, bump and swelling, e.g. osteoma and water oedema.
- The naturally occurring lumps, bumps and swellings found in the body, e.g. bursa.
- An understanding of the natural fluid content of the body's tissues and their secretions and excretions and how excesses of such can accumulate.
- A basic scientific knowledge of the active and passive fluid transportation mechanisms of the body, i.e. diffusion, osmosis, filtration etc.
- An understanding of the body's natural responses and healing and repair processes, i.e. inflammation and the complications of such (*see Chapter 3, Parts 1–5*).

Only then will the sports therapist be able to both safely and effectively deal with most of the lumps, bumps and swellings that he/she will come across. Also having identified these, does the therapist refer, treat or ignore?

NOTE: It should go without saying that medical conditions as such do not fall within the sphere of treatment by a sports therapist unless under the supervision of a medical practitioner.

Swellings can be considered under the following headings:

- **INFECTIONS**.
- **INJURY**.
- **NEOPLASMS/TUMOURS**.
- **OBSTRUCTIONS**.
- **MISCELLANEOUS**.

Infections

Most swellings found as a result of infections are those of the lymphatic system where toxic waste material has affected the glands/nodes. This may be as a result of fungal, viral or parasitic invasion. **Mumps** are swollen, infected cervical glands. **Glandular fever** is a serious infection of the lymph nodes that become swollen and sore and cannot filter. The person becomes generally run-down. Should a gland be infected by **tuberculosis**, it has no tenderness or heat, but is a hard swelling which breaks down and forms pus and has to be drained. **Lymphangitis** is acute inflammation of lymphatic vessels. **Adenitis** is acute inflammation caused by infection of a lymph node.

Injuries

Swelling can occur as a result of the body's natural response to the initial injury, whether that be caused by trauma or overuse (*see Chapter 1, Part 5 and Chapter 3, Part 3*). **Adhesions** can occur if the fluid, which has accumulated in response to the injury, is allowed to remain in the lymph spaces. This sticky and tacky fluid adheres to the surrounding tissues, resulting in a fibrous, 'knotted' mass. In this state the fibres need to be separated and the fluid made less viscous, as in its present consistency it will not return to the lymphatic vessels. Therefore much deep friction, by a qualified, experienced therapist is necessary to reduce the adhesion so that it can be absorbed and the fibres can re-align themselves along lines of stress. **The aim being to break down its mechanical properties** (*Hunter, 1997*). Which is in contrast to the earlier view that there is:

> **"No support for the hypothesis that frictions promote the repair of sprained ligaments."**
> *Walker, J. M., 1984*

Neoplasms/Tumours

Neoplasms are growths in their early stages and can be **either simple/benign or malignant**. Tumours are abnormal swellings that relate to the type of tissue affected and are identified by the suffix **OMA** and can sometimes be categorised according to size, shape, colour etc. **Tumours can also be simple/benign**, which are a less serious form, slow growing, non-active and restricted to one area of the body. **Malignant** are a more serious than usual form, very active, fast growing and spreading to other parts of the body.

NOTE: A 'red flag' to suspect a tumour would be unremitting night pain.

- **Skeletal neoplasms/tumours** can be **primary or secondary (metastatic)**, the latter resulting from a primary tumour elsewhere in the body.
- **Carcinoma** (epithelial tissue) **and sarcoma** (connective tissue) are general names for malignant tumours.
- **Chondrosarcoma** is a malignant tumour affecting hyaline cartilage arising from chondroblasts. The common bones affected are femur, spine, pelvis, ribs or scapula.

- **Osteochondrosis** is a temporary softening of growing bone, e.g. Perthe's disease affecting the femoral head. Scheurmann's disease affecting the thoracic spine. Scheurmann's disease is one of the most common primary, malignant tumours of skeletal tissue and is a condition which occurs during bone growth.
- **Osteosarcoma** is the most common type of skeletal tissue tumour. Common bones affected are tibia, femur and humerus.
- **Lymphoma** is a tumour of the lymphatic cells/lymphoid tissue.
- **Hodgkin's disease** is cancer in the lymph nodes.
- **Leukaemia** is cancer of the white blood cells.

Obstructions

These are numerous and appear in many forms i.e. aneurism, hernia, rupture etc. **Lymphoedema** is caused by the blockage to the lymph nodes causing oedema.

Miscellaneous

This heading can include: acne, blisters, boils, carbuncles, calluses, corns, cysts, ganglions, goitres, moles, pimples etc. Many of these relate to skin eruptions and therefore require referral to a medical practitioner. **Cysts** are either bursae or tendon sheaths distended by fluid or protrusion cysts from joint capsules herniated by hydrostatic pressure. **Bursitis** is an inflammation of the bursa.

Differential Diagnosis

- Swelling in the glands may have **NO HEAT OR TENDERNESS**.
- Bursitis when compared to synovitis tends to be very localised and not just in the joint.

Three types of swelling with particular relevance to sport are:

1. **HAEMARTHROSIS**. This is blood in a joint and is a serious injury, considered **CLINICALLY SIGNIFICANT AND SHOULD BE MEDICALLY REFERRED**. There is immediate swelling, usually within a few hours, resulting in a hot, tight, large, painful, swollen joint. It is usually the result of direct trauma, e.g. a blow, kick or an excessive twisting or tortioning of the affected joint tissues, e.g. anterior cruciate ligament disruption, intra-articular fracture, meniscal damage. There would be reduced range of movement and ease of movement, with a reluctance on the part of the athlete, to move the affected joint.

2. **SYNOVIAL EFFUSION/TRAUMATIC SYNOVITIS.** There is increased synovial fluid within a joint as a result of inflammation to the synovial membrane or injury. The excess fluid takes longer to accumulate than a haemarthrosis, up to 24 hours post injury.

3. **OEDEMA** (Inflammatory Exudate). This is an abnormal accumulation of fluid (synovium and blood) beneath the skin or in one or more cavities of the body. It is a general term but can be specific in certain places when used medically, i.e. Ascites – Abdomen. Oedema can be caused by:

- Disturbance of the permeability of the capillary vessels by injury, ill-health (infection), 'poverty of the blood', (dietary deficiency), and poisonous materials in the blood.
- Obstruction of the blood flow through the blood vessels or obstruction to lymph flow through its channels. Cardiac failure, blood and osmotic pressure problems, gravitational problems can all effect body fluid dynamics (*see Chapter 3, Part 2*).

In the case of disruption to the semi-permeable membrane the fluid swelling may involve blood and tissue fluid as a result of damage to local capillaries resulting in an outflow of blood into the tissue spaces. The blood plasma that leaks out is high in plasma proteins which 'draws' watery tissue fluid out from the cells into the tissue space. The main plasma proteins being fibrinogen, prothrombin, albumin and globulin.

Chemical substances released as a result of tissue damage and inflammation add to this effect by increasing blood flow and membrane permeability, e.g. bradykinin and seratonin. As a result there is associated heat and pain with initial swelling which takes place in the acute stage (0–48 hours). Reduced muscle activity may cause further accumulation in the lymphatics and the fascial sheaths, especially in those limbs under greater gravitational pull, e.g. ankles. Swelling can therefore be graded as:

1. **Minor/Grade 1**. This is when the joint bony points can still be identified.
2. **Moderate/Grade 2**. With a moderate swelling, bony points cannot be distinguished. There is significant fluid presence that can be massaged/moved from one side of the joint to the other.
3. **Severe/Grade 3**. There is a large, hot, tense swelling. Fluid cannot be massaged from compartment to compartment and the bony points cannot be distinguished.

References

1.   Association of Chartered Physiotherapists in Sports Medicine (ACPSM): 1998. Guidelines for the management of soft tissue (musculoskeletal) injury with Protection, Rest, Ice, Compression and Elevation (PRICE) during the first 72-hours. Association Chartered Physiotherapists in Sports Medicine.

2.   Acta Chir. Scan., 1977. Local Hyperalimentation of Experimental Granular Tissue. 143, 201.

3.   American Journal of Surgery, 1991, Nutrient Modulation of Inflammatory and Immune Functions. 161, 230.

4.   Arnheim and Prentice: 2000. See Smith, G. N., 2001.

5.   Brukner, P., and Khan, K.: 2001. Principles of Treatment, Chapter 8, 127. Clinical Sports Medicine. 2nd. Ed. McGraw Hill.

6.   Bucci, L.: 1995. Pain Free. Fort Worth, The Summit Group.

7.   Bucci, L.: 1997. Introduction in: Sports Nutrition. Wolinski, I., and Driskell, J., eds., 1–28, CRC Press.

8.   Burke, E. R.: 1997. Nutrients that accelerate healing, strength and conditioning. National Strength and Conditioning Association, 19–23, October.

9.   Burrough, P., and Dahners: 1990. The effect of enforced exercise on the healing of ligament injuries. *American Journal of Sports Medicine*, 18, 4, 376–378.

10. Cyriax, J.: 1984. Textbook of orthopaedic medicine, volume 2. Treatment by massage, manipulation and injection, part 1.

11. Davidson, et al: 1979.

12. Dekkers, J. C.: 1996. The role of anti-oxidant vitamins and enzymes in the prevention of exercise induced muscle damage. *Sport Med*. 21: 213–238.

13. Dietrich, R.: 1965. Oral proteolytic enzymes in the treatment of athletic injuries: a double blind study. *Pennsylvania Medical Journal*, 68: 35–37.

14. Dodds, Dr. G.: 1989. Body chemistry and its effects on soft tissues. NIM lecture, 8.4.89.

15. Donaho, C., and Rylander, C.: 1962. Proteolytic enzymes in athletic injuries. a double blind study of a new anti-inflammatory agent. *Delaware Medical Journal*, 34: 168–170.

16. Dyson, Dr. M.: 1992. FA Medical Conference, Lilleshall, 4.10.

17. Green, E.: 1987. Tissue healing and massage therapy. *Massage Therapy Journal*, Summer, 1987.

18. Ho, S., et al.: 1994: Comparison of various icing times in decreasing bone metabolism and blood flow in the knee. *Am. J. of Sports Medicine*, 23, 174–176.

19. Hunter, G.: 1997. The timetable of soft tissue healing. OCPPP Seminar, Dynamic tissue healing and the effects of physiotherapy, Manchester.

20. Jarvinen, M. J., and Lehto, M. U. K.: 1993. The effects of early mobilisation on the healing process following muscle injuries. *Sports Medicine*, 15, 2, 78–89.

21. Karlsson, et al.: 1996. Early functional treatment for acute ligament injuries of the ankle joint. *Scand. J. Medicine and Science in Sport*, 6, 341–345.

22. Knight, K, L.: 1995. Cryotherapy in sports injury management. Human Kinetics.

23. Knight, K. L.: 1989. Cryotherapy in sports injury management. *Int. Perspectives in Physiotherapy*, 4, 163–185.

24. Komi, P., and Buskirk, E.: 1972. The effects of concentric and eccentric muscle activity on tension and electrical activity of human muscle. *Ergonomics*, 15: 417–434.

25. Lederman, Dr. E.: 1998. Active technique workshop, Huddersfield, 14–15 November, 1998.

26. Levin, S.: 1993. Early mobilisation speeds recovery. *Physician and Sports Medicine*, 21, 8, 70–74.

27. Low and Reed: 1994. See Smith, G. N., 16.6.2001.

28. Macdonald, et al.: 1995. See Smith, G. N., 16.6.2001.

29. McMaster, et al.: 1978. Laboratory evaluation of various cold therapy modalities. *Am. J. of Sports Medicine*, 6, 5, 291–294.

30. Noyes, et al.: 2000. See Smith, G. N., 16.6.2001.

31. Passwater, R. A.: 1985. The new super antioxidant – plus.

32. Peterson, Dr. L., and Renstrom, Dr. P.: 2000. See Smith, G. N., 16.6.2001.

33. Prentice: 1999. See Smith, G. N., 16.6.2001.

34. Read, Dr. M.: 1992. 'The Achilles Tendon.' Society of Sports Therapy Annual Conference, Solihull.

35. Reider, B., et al.: 1993. Treatment of isolated M.C.L. injuries in athletes with early functional rehabilitation. *Am. J. of Sports Medicine*, 22, 470–477.

36. Rucinski, T. J., et al.: 1991. The effects of intermittent compression on oedema in post-acute ankle sprains. *J. of Orthopaedic Sports Physical Therapy*, 14, 2, 65–69.
37. Scheffler, et al.: 1992. See Smith, G. N., 16.6.2001.
38. Schmidt, R. A.: 1982/91. Motor learning and control: a behavioural emphasis. Human Kinetics.
39. Shelbourne and Rask: 1998. See Smith, G. N., 16.6.2001.
40. Smith, G. N.: 1997. Stages of tissue repair and implications for treatment. Annual Conference of the Society of Sports Therapists, 11.5.97.
41. Smith, G. N.: 2001. Current trends and philosophies in the treatment and rehabilitation of the injured knee. Body and Soul Conference, Birmingham, 16.6.2001.
42. Sports Therapy Education Services. 1990. Module 9 course notes.
43. Surgery, 1990, Argnine enhances wound healing and lymphocyte immune response in humans. 108, 331.
44. Troop, R.: 1999. Sports injuries, *Peak Performance*, 117.
45. Tuber, C.: 2001. Measurement of reactive vasodilation during cold gel application to non-traumatised ankles. *Physical Therapy*, 72, 4, 294–299.
46. Walker, J. M.: 1984. *JOSPT*, 6:2, 89–94.
47. Whitelaw, G. P., et al.: 1995. The use of cryocuff versus ice and elastic wrap in the post operative care of knee arthroscopy patients. *Am. J. of Knee Surgery*, 8, 1, 28–31.
48. Zaffaganini, et al: 1998. See Smith, G. N., 16.6.2001.
49. Zuluaga, M., Briggs, C., Carlisle, et al.: 1996. Sports physiotherapy, applied science and practice. Churchill Livingstone, Melbourne.

Bibliography

1. Injury and repair of the musculoskeletal soft tissue. American Academy of Orthopaedic Surgeons Symposium.
2. Oxford concise medical dictionary, 4th ed. 1994. Pages 166 and 501.

Chapter 4
Examination, Assessment and Diagnosis

A man who asks is a fool for 5 minutes.
A man who never asks is a fool for life.
Chinese proverb

Part 1

An Overview of First Aid and the Immediate Care of the Sports Person in the Sporting Environment

It is important to emphasise the importance of a first aid qualification for anyone working with, and responsible for, other people. In this respect the sports therapist is no different to anyone else. They are also no different in that when called upon to use such knowledge, skills and expertise it has to be done, at times, under extreme pressure. Therefore the need to update, practise and regularly assess this knowledge, skill and expertise is vital not only in terms of continuing professional development but also to protect, in case of litigation, the therapist and the patient. This can only be achieved by attending, in the first place, a recognised first aid course, preferably one geared to sport. Secondly, by regularly practising the active elements of such a course and thirdly, by regularly, at least every three years, updating such knowledge, skills and expertise.

For this reason, the author has deliberately not detailed this section on first aid by trying to produce a pseudo first aid course. Instead, an overview of the

subject is preferred by highlighting key areas and leaving the details to the experts by referring the reader to the many practical texts/courses on the subject. The FA and NSMI are two such organisations who run courses with the sporting environment in mind.

The roles and responsibilities of the sports therapist are to preserve/maintain life; prevent the condition worsening; promote recovery and pre-empt the correct treatment on the field of play/sporting arena. An ounce of correct examination/assessment on the field is worth a kilo of work in the treatment room afterwards.

This carries with it, amongst other things, a paralegal responsibility, a moral responsibility and a duty of care and involves knowledge of/familiarity with, amongst other things:

- Primary and secondary surveys and the difference between and the significance of signs and symptoms.
- Cardiopulmonary resuscitation.
- Recovery position.
- Bleeding.
- Strokes.
- Heart attacks.
- Choking etc.

There is a definite chain of survival where by doing the correct thing early enough lives can be saved, and less life threatening injuries are assessed quickly, therefore potentially cutting down recovery times/rates. In a sporting scenario the first aider is in a competitive environment, and not only has to deal with the injury but also the problems that might go with being in such a situation, i.e. sporting mentality (*see Chapter 1, Part 2*).

Dealing with an acute injury scenario involves the use of common sense and engaging the eyes and the ears before the hands. The only time a player is initially handled is if he/she is unconscious, when they are **in a potentially 'life threatening' situation and a primary survey is called for**. This will involve what is known as the **DRABC scenario: Danger, Response, Airways, Breathing and Circulation.**

Mouth To Mouth Resuscitation

A secondary survey is 'non-life threatening' and would involve: seeing what happened, asking what happened, looking at the site of injury, touching relevant

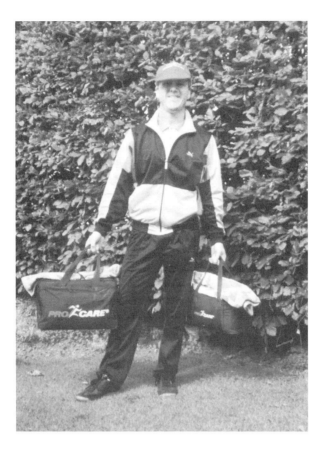

◄ *Figure 38.*
Always carry the
relevant equipment
for possible
treatment on the
field of play.

structures, getting the injured party to move the injured joint and moving the injured limb for them. Then you must ascertain if the limb/joint is strong enough and can bear weight. **After such an examination the therapist needs to make a clinical judgement/decision based on objective criteria not subjective opinion.** The decision can be:

• To let the player continue with no treatment.
• To let the player continue after on the spot treatment.
• To temporarily stop the player continuing whilst further assessments and/or treatment is made or given.
• Inform the player that they cannot continue.

Fundamentally, if the injured party can't and/or won't then they are removed from the field/area of play. In other words off they come! Obviously the practicalities of this involves playing, 'what if', which will be covered on first aid courses. Any treatment that is administered at this time is based on the initial signs and symptoms. This may involve referral to medical personnel and/or discharge to a hospital. **Signs are what are seen and perceived using ones' senses and symptoms are what the injured party tells you.**

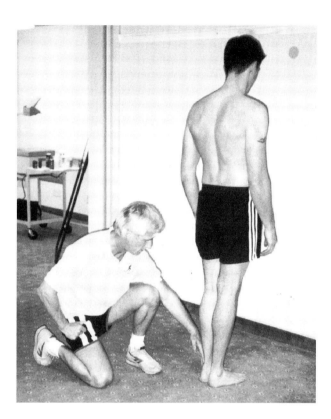

► *Figure 39.*
Principles of
examination.

Part 2

Principles, Procedures, Protocols and the Practice of Examination

Reference to the numerous examination and assessment texts will elicit the best way to examine but as with most things these depend upon from which perspective the examination is to be viewed. A neurologist will be keen to find neurological disturbance, a general practitioner signs of pathology, a manual therapist postural imbalance/restricted movement etc. Ideally a procedure including all of these perspectives and those not mentioned would hopefully provide us with enough information to arrive at a valued judgement/hypothesis. A true medical diagnosis only being possible when all the relevant medical data has been collected. However, the problem with trying to include everything, even if trained and qualified, is one of practicality. Whilst there should be no time limit on the examination and assessment, practical constraints will always determine what is possible in the time available. What is important is to have a definite, clear, logical procedure to follow. **WHEN, HOW** and **WHERE** this is done is important, not only for its effectiveness but also because of the legal implications. The legalities should never be ignored. **INFORMED CONSENT IS VITAL** (*see Chapter 7*).

Assessment, Evaluation and Diagnosis

The following principles, procedures and protocol will ensure the sports therapist will be able to practically demonstrate safe and effective competence in examination and assessment. However, these are not definitive prescriptions but guidelines to help the sports therapist arrive at a considered opinion, valued judgement, hypothesis and working diagnosis. As with everything related to the body the areas are interrelated and interdependent. **You don't get a second chance to make a first impression.** The therapist needs to quickly establish a rapport with the patient/athlete as it is during this initial contact that impressions are made. During examination and assessment communication is vital (*see Chapter 1, Part 2 and Appendix 1*). The examination and assessment begins as soon as eye contact is made.

History Taking and Consultation

What do we need to know?

It is vital during consultation to look and listen, whilst asking the right kind of questions. Reference to a variation of the Chinese proverb is very apt here.

'I look but I don't see.'
'I hear but I don't listen.'

The patient holds the key to arriving at a correct diagnosis. **If we don't train ourselves to actively listen and observe what we see all the relevant clues will be missed.** The following should be observed:

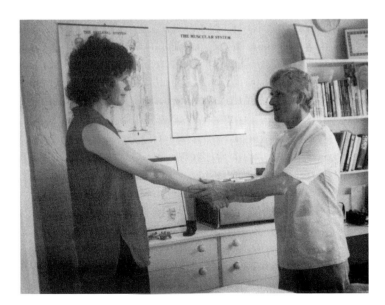

◄ *Figure 40. You don't get a second chance to make a first impression.*

- Talking is sharing but listening is caring.
- Control the conversation with body language/voice tone/non-verbal response.
- Generally ask relevant open questions as opposed to closed questions, i.e. "Tell me about the pain", as opposed to, "does it hurt?" (*see Chapter 5, Part 2*).
- Actively listen – keep writing to a minimum (*see Chapter 7, Part 3 and Appendix 4*).
- Let the athlete talk – the skill is when to stop them.
- Make eye to eye contact.
- Don't lie the person down.
- Create a relaxed but professional atmosphere. '**THE FAMOUS FIVE**' can be used as a basis for questioning. **WHEN**, will elicit at what stage the injury is presenting, i.e. acute, sub-acute, chronic. **WHERE**, will give insight to the area of the body that is injured. **WHY**, will give a clue to the cause. **HOW**, will give an insight to the mechanics of the injury. **WHAT**, will give information to what tissues may be affected.

Observations

To do, 'a quick postural check' we need to have the person undressed down to their underwear and then to observe their symmetry related to the spine. Skin colour, blemishes, scars, varicosity and weight distribution etc. can be observed. **Look at all aspects of the person, someone may have left the label on!** This initial check gives a first impression and indicates where potential, as well as obvious, problems may lie. During consultation and observation **look at body language**, i.e. finger pointing is specific and hand gestures are general. The use of **dermatomes** (cutaneous, segmental areas of skin that are supplied by a single spinal nerve) is a useful guide for neurological disturbance. Reference can be made to most standard neurology texts.

Postural Check (*see Part 5*)

With the person standing the following should be considered/observed:

- Anterior/posterior view (front to back and vice versa).
- Lateral/medial, non dominant to dominant side, injured/non injured side.
- Weight-bearing/non weight-bearing effect.
- Dressing/undressing, removing/putting on articles of clothing.
- One limb compared to the other. What is the norm for that person?
- Body types – consider a three figure Sheldon somatotype ratio (*see Chapter 1, Part 5*).
- Gait as the person enters vision (*see Part 4*).
- Alignment/balance (*see Chapter 4, Part 5*).
- Swelling, scar tissue, marks etc.
- Skin colour, fascia and general skin conditions.

Observation of skin colour can be helpful during examination and assessment:

- Blue colour, may suggest lack of oxygen (cyanosis).
- Yellow colour may be indicative of liver problems, i.e. jaundice, redness, fever, alcohol intake, trauma or inflammation.
- Red streaking may be as a result of blood poisoning, lymphatic infection, deep vein thrombosis. Bruises should be noted and pointed out to the patient. This serves several purposes in that it tells the person that the sports therapist didn't cause it and, depending on the reply indicates if the person bruises easily.

Obviously any skin colour change that raises doubts or suspicions should be referred to a doctor but commonsense should be used. Reference to the doctor should not be made just because the person looked red after running or because they have a bruise. **Medical diagnosis should not be given by a non-medically trained personnel**.

Always make comparisons with the opposite side of the body not the book, i.e. dominant side/non dominant, injured/non injured. **The use of the dominant eye, centrally aligned**, will give a balanced picture. The following landmarks can be noted:

- **WHOLE BODY**. Body type? Overweight/underweight?
- **HEAD**. Is it tilted?
- **EAR LOBES**. Are they level/anterior/posterior?
- **NECK CURVATURE**. Are the slopes symmetrical?
- **SHOULDERS**. Are they level/anterior/posterior?
- **SCAPULA**. Are they level/prominent/winged?
- **ARMS**. Do they hang level? Are they equidistant from the side of the body? Where do the fingertips reach?
- **HANDS**. Heberden's nodes are tiny nodules that appear at the sides of the dorsal aspect of the distal, interphalangeal joints and are indicative of osteoarthritis. Bouchard's nodes, which are indicative of rheumatoid arthritis, are found on the proximal, interphalangeal joints.
- **SPINE**. Is it excessively scoliotic/kyphotic/lordotic. If so, where? Are the natural curves reduced? Does the chin jut out?
- **POSTERIOR SUPERIOR ILIAC SPINE**. Are the dimples level?
- **ILIAC CRESTS**. Are they level?
- **SKINFOLDS**. Where are they and are they the same on both sides?
- **GLUTEAL CREASES**. Are they obvious/level?
- **POPLITEAL CREASES**. Are they level?
- **KNEES**. Is the person hypo/hyperextended/knock-kneed (**VARUM**)/ bowlegged (**VALGUS**)?

- **ACHILLES**. Does it lie vertical to the heel/foot?
- **FEET**. Is the weight equally distributed? Have they an apparent arch problem?

At this stage only observation should be done, the patient should not be encouraged to be active or functional other than what they do themselves, as this may knowingly exacerbate the problem.

Touch

> "The hand has the greatest concentration of exteroceptors and proprioceptors in the whole body."
> *Montague-Cook, B., 2000*

At this stage in the examination touch involves using the **DORSUM** of the hand to detect temperature variations or to detect if the skin is dry or damp. The **PALMAR SURFACE** is used to sense contour (**STEREOGNOSTIC**). Touch is light and superficial, more intensity and depth comes later under palpation. Levels 1 and 2 of Sandy Fritz's palpatory levels can be included here (*see palpation, page 203*).

The Significance of Touch

Touch sense is extremely complex and the subtle language of touch is important as we feel our way from childhood to death. Every person, every group is a unique product of their sensory experiences. It is critical for health and well being **but sadly there are many taboos against touch and now it has even greater significant implications, in the 'compensation culture world' in which we live. Intent and assault and battery are all issues that are very real. A manual therapists' hands are their eyes and as such, are sensitive valuable tools which need to be protected, insured and cared for** (*see Chapter 7*).

Range of Movement (ROM)/Ease of Movement (EOM)

This involves comparing joint ranges of movement looking for how far they move (ROM) and how easily they move (EOM) (*see Chapter 1, Part 3*). Both are significant. **Consideration should be given to 'the level of irritability', which may give guidance as to how much physical examination may be possible. Repetition of movement will give a clear picture, with alterations in movement patterns being a good clinical indicator during repetition.**

- **ACTIVE**. The patient moves the limb and tests muscle/neurological integrity. This is known as the **PHYSIOLOGICAL RANGE OF MOVEMENT**.

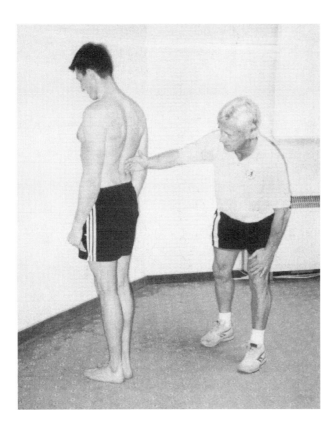

◄ Figure 41.
Significance of touch.

- **PASSIVE**. The sports therapist moves the limb for the person and this tests the integrity of the joint capsule/ligament. This is known as the **ANATOMICAL RANGE OF MOVEMENT**.
- **'END FEEL/PASSIVE SPRING'** are important components of the range and ease of movement and relate to when the person moves the limb as far as it will go and then the sports therapist exerts pressure to take it a little further. The sports therapist is looking for tissue response. 'Passive spring' is what it feels like at the end of the range. 'End feel' tests the joint's ability to protect itself at the end of the range.
- **RESISTIVE**. Related to the end feel and is the ability of the joint to protect itself during static and dynamic activity at the limit of range available. It is **not** specific muscle testing as this follows next.

Muscles/Myotomes

These take the form of isometric or isotonic testing to check the muscles strength and neurological integrity. Isometrically, the mid to inner range is the strongest range and therefore is considered the safest (*see Chapter 1, Part 4*). In spinal

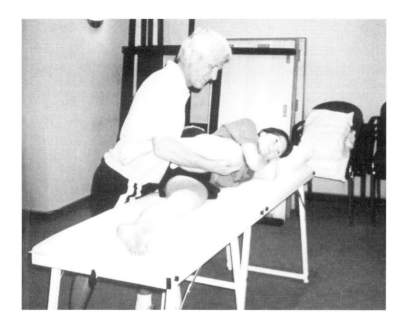

◄ *Figure 42.*
Passive range of
movement.

assessments, muscle testing is generally considered myotomal. Myotomes are not fixed territorial or anatomical entities as some dermatomes extend more distally than relevant myotomes, e.g. supraspinus tendonitis can extend to the radial border of the hand whereas C5 myotomes end at the elbow. The following are general guidelines:

Cervical flexion	**C2**	Interossei	**T1**
Cervical extension	**C3**	Hip flexion	**L2**
Shoulder elevation	**C4**	Knee extension	**L3**
Abduction	**C5**	Dorsiflexion	**L4**
Elbow flexion	**C6**	Toe extensor	**L5**
Elbow extension	**C7**	Plantar flexor	**S1**
Thumb extension	**C8**		

Ligaments need to be put on stretch and stressed to test their integrity.

Palpation

Touch and palpation of the skin and underlying tissues are helpful during examination and assessment feeling for elasticity, texture, dryness, dampness, thickness and thinness etc. Flashing during palpation (a sudden reddening and blushing) and tacky, damp skin (sudomotor as opposed to vasomotor reflex response) can be indicative of underlying pathology. Fascia can be palpated in sheaths or planes running on the surface of the body (iliotibial band) perpendicular to the body or bone (linea alba and nuchal ligament) and horizontally (diaphragm and pelvic floor). Muscle palpation should be in a natural resting position and not elongated as this will cause the muscle to feel tight because of increased intra muscular pressure. **Palpation can be used not only as a diagnostic tool but also a therapeutic tool**. Information collected through touch/palpation is added to information received and interpreting the information, via tactile sensitivity, so it is **VITAL** that we concentrate.

The phases of palpation can be considered as:

1. **RECEPTION** where mechano and proprioreceptors are activated and send messages.
2. **TRANSMISSION** when the peripheral and central nervous system send the impulses to the brain.
3. **INTERPRETATION** is the brain making comparisons. Dr. Lederman, 1998, reminds us that the peripheral mechanoreceptors (afferent) and proprioceptors provide information to the brain but do not control the motor system. This is centrally controlled.

- **PALMS** can be used to sense contour.
- **DORSUMS** of the hand – temperature.
- **FINGER PADS** – fine discrimination of textural differences.
- **TIPS OF FINGERS AND THUMBS** can be used as depth probes.
- **FINE LIGHT TOUCH** is using superficial light pressure.
- **DEEP TOUCH** is the result of additional pressure.
- **COMPRESSION** is palpation through multiple layers.
- **SHEAR** is movement through layers.

During palpation, temperature variations, body rhythms, patterns and pulses, i.e. breathing and circulation, can be detected. Obviously these subtle skills require many hours of practise and for some are more instinctive than others. Sandy Fritz, 1995, highlights thirteen levels of palpation. These thirteen levels are included here for completeness and to highlight the complexity and importance of palpatory skills.

LEVEL 1   Detects hot and cold but without touch.
LEVEL 2   Involves light touch determining if the skin is dry or damp; possesses goose or 'ducky' bumps/pimples (pilomotor reflex). **OBSERVATION** of hair, nails, growths, skin conditions is also included at this point.
LEVEL 3   Light touch to skin itself involving small stretching, comparing elasticity, texture, roughness or smoothness.
LEVEL 4   Assesses skin and superficial fascia for tightness, looseness and restrictions.

LEVEL 5   Actual superficial connective tissue that holds fluid, superficial blood vessels, lymph vessels and nodes. At this level we are feeling for a 'water balloon', resistant and springy effect. The vessels feel like soft tubes. The pulses can be felt and the nodes feel like small soft gel caps. Sometimes small nodules of adipose tissue can be felt more when touched. The issue and significance of lumps, bumps and swelling is acknowledged (*see Chapter 3, Part 6*).

LEVEL 6   Skeletal muscle which is fibrous to palpate. Muscle bulk and tone should be noted.

LEVEL 7   Tendon that feels more pliable and less ribbed than muscle. The musculotendonous junction is where muscle fibres end and connective tissue continues. It is an area of susceptibility.

LEVEL 8   Fascial sheaths or planes. These run relative to the surface of the body, perpendicular or horizontally. Fascial sheaths separate muscle groups.

LEVEL 9   Ligaments that are not very pliable.

LEVEL 10   Joints which will be discussed later in the examination procedure.

LEVEL 11   Bones.

LEVEL 12   Viscera/internal organs.

LEVEL 13   Rhythms and pulses.

Obviously experienced practitioners are able to work on more than one level at once because of their anatomical surface awareness, e.g. joint lines, bony points, attachments or origins and insertions etc.

NOTE: During examination, levels one and two would follow observation, whilst levels three to thirteen would be specific palpation prior to examination of the joints above and below.

Joints Above and Below

This is because pain can be referred from other areas. The body **COMPENSATES** when there is imbalance that throws extra loading onto other structures, areas and joints. This can sometimes be due to **leg length discrepancy** as a result of:

- Anatomical i.e. trauma, growth – poliomyelitis.
- Physiological i.e. sagittal innominate rotation.
- Hip contracture.
- Vertical shear.

With all leg length discrepancy it has to be ascertained if the discrepancy is structural or functional, apparent or real. One way to ascertain if it is apparent or real is to take measurements to both legs and compare.

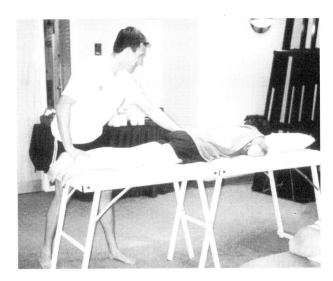

◀ *Figure 43. Leg length discrepancy.*

1. Measure from the anterior superior iliac spine to the tip of the medial maleoli, and if not equal do (4).
2. Measure from the anterior superior iliac spine to the tibial tuberosity.
3. Measure from the tibial tuberosity to the tip of the medial malleoli.
4. Measure from the greater trochanter to the tip of the lateral malleoli.

Also the nerve supply coming from the spine can be compromised and this can **REFER PAIN** into the periphery. In examination and assessment familiarity with upper and motor neurone disturbance should be learned. **As a general guide referral to a medical practitioner would be indicated if the patient had unremitting pain even at rest, inequality of pupil size, diplopia (double vision), abnormal Babinski's reflex, unremitting headache, vomiting, temporary loss of function, i.e. speed visions, motion, seizures.**

CORD SIGNS

Bilateral
Not dermatome related
Constant
Dizziness
Diplopia – double vision
Drop attack
Dysphasia – difficulty swallowing
Dysarthria – disturbed joint sense
(*see Chapter 5, Part 3*).

ROOT SIGNS

Unilateral
Referred
Dermatomal
Proximal myalgic tenderness
Provoked by coughing, sneezing

Specific/Special Tests

These relate to objective tests which are normally related to a specific body part. **They are repeatable and comparable.** These tests can be used to see if specific structures are injured. They are used at the relevant time and depending on what they are testing can be included anywhere in the protocol – although most will be done during the functional stage. These tests can relate to **orthopaedic,** e.g. leg length discrepancy; **neurological**, over-activity/deficit, e.g. reflexes etc; **specific muscle tests**, e.g. vastus medialis; **ligament stress tests**, e.g. valgus/varus stress, anterior draw etc.

The following are just a few of the many orthopaedic and neurological tests that can be performed to assist differential diagnosis during examination and assessment. Referral to the relevant texts will explain the procedure and significance of such tests.

The Foot and Ankle

- Homans sign for deep vein thrombosis.
- Passive dorsiflexion as reduction can lead to gait problems (*see Chapter 4, Part 4*). Demi Plie (L4, L5).
- Calf strength/stretch necessary for concentric and eccentric propulsion/balance and S2 integrity.
- Proprioception (eyes open/closed). Closing the eyes will take away the visual information emphasising a greater usage of other mechanisms/reporting stations (*see Chapter 6, Part 2*).
- Achilles reflex (S2), (x 6). Absence of which could also be indicative of disc pathology.
- Achilles pathology, socks off/shoes on PF/DF to locate possible area of problem.
- Campbell's, Thompson, Flipper, Simmond's tests to identify Achilles rupture.

Knee

- Lachmann's test for anterior cruciate ligament laxity.
- Posterior and anterior cruciate (draw sign).
- Valgus and varus stress tests to identify possible medial and lateral collateral (+ capsule) problems.
- Apprehension test to patella.
- Knowledge of McMurray and Apley tests for meniscal damage but medical advances have questioned the validity and use of such tests, e.g. arthroscopy.
- Knee jerk reflex (L4), (x 6).

Hip

- Psoas/Thomas test to identify psoas and rectus femoris tightness.
- Trendelenburg test for pelvic dynamism and muscular instability.
- Quadrant test for potential hip pathology.
- Piriformis test which is not only related to rotational problems of the hip but sciatica type pain.
- The iliofemoral, (capsule) ischiofemoral, pubofemoral ligaments.

Sacroiliac (S/I) or Lumbar?

The following three tests can be performed and if pain/limited movement is noted in two out of three then an S/I problem may be indicated, otherwise a lumbar lesion may be suspected:

1. **SUPINE.** Flex the knee and adduct to the opposite shoulder. Compare both legs.
2. **SUPINE.** Test adductor muscles by putting them on stretch.
3. **PRONE.** Knees together and test V as the feet drop out.

Consideration can also be given to:

- Waist to hip ratio.
- Body mass index.
- Skinfold-caliper test (*see Chapter 4, Part 6*).

Shoulder

- Abduction of the arm to test:
  - Glenohumeral/humeroscapula rhythm.
  - Trick movements to avoid pain.
  - Painful arc/impingement.
- Combing hair.
- Fastening bra strap.
- Putting on coat tests.
- Rotator cuff integrity.
- Yergasson's test (biceps).
- Drop arm test.
- Shoulder apprehension test.
- Anterior scalene syndrome test.
- Pectoralis minor hyperabduction test.
- Shoulder girdle movements.
- Neck movements.

Elbow

- Resisted wrist extension.
- Darol test: active, resistive, digital test.
- Power grip + resisted elbow flexion (lift a chair).

Wrist/Hand

- Active passive/passive spring.
- Prayer test.
- Scaphoid/anatomical snuffbox – 'Chen', 'Clamp' signs.
- Grips – power/hook/key/pen.
- Thumb movements.
- Darol test: active, resistive, digital test.

Spine/Trunk

- Leg length discrepancy – is it real/structural or is it apparent/functional? (*see Joints Above and Below*).
- Keynote position for scoliosis – is it structural or functional?
- **Vertebral artery test prior to cervical manipulation/mobilisation – vital.**

REFLEXES test the anterior spinal horn and the integrity of the motor pathway and these need to be repeated six times to check the cumulative effect:

1. **VITAL REFLEXES CENTRES** are found in the brainstem in the nuclei of the medulla oblongata, i.e. cardiac, vasomotor and respiratory. They work on a mechanism of 'positive and negative feedback', responding to increases/decreases in blood constituents.
2. **SPINAL REFLEXES** refer to the spinal cord and spinal reflexes.
3. **CLONUS**. If the reflex decreases, a lower motor neuron (LMN) problem can be suspected. If the reflex increases, an upper motor neuron (UMN) problem can be suspected, as there is reduced or no inhibition.

Knee jerk	L4		Bicep	C6	
Achilles	S2		Brachioradialis	C7	*Babinski*

However, Dr. Lederman, 1997, tells us that the stretch reflex is a physiological artifact that doesn't happen in real life, and tells us very little about the central nervous system.

Functional

Coming at the end of the examination and assessment this is only done if the therapist has failed to find anything and feels the patient can do it, without causing further injury. This is extremely important with regards to litigation. Here the examination consists of replicating the problem if other testing has failed to elicit the problem, i.e. if running upstairs hurts then the patient is asked to run upstairs.

The athlete is only asked to do what they and the therapist feel they can. Things to consider are **GAIT** analysis and anything related to the patient's lifestyle (*see Chapter 4, Part 4*).

Differential Diagnosis

As previously mentioned the purpose of an examination and assessment is to arrive at a valued judgement, informed opinion, working diagnosis, hypothesis. When presented with an athlete with a problem many questions can arise:

- Is it lumbar or sacroiliac?
- Is it neck or shoulder?
- Is it disc?
- Is it true sciatica or is it piriformis etc?

By trying to objectively decide what the problem can and cannot be is known as differential diagnosis and allows the examiner to:

Repeat, Confirm and Define

This is the conclusion to the examination when the sports therapist re-iterates what they have found and the athlete confirms. This ensures that both the athlete and therapist are aware of the same problems. It is at this stage that the therapist has to make decisions:

- Has a 'working diagnosis'/hypothesis been reached?
- Is a second opinion required?
- Is there a need to refer for further investigation?
- Is this person going to be accepted for treatment and if so what treatment is going to help them?

NOTE: An expert is NOT the one who thinks they know everything and can treat everyone but the one who knows when to refer.

Record Keeping

Having personal data records that the therapist and the patient fill in helps to follow a logical pattern of enquiry (*see Chapter 7, Part 3 and Appendix 4*). To re-cap on some of the important issues concerned with examination and assessment:

1. **ALWAYS** remember you are treating people not labels. Don't examine symptomatically!
2. **USE YOUR COMMONSENSE!**
3. **ESTABLISH** a rapport with your patient – you won't get a second chance to make a first impression!
4. **COMMUNICATE** effectively with the patient, i.e. ask relevant questions, actively listen, be positive.
5. **LOOK** at the identified site of injury.
6. **MAKE COMPARISONS** with other parts/limbs especially above and below.
7. **HANDLE** the tissues/limbs in a safe, effective manner.
8. **TOUCH/PALPATE** the appropriate tissues.
9. **MOVE** the relevant joints, **ACTIVELY, PASSIVELY, RESISTIVELY**.
10. **PERFORM** the appropriate **OBJECTIVE TESTS** for the joint/tissue involved, muscles and ligaments.
11. **GET THE PATIENT** to perform any relevant functional movements if they feel they can.
12. **REPEAT, CONFIRM AND DEFINE** what you have found and intend to do.

At this point:

- List and prioritise your problems.
- State the aims and objectives of treatment. In other words:

> **"Plan your work, then work your plan."**
> *Pook, M., 1995.*

Part 3

Hypermobility

> **HYPER** – means more than the norm.
> **HYPO** – means less than the norm.

HYPERMOBILITY (*'loose limbed'* – *'double jointed'* – *'joint laxity'*) is where there is mobility at a 'joint' beyond the normally acceptable range of movement. Just as restriction to a joint's full range of movement (hypomobility) can cause problems, too much mobility (hypermobility) can be equally problematic. It must be borne in mind that mobility decreases with age and is greater in females (except for the back).

Whilst hypermobility could be considered an advantage in certain pastimes, sports professions, e.g. dancing, gymnastics, it is also potentially hazardous causing orthopaedic and numerous rheumatological problems. In certain cases it can be considered as a pre-cursor to premature arthritis. In the USSR hypermobility used to be an exclusion factor in the selection of ballet dancers because the subsequent risk factor for potential injury and problems outweighed the advantages.

Neurological disease (polio), anatomical abnormalities (defects of the acetabula cup) and connective tissue defects (ligament laxity) may give rise to hypermobility. Awareness of hypermobility and its significance can help the sports therapist not only in their examination, assessment and evaluations, but also in their choice of treatment modality, i.e. hypomobile joints require stretch and deep, soft tissue massage; hypermobile require strength and superficial, soft tissue massage.

As outlined, body mobility can be affected by many factors but in essence it is the interrelationship of the joints (serving as pivots/fulcrums), the bones (providing the leverage) and muscles (providing the effort/pull) working as an integrated, functional unit that has the greatest effect.

Measurement of Hypermobility

Hypermobility may be measured by a nine-point scale, a global index or by a hyperextension meter. The scale most often used to quantify hypermobility is Beighton and Horan's (1970) modification of the Carter and Wilkinson index (1954). It gives a maximum score of 9. Scores of two or less could be regarded as normal.

1. Passive dorsiflexion of the fingers, especially the little finger beyond 90° (one point for each hand) – two points.
2. Passive apposition of the thumbs to the flexor aspects of the forearm (one point for each thumb) – two points.
3. Hyperextension of the elbows beyond 10° (one point for each elbow) – two points. The 'carrying-angle' at the elbow is caused by the obliquity of the ulnar and humeral joint. In men the norm is 5°–10° and in women 10°–15°.
4. Hyperextension of the knees beyond 10° (one point for each knee) – two points.
5. Anterior flexion of the trunk with knees fully extended so that the palms of the hands rest flat on the floor – one point.

Part 4

Gait Analysis in Walking and Running

An area of study that requires specialist training and is of interest not only to sports therapists but also to manual therapists, physiotherapists, chiropodists and podiatrists. Analysing how sports people balance, walk, run and move can give indications to not only why they have faulty posture but also the cause of many of their injuries. It requires a sound anatomical, biomechanical knowledge of the lower limb and unless qualified, the sports therapist should refer suspected biomechanical problems to a sports podiatrist for further investigation. The following is included to provide a little insight into the subject.

The foot is a masterpiece of biomechanical engineering, integrating one structure into two opposing functions; propulsion and weight transfer. It is multi-segmented with the most important segments biomechanically being the ankle (tibia/fibula/talus), subtalar (talus/calcaneum) and midtarsal joints (calcaneum/cuboid/navicular). Collectively these allow a triplane motion involving plantar flexion/dorsiflexion; eversion/inversion; and adduction/abduction to allow the foot to adjust and adapt to the varying terrains as well as compensate for any postural changes made by the body. Gait is influenced by the rate, rhythm and character of the movements employed in walking. Any deviations from 'the norm' will cause abnormal, as opposed to normal, compensations. In the foot this usually means over pronation (abduction, dorsiflexion and eversion) or supination (adduction, plantar flexion and inversion).

> **"The subtalar joint plays a crucial role in human locomotion. Subtalar joint pronation unlocks the midtarsal joint, allowing the foot to become a mobile adaptor while subtalar joint supination locks the midtarsal joint allowing the foot to become a rigid lever."**

> **"Without intervention abnormal compensation is likely to be permanent, repetitive and destructive."**
> *Padhiar, N., 2000*

Such is the complexity of the body that problems at its base, the foot, can lead to problems anywhere above. As for the soft tissue component, from the tip of the toes to the pelvic girdle and above, there is a kinetic chain of reciprocal parts where a fault at one end of the chain can affect the whole chain. For example, weak gluteals and hamstrings can cause too much hip flexion during the stance phase. This induces excessive knee flexion.

These problems can range from plantar fasciitis, Achilles problems, 'shin splints', sprains, strains, iliotibial band syndrome, to stress fractures, knee pain, osteoarthritis and stiff necks. During walking, one full gait cycle is considered as the interval of time from heel strike of one foot with the ground to heel strike of the same foot at the next step and spans 0.2 seconds. This consists of two phases:

1. **STANCE**. The foot is on the ground and represents 60–62% of the cycle, and is the phase between heel strike and 'toe off' for each foot.
2. **SWING**. The body is moving forwards, which represents the other 38–40%, and is the phase when the foot swings from one step to the next.

During running between the stance and swing phase and before the heel strike there is a **FLOAT PHASE**, when both feet are off the ground – this represents 30% of the whole cycle. Stride length and rate are affected by not only speed but by running up and downhill. Running uphill tends to shorten the former and increase the latter, whilst going downhill reverses the effect. The **STANCE PHASE** can be greatly affected by inadequate footwear and can be divided into:

1. **HEEL STRIKE**, which is equivalent to hitting a brick wall at 30 mph, with this ground reaction force being increased with speed. Athletes may strike the ground with either their fore foot or mid foot. During this phase the pelvis rotates, there is a lateral pelvic shift, the tensor fasciae latae muscle works antagonistically with the quadratus lumborum and the gluteus medius becomes involved. This stresses the anterior cruciate ligament in the knee because with the leg straight, the femur is posterior to the tibia. With the knee bent the tibia is posterior to the femur and therefore the posterior cruciate ligament can be affected. The hamstrings help to decelerate forward forces just before heel strike.

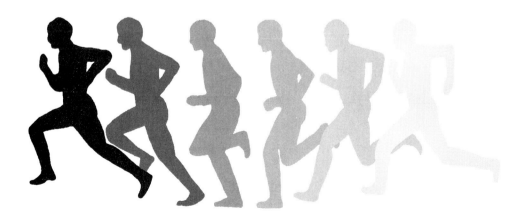

▲ *Figure 44. Running Gait Analysis.*

The calf muscles are most active just before heel strike, to eccentrically control/position the foot for heel strike; at initial foot strike and during initial foot strike. Any weakness in this eccentric control can lead to Achilles problems.

2. **MID-STANCE**, which constitutes 40% of the stance phase, begins with toe off of the opposite foot and ends with heel lift of the same foot. There is weight-bearing and transference from the heel to the little toe and then to the big toe as the foot changes from a 'closed packed position' (calcaneum everted, talus inferior with the navicular being rotated on the cuboid to the same level) to an 'open packed position' (the calcaneum being inverted, the talus moving upwards and outward and the cuboid rotating on the navicular down and in). The muscle involvement here concerns gluteus medius, minimus and quadratus lumborum.

3. **FOOT FLAT**. The muscle involvement here concerns gluteus medius, minimus and quadratus lumborum. Weak dorsiflexors cause foot drop (L4) after heel strike. The function of the calves during the stance phase being to control dorsiflexion, pronation and stop the foot collapsing with a reduction of the longitudinal medial arch.

4. **TOE/PUSH OFF**, is the propulsion phase and starts with heel lift and ends with toe off and constitutes 30% of the stance phase. The heel lift is the point at which the foot must be most stable (*Lindy, M., 1999*). It finds the femur anterior on the tibia. Gluteus maximus, minimus and hamstrings are involved with push-off initiated by flexor hallucis longus and assisted by the elastic recoil of gastrocnemius and soleus which have been stretched to eccentrically control the foot (S1, S2 nerves supply).

During the **SWING PHASE**, the innominate medially rotates backward as the lead leg goes forward. The other innominate does the opposite. The dorsiflexors, tibialis anterior, extensor hallucis longus and extensor digitorum longus are active throughout the whole phase.

1. **ACCELERATION** (concentric action). If there is a weakness to the quadriceps (L2, L3, L4) acceleration is affected.
2. **MID-SWING**. A steppage gait can occur if the dorsiflexors are weak and the shoe scrapes the ground.
3. **DECELERATION** (eccentric action). If there is hamstring L5, L2 weakness deceleration is affected just before heel strike. Any abnormality related to these phases especially the stance phase leads to an **ANTALGIC GAIT** whereby the body compensates by trying to avoid the painful component.

This overview should emphasise the significance of gait analysis and its importance to injury. Treatment of such problems can include injections, physiotherapy, manipulation, mobilisations and foot orthotics, which are meant to re-align the foot, which in turn will have a compensatory effect on the joints above. The key to orthotic treatment is the position of the midtarsal joint as it provides a lever (*Lindy, M., 1999*). It would appear that a combination of all modalities is the best course of treatment.

Certain sports people can be seen to adopt their own personalised, exaggerated gait, which may or may not be the result of poor posture, co-ordination, control and/or proprioception. On the other hand it may be a psychological ploy to convey certain messages about their sporting image/prowess. Historians may use such behaviour to highlight the fact that in spite of much development some elements of society can't shake off its primitive roots.

Part 5

Postural Analysis

Posture is far more complex than just standing or sitting up straight. It is not a static quality and is constantly changing as a result of responses by the body to sensory inflow and resultant adjustments in position of various segments relative to each other. Newton's Third Law of Spinal Motion implies that for every action there is an opposite and equal reaction. Because of this constantly changing quality we find the term posture can project different images ranging from lifeless to obese and strained to healthy. It is affected by factors such as heredity, disease and habit. Habit is the easiest to adjust. Posture can be considered as:

> "The relative disposition of the body at any one moment and a composite of the position of the different joints of the body at that time."

> "It is an expression of one's personality, sense of well being and self-esteem."
> *Magee, D., 1987*

> "Posture equals the sum of the mechanical efficiency of the body. Good body mechanics being essential for efficient movement and defence against injury."
> *Chaitow, L., 1988*

> "Posture refers to the alignment of the body segments anterior, posterior and laterally."
> *NCF, 1986*

> "Good posture is when the head is centred over the pelvis, the face is directed forward and the shoulder girdle is on the same plane as the pelvis. Poor posture is when the head is carried forward, the scapula is

held in abduction and the shoulders are rounded. The thoracic curve is increased and the chest is flattened (the round back). There is a prominence of the anterior abdominal wall below the level of the umbilicus accompanied by an anterior tilt of the pelvis with the knees slightly extended (corporation)."
Chaitow, L., 1988

The Sports Council, 1986, described efficient posture as one where maximum efficiency is achieved with minimum effort, i.e. the position of the body at any one instant is perfect for the next movement to take place and the transition can take place without any extraneous movement. The relative position of the joints is due, in part, to muscle strength or lack of it. David Magee, 1987, adds more to the imagery by stating that:

"Correct posture is the position of which minimum stress will be applied to each joint. Faulty posture being any position that increases the stress to the joints."

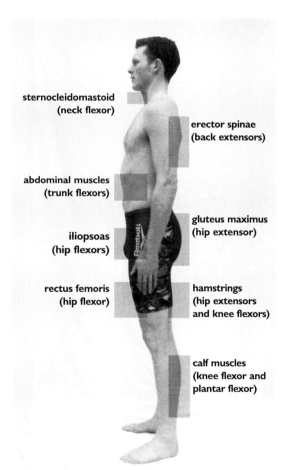

► *Figure 45. Muscles governing postural balance.*

sternocleidomastoid (neck flexor)

erector spinae (back extensors)

abdominal muscles (trunk flexors)

gluteus maximus (hip extensor)

iliopsoas (hip flexors)

rectus femoris (hip flexor)

hamstrings (hip extensors and knee flexors)

calf muscles (knee flexor and plantar flexor)

By accepting these definitions it can be seen that posture has got something to do with body:

- Positions.
- Composition/parts.
- Mechanics.
- Relationships.
- Homeostasis.

In simplicity, the **BALANCE** of all the internal and external factors affecting the body structure and functioning. **STRESS** can be seen as the failure of the body to normalise tissues or function after a response effort that is almost constant. As a result of poor posture, dysfunction occurs with shortening, thickening, calcification and tension in the soft tissues. Fascia is one of the first tissues to show signs along lines of stress. These changes in turn can affect the circulatory, nervous and endocrinal systems. *Homosapiens* have often been described as two legged creatures with backache and the problems associated with postural evolution are there for all observant therapists to see.

> **"The spine of a man is a perfect example of a cantilever bridge, when in the all fours position, which has been turned through a ninety degree angle and is now an unstable skyscraper."**
> *Professor I. Korr, 1995*

The Development of the Postural/Spinal Curves

The body starts life in the foetal position, concave-forward flexed. Once born the child starts to lift its head, thus creating the start of the cervical lordosis, with a neck curve developing after about three months. As it starts to sit, stand on two legs and walk, the lumbar lordosis appears between six to eight months.

Thus we have the 's' shaped vertebral column, as viewed from the side, with the four spinal areas of cervical, thoracic, lumbar and sacrococcygeal. The thoracic and sacral being known as the primary curves, as they were present at birth and the cervical lumbar known as the secondary curves, as they developed as a result of adopting an upright posture.

Military posture (*Calliet, R., 1984*) or image posture (*Latey, P.*) is the one that is adopted when being observed and can be compared to anatomical posture. **Slump posture**, which can be compared to slack standing, is the posture adopted when not on show or being observed. Calliet refers to this as depressed posture, which can be related to emotional strain, dissatisfaction, apprehension, anxiety and depression.

On a practical level, posture can be observed from the point of view that our individual posture, which can be known as **residual posture**, is the result of the difference between military and slump posture.

Lines of Gravity

With the knees fully extended **the anatomical line of gravity** falls through the head of the femur, slightly in front of the knee joint and through the middle of the tarsus. In strict anatomical terminology it passes through the tip of the odontoid process (C2), emerges from the promontory of the pelvis and bisects the transverse axis of the hip, knee and ankle.

With the knees slightly flexed, **the slack standing line of gravity** is behind the ears, behind the centre of the hip and knee joint and through the middle of the tarsus. The tilt of the pelvis will be slightly diminished in this position. In other words, slightly posterior to the anatomical line.

The fundamental line of gravity is in front of the ears, cervical and thoracic vertebrae, through the lumbar vertebrae, through the hip and ankle joint. However, this varies due to individual somatotype, lifestyle, occupation, asymmetrical development, specificity of training, habit and genetic disposition.

An efficient posture is one where the line of gravity would pass just behind the ear, behind the cervical lordosis, in front of the thorax, behind the lumbar lordosis, continuing through the hip just behind the knee and just in front of the ankle. For correct posture the anterior superior iliac spines should be in the same vertical plane as the symphysis pubis.

Part 6

Body Weight and Fat Assessment

Various tissues can affect our body weight. Blood weight can increase by approximately 0.9 kg as we get more aerobically fit and bone may increase on exercise too. However, the most significant tissues to affect weight are muscle and fat (*Sharp, C., 1994*).

Muscle which contains glycogen (stored glucose) can sustain about three hours of jogging before these supplies are depleted. Muscle weighs approximately 1.3 times more than fat and so if people exercise and change their fat/muscle, body composition ratio they may not lose weight and may actually put on weight. During the first few weeks of aerobic exercise muscle weight increases, bone weight increases, blood weight increases but fat weight decreases. An acceptable fat content is essential for the body to carry out its vital functions. Fat protects, stores vitamins, helps the body to regulate temperature and regulate itself when food is in short supply.

The body relies on two types of fat: **STORED (ADIPOSE TISSUE) AND ESSENTIAL**. The former being primarily a fuel store and energy producer, providing enough energy to stay alive for a week or 5–10 days of exercise. The latter is that which can be found in the myelin sheath and protecting/insulating organs. The percentage of each on average is:

	STORED	**ESSENTIAL**
MALE	12%	3%
FEMALE	15%	13%

The average 18+ male: 15–18% in total.
The average 18+ female: 25–28% in total.
Male athlete: 10–15%.
Female athlete: 16–20%.
Elite athlete: 5–8%.

Obviously these figures are dependant on many variables but because of genetics, hormones, child bearing potential etc. women have approximately 10% more essential fat than men. This is one of the main reasons for women generally being slower than men by about 8–10 % (*Sharp, C., 1994*).

Excess fat can lead to obesity that can have serious health risks of diabetes, high blood pressure and high cholesterol. Fitness, fatness and appearance can sometimes be confused. A person can be fat and fit, e.g. a sumo wrestler. Appearances are also deceptive in that a slim person can possess a high percentage of body fats whilst quite plump looking people can be quite muscular. Low body fat can lead to loss of vital nutrients, essential for body functions, amenorrhea and dysmenorrhea. In sport, female marathon runners may not have periods for years, which, I have been informed, can be a blessing on the morning of a major championship (*see Chapter 2, Part 2; Chapter 1, Part 5*).

In assessing body fat, several tests can be carried out to give a general guide:

1. The waist to hip ratio.
2. The body mass index.
3. The skinfold-caliper.

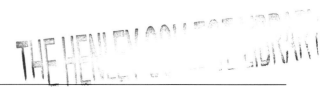

These could be added to any examination and assessment sheets that the sports therapist devises for patients and sports-type personnel just love having measurements to relate to, especially if it relates to fitness.

1. THE WAIST TO HIP RATIO TEST

The hips are measured at the widest point around the buttocks. The waist is measured around the umbilicus. The waist measurement is then divided by the hip measurement.

e.g. 85cm/95cm = 0.89cm.

If the ratio is above 1 for men and 0.8 for women then these types are at risk of disease. In men the risk factor appears if the waist exceeds the hip size and in women, if the waist exceeds 80% of the hip size.

2. THE BODY MASS INDEX (BMI)

The metric height of the person is measured in bare feet and the weight is taken in kilograms. The weight is then divided by the square of the height (H^2).

e.g. A person weighing 66kg and measuring 1.672m in height. The weight squared equals 2.79m, therefore 66 divided by 2.79 = 23.66. Therefore, the person has a BMI of 23.66 and would be considered as having an ideal weight–height ratio.

- 30+   – obesity.
- 25–30   – overweight.
- 20–25   – ideal weight–height ratio.
- < 20   – underweight and possibly anorexic/bulimic.

Obviously these are general guidelines but do provide factual evidence that a person may be at risk.

3. SKINFOLD-CALIPER TEST

This test requires that skinfold measurements, pinched between thumb and index finger are taken at various sites throughout the body. Millimetres are used. The site should always be relaxed:

- **BICEPS**. The lower arm is supinated, halfway between the elbow and shoulder.
- **TRICEPS**. Midway between the shoulder and elbow.

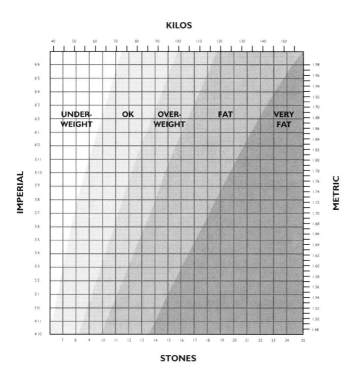

◀ *Figure 46. Body mass index chart – applies to both men and women. Reproduced with permission of Health Education Authority.*

- **THIGH**. Middle, front, lateral aspect of the thigh between the knee and hip.
- **ABDOMEN**. A vertical skinfold at a point adjacent to the umbilicus.
- **SUBSCAPULARIS**. At the inferior angle of scapula.
- **SUPRA ILIAC**. Above the iliac crest on the lateral side of the body.
- **CHEST**. Over the pectoralis major near to the axilla use a diagonal skinfold, i.e. shoulder to the opposite hip.

This is done with the left hand but their appears to be some disagreement between English and German methodology, with the English taking measurements on the right, the Germans the left. The former suggests taking three measurements and averaging. Nomograms are then used for boys and girls and males and females (*see Appendix 5*). The sites for boys and girls are triceps/subscapularis, whilst for men thigh/abdomen/chest are used and for women triceps/thigh/supra iliac.

Tancred, 1987, says that although the skinfold-caliper test is not perfect it does provide an estimate of body fat although in these days of technological advancement, body fat monitor/scales can be used. These determine the composition of body fat by transmitting a low electrical current through the tissues to measure the bioelectrical impedance. The current passes freely through fluids and muscle but finds more resistance passing through fat. Bioelectrical impedance analysis (BIA) is reported to be 95% accurate, with some variations due to body water content, which may fluctuate with exercise, diet, sweating, and use of alcohol or drugs (*Mosby's Medical Dictionary, 1990*).

References

1. Beighton and Horan: 1970. Hypermobility index.
2. Calliet, R.: 1984. Understanding your backache.
3. Chaitow, L.: 1988. Soft tissue manipulation. Chapter 4.
4. Fritz, S.: 1995. Assessment with palpation, fundamentals of therapeutic Massage. Chapter 11: 302–309.
5. Korr, Professor, I.: 1995. Osteopathy 2000 conference, London.
6. Latey, P.: Muscular manifesto. Osteopathic Publications.
7. Lederman, Dr. E.: 1998. Active Techniques Workshop. Huddersfield.
8. Lindy, Dr. M.: 1999. Entering the foot zone. 1 day workshop, Haydock, 6.11.99.
9. Magee, D.: 1987. Orthopaedic physical assessment. Chapter 14.
10. Montague-Cook, B.: 2000. Osteopaths: unconscious manipulators of the unconscious? *Osteopath*, April, 2000.
11. Mosby's Medical, Nursing and Allied Health Dictionary, 3rd ed.: 1990.
12. National Coaching Foundation: 1986. Physiology and performance. Handbook 3.
13. Padhiar, N.: 2000. The biomechanics of gait and running. *SportEX*, 4, March, 2000.
14. Pook, M.: 1995. Competencies required for osteopathic practice – CROP weekend. Haydock, June, 1995.
15. Sharp, Professor, C.: 1994. Exercise, weight loss, health and fitness. *SportsCare Journal*, 1, November, 1994.
16. Tancred, W.: 1987. Health-related fitness. Hodder & Stoughton.

Bibliography

1. Artfile Sport, Phaidon Press Ltd. Oxford, ISBN 0–7148–2667–7.
2. De Gowin, and De Gowin: 1994. Diagnostic examination, 6th ed. McGraw Hill.
3. Goodman, and Snyder: 1995. Differential diagnosis in physical therapy, 2nd ed. Saunders
4. Hoppenfield, S.: 1976. Gait analysis, physical examination. Chapter 5.
5. Fuller, G.: 1993. Neurological examination made easy. Churchill Livingstone.

Chapter 5
Treatment

Give me the facts, but above all,
Give me the understanding.
Solomon

Part I

Aims, Objectives, Priorities, Principles, Procedures, Protocols and Practicalities

"The person who discovers a way to increase the normal speed of healing of the body will win a Nobel Prize."
Quigley, T. B., 1981

Chapter 2, Part 4, considered exercise and its use in treatment, training and rehabilitation and Chapter 3, Part 3, considered treatment implications regarding the physiology of injury, inflammation, healing and repair. The following looks at the overall principles that need to be adopted in treatment generally.

General Considerations – Priorities

- Symptomatic treatment is not good enough. The cause **must** be addressed.
- The approach needs to be individualised. If predictable, the therapist is not doing their job.
- Think body/person not injury. Each athlete possesses individual knowledge, needs, demands, beliefs, faith, expectations, anticipations and perceptions that must be addressed.

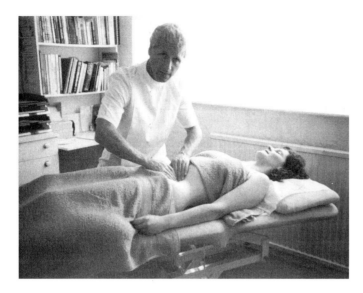

◄ *Figure 47. Appropriate methods and modalities must be selected. (model: Karen Probert).*

- What level is their participation; recreational, amateur or professional?
- Do they have another job if they are only semi-professional? What is it?
- What sport/position do they play?
- What training methods, techniques and tactics do they use?
- What is their perception of the injury?
- How do they view the time they are not involved?
- How do they believe the injury will respond?
- Are their expectations the same as yours, etc.?
- You need to work with athletes not in spite of them and vice versa.

If these issues are not addressed then problems can arise and full recovery can be delayed (*see Chapter 5, Part 2*).

BEFORE INITIATING TREATMENT there is a need to **EXAMINE** and **ASSESS**. Examination and assessment are vital prior to instigating any treatment, exercise, training or rehabilitation regime. Because of the legal implications all decisions must have an objective input.

CLASSIFY the injury – at what stage has the injury presented?

- **ACUTE**.
- **SUB-ACUTE**.
- **CHRONIC**.

Consider these classifications physiologically rather than on a timescale and remember injuries don't always follow nice easy patterns – they are all shades of grey. The acute treatment is the same for all injuries. Further down the line treatment/rehabilitation is much more specific:

Prioritise the Aims and Objectives

Aims (long-term) and objectives (short-term) must be clearly thought out and prioritised at each stage of the process. Don't forget that if we aim at nothing we hit it every time giving a false sense of success. Are the body's natural healing processes being assisted or interfered with? It must be known what is happening inside the body, i.e. injury – inflammation/haemostasis – repair – remodelling.

Short-term Aims

Clinical/injury specific, i.e.:

- Pain.
- Swelling.
- Heat, etc. (*see Chapter 3, Part 3*).

Long-term Aims

Fitness and function, i.e.:

- Range of movement/ease of movement.
- Strength/power/speed.
- Stretch, proprioception, balance, co-ordination.
- Function, etc.

ADAPTABILITY/FLEXIBILITY is the key to successful restoration of full functional fitness. These need to relate to **FUNCTIONAL CAPACITY v PHYSIOLOGICAL PROCESSES**. By understanding the physiological processes involved we can optimise such processes by changing the environment in which repair takes place so that the tissues are capable of meeting the functional demands placed upon them. This should ensure that treatment and rehabilitation protocols are safe and effective. Safety is a key issue and there will be considerable pressures to take 'short cuts' both from the athlete and or other personnel involved in their sport. Be guided by **'P' PRINCIPLES** (*see Chapter 1, Part 7*). Appropriate modalities/methods for which the therapist is trained and qualified to administer must be selected and used.

Treatment and rehabilitation must be **INJURY PHASE CLASSIFIED** and **SPORTS SPECIFIC**, e.g. acute, sub-acute, chronic; tennis, rugby etc. Recovery is dependent on many factors not only those outlined regarding Factors Affecting Repair (*Chapter 3, Part 4 and Chapter 5, Part 2*) but also:

- **Early bonding, trust and co-operation are essential** – a positive relationship is a must.
- **Communication, explanations and reasons are an important** part of the role of a sports therapist during treatment/rehabilitation (*see Chapter 1, Part 1 and Appendix 1*).
- **Discipline is vital** so that the athlete knows what to do? when to do?; how to do?; and what not to do, etc.

Intensity and Degree/Duration Needs Controlled Overload

There are **CRITICAL PERIODS**, i.e. the lag phase, 36–42 hours and the middle to end of rehabilitation are when problems can be encountered. There are also **STAGES** that must be gone through **NON-WEIGHT BEARING** to **PARTIAL WEIGHT BEARING** to **FULL WEIGHT BEARING** etc.

- **Enthusiasm/stimulation** is necessary especially the longer the athlete is 'out of action'.
- **Team-work is essential** which will involve a great deal of positive interaction between all concerned so that each knows what the other is trying to achieve.

This is one of the most demanding roles of the sports therapist, as they have to cope with not only sporting mentality but also exaggerated egos. Sometimes people in sport find it difficult to 'let go' and share (*see Chapter 1, Part 7*).

Surgical Intervention/Operative Procedures

As a sports therapist there may be times when you are asked or may need to consider an operation. Obviously it goes without saying that one has to be very careful about how to handle such situations. **Engage the brain before opening the mouth!** The implications of any decisions made in this respect are enormous and must be made in consultation with all the parties concerned; athlete, coach, trainer, doctor, orthopaedic specialist/consultant, physiotherapist, masseur/masseuse, sports therapist etc., based on sound, objective, medical decisions. As a general guideline, certain questions and issues need to be addressed:

1. Does the injury affect the person's quality of life and would surgery ensure and improve this?

2. What are the pro's and con's of such intervention?

3. Does the patient **need** to have surgery or would they just **like** to have it or just **want** it believing it to be the answer to all their problems?

Where there is a genuine **need**, for example, if the situation is career threatening, this can be considered a higher priority than just **wanting** or **liking** to have the surgery.

Part 2

Improving Effectiveness

1. Why do some people get better going to one practitioner/therapist but not another, when they both **appear** to be offering the same?

2. Why are some people healthy and others not?

3. Why do some people seek to improve their level of health, whilst others don't?

The answers to these questions lie in looking at multi-factorial models of illness, disease and an individual's health beliefs. Whilst this is part of a much wider consideration of health in general and not specific to sport, awareness of such, will in many ways help sports therapists improve their effectiveness. To reiterate what has already been mentioned in Chapter 1 because it is again relevant; **how to be safe, effective, efficient, caring, compassionate, communicating, problem solving sports therapists is about questioning, reviewing, and analysing HOW, WHAT AND WHY they do what they do. Continuing professional development should be about quality of experience, including reviewing, questioning, analysing and reflecting upon practice, not necessarily quantity, by attending another course/workshop. Reflection should be an essential part of personal and professional development and all therapists, allopathic and complementary, must engage in it from time to time. This should increase their awareness of why they do what they do without causing, 'paralysis from analysis'.** (*Dr Simon Jenkins, 2000*). However:

> **"If people go on believing that they 'know' it makes it impossible to teach them."**
> *Alexander*

Is this arrogance or ignorance? (*see Convention, page 62*).

Not that change should be introduced just for the sake of it but innovation does take time. As with all therapies, sports therapy is no different in that practitioners can be exposed to a wide range of sometimes bewildering philosophies, terminology, approaches and techniques to deal with what basically is the same thing; an injury/abuse as a result of involvement in sport. So when it comes to treatment do we go for manual therapy, exercise therapy, lotions, potions, creams, supplementation, electrotherapy, operative procedure, psychology, etc.? Obviously the answer is that **the therapist gives the best possible treatment for which they are trained, qualified and capable of giving, irrespective of race, creed, colour or social status. For the patient it is what is best for that particular person at that moment in time.**

But how do we know what is best for any one individual when each will have his/her own perception, expectation and need related to his/her own health belief model? By looking at the way practitioners/therapists work may help to clarify the issue.

Different Approaches

On the topic of different approaches to treatment:

> **"It's not only what you do, it's the way that you do it."**
> *Roberts, J., 1996*

> **"Most of these differing treatment approaches can be crudely divided into major groups according to the degree of physical contact involved."**
> *Roberts, J., 1996*

These, although referring to osteopathy, provide an excellent, 'tongue-in-cheek', some might even argue doubting, perhaps cynical, consideration of the possible methods adopted in sports medicine. The author has 'doctored' the original text to make the content less specific to osteopathy.

The 'Hands-off' or Cerebral Approach

Here the treatment consists almost entirely of advice, electrotherapy, medication or sometimes a lecture on diet, exercise and posture. 'Run it off lad you'll be alright,' could be one piece of advice. 'Stop playing sport', is another. Such an approach is recommended for those who are not keen on touching the naked skin of near strangers, or who prefer a less physical approach.

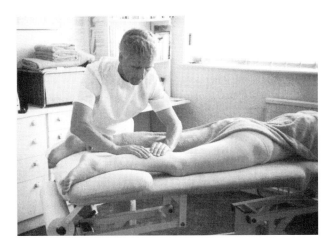

◀ *Figure 48. Light massage – laying-on of hands. (model: Karen Probert).*

The Very Light Touch or 'Laying-on-of-Hands' Approach

This would include such techniques as light massage, cranial and just the laying-on of hands. It is perhaps best suited for those who know themselves to be endowed with healing gifts, or for those who are in touch with higher forms of intelligence and life. Did not a certain English football manager, in the late 1990's, get into trouble for believing in this even to the extent of employing such a person as part of his backroom staff?

The Deep Touch or 'Get-stuck-in' Methods

These could include deep soft tissue, neuromuscular techniques, and let's send the team to a remote Scottish island, with limited rations, in the middle of winter, with an ex-SAS officer, to help bonding and team morale. This approach, which is quite prevalent in sport, works on the long held belief of no pain, no gain. Such methods are likely to appeal to would-be sadomasochists, master bakers or those who, as children, were deprived of plasticine by house proud-parents!

The Heroic, Kung Fu/Martial Arts, or 'I've Got a Good Lawyer' Group of Methods

These could include high velocity thrust and long lever thrust techniques, impact therapy etc. 'Let's give it a go and see,' may be the aim here. This approach possibly is sometimes guilty of making too many assumptions.

Anyone for a Spot of Bodily DIY Methods

The final recourse in most people's eyes is that of operative intervention. Sometimes after abusing the body during a lifetime of sport the thought processes here would appear to be, "surgeon wave your magic wand and put it right, so that I can carry on as before." However, the questions of, I'd like it and I want it, must be considered and addressed in terms of priority with, I need it. Is such a course of action necessary or are there alternative, less invasive methods? (*see page 218, Surgical Intervention/Operative Procedures*).

Most practitioners/therapists of course use a mixture of techniques/approaches that they have been trained and qualified to use but I'm sure many have tried and tested favourites that fall into one of the above categories. To take these thought processes further we could say that the approach should also be: **'It's not what you say but the way that you say it'**. With informed consent and intent (*see Chapter 7*) very much to the fore here and very much: **'It's not what you think you're doing but why you do it and what you're actually doing.'** Has the receiver/responder got what the sender has sent?

> "Some evidence points to the concept that it is not only the physical treatment advocated but also the psychological qualities of the patient/therapist/practitioner relationship which can be a major mediator for improvement. The practitioner/therapist has considerable power to influence and define outcomes of treatment."
> *Robin Kirk, 2000*

The Psychophysiological Connection

Dr. Lederman, 1997, refers to two types of manipulation:

1. **EXPRESSIVE.** Involves considering the whole body and is to do with intent, empathy and awareness of a person's needs.
2. **INSTRUMENTAL.** Highly specific and physical and is used to correct mechanical failure.

Studies such as these have shown that not only is the choice of technique important for treatments to be safe and effective but also how the technique is administered.

> "Treatment that is highly mechanistic and detached may fail to meet the patient psychologically. Efficacy of treatment is related to the ability of the therapist to communicate through touch, messages of support, comfort and compassion, and to the ability of the patient to comprehend these messages. Techniques at this level have no true form but, like other forms of interpersonal communication, reflect interactions between two individuals, the effects of manipulation being

related to the whole treatment event rather than a specific technique. At this level, one can only speak of 'manual events' rather than specific manual techniques."
Lederman, Dr. E., 1997

How often are we reminded that we are treating a person with a problem not an isolated problem? **The cognitive therapist may also add that it's not the problems themselves that distress us but the views we take of them**.

"The way one considers the elements of diagnosis, prognosis and treatment is altered according to the gaze."
Foucault, M., 1973

There is a large body of research into the interaction between patient and practitioner looking at patient response, other than what is obvious and expected. Kane, 1995, researching back pain factors in successful treatment included **touch, the act of listening, explanation of condition, monitoring of progress and co-operation between patient and practitioner as all having some bearing on successful outcomes**. Hammond, 2000, looked more at the mind-body connection showing what a significant effect on the success of any treatment such interaction can have. This is based on **a person's knowledge, faith, perceptions, anticipations, expectations, needs and beliefs, and gives an explanation as to why a person can respond more positively to one therapist's intervention and not another. Confidence in ones beliefs**, for both therapist/practitioner and athlete/patient, **is also another strong factor**, if for no other reason than via **PLACEBO**. Reflective practice is about challenging these beliefs.

There is a considerable literature on patient's perceptions of health, illness and injury (*Rogers, W. S., 1991*), which in the main tend to be influenced by **AGE**. **The older the patient, especially the male, the less likely they are to connect their health/illness/injury to their lifestyle**. How true is this of the 35+ sporting person who thinks they still can perform and steadfastly refuse to acknowledge their persistent injuries are as a result of still training seven days a week at an intensity of a 21 year old? Of course there will always be the exception to the rule, for example, Steve Redgrave.

Health beliefs, health promotion, public health and preventative medicine are all important issues to consider but because of the subjective nature of the issues/ideas that need to be examined they are difficult to objectively measure (*Stapleton, 1997*). How can we measure relative concepts such as 'health' or 'illness'? The term injury has also been shown to have numerous definitions (*see Chapter 1, Part 5*).

"Health promotion as a concept first became prominent in the 80's when the focus of attention became the patient rather than the practitioner and endeavours were made to make the patient more responsible for his/her own level of health."
Kirk, R., 2000

It differs from public health and preventative medicine in that it seeks, according to Kirk, to empower the individual and the community to take a far greater or lesser degree of responsibility for his/her own health from the grass roots. **EMPOWERMENT AND AUTONOMY** are the determinant factors. Natural therapy looks at not only the patient as a whole but relates such an individual to the environment in which he/she lives. **Of recent times this has been seen as a multi-factorial, biophysical/psychosocial, economic model of health care** and whilst the author is unaware of any definitive research into its relevance to the sports person, as they are also individuals, it is still appropriate.

If a patient is aware of their health status/condition then it follows that they have an idea of what needs to be done about it. **It has been suggested that patients will choose and respond best to practitioners/therapists, whose models of lifestyles, illness, diagnosis and treatment fit the patients' own theories of lifestyles, health and illness** (*Hopwood, 1997*).

Adopting an attitude of: 'well it's your own fault, you shouldn't play sport,' will not endear a person to the populace who are being encouraged to exercise because it's supposedly good for you. Therefore it is important to address this issue of expectation in any verbal contract of agreement when dealing with sports people.

Holistic medicine involves considering not only the parts in isolation but also how those parts relate and interact and involves the potential influence of **COGNITIVE, SOCIAL AND CULTURAL FACTORS** in a patient's experience of illness which should be recognised (*Greenwood, H., 1999*).

Whilst some practitioners/therapists advocate an holistic approach to their work, which would address such issues, "Do as I say not do as I do", would appear to be the reality in some cases. Obviously we don't all live in an ideal, theoretical world where individuals fit neatly into nice little niches where the pressures of getting people fit and the numerous constraints that can be brought to bear cannot be overlooked. It must not, however, be overlooked that a practitioner must satisfy certain needs, via a code of conduct, as failure to do so can lead to a charge of neglect (*see Chapter 7*). This will involve accepting that sports people are individuals in more than just a physical sense.

Placebo/Responders – Nocebo/Non-responders

The Mind–Body Connection

Placebo, the Latin derivative of which has numerous translations, ranging from, 'I shall/will please', 'to humour', to, 'do nothing', has shown to be successful, on average, for 30–35% of people and as high as 90% for some, in both allopathic and complementary medicine. It has also been shown that **placebo can drastically alter physiology** (*Holden, C., 1978*). According to US studies and in particular work by Professor Herbert Benson of the Mind and Body Medical Institute of Harvard Medical School has shown the mind-body connection relates to eliciting a 'relaxation response', a mental state that triggers physiological changes. It can follow a patterned response similar to the response from drug treatment. **Everything has a placebo**; colour, size, type of machine, capsule, tablet, hands-on, hands-off, etc. **but its power is related to various things, not least of all the relationship between the giver/sender and the receiver/responder**. In sports therapy, the giver/sender is the therapist, coach, trainer, etc. and the receiver/responder, the athlete/patient. It is closely linked to **expectation and anticipation**, with people learning to be placebo responders via expectation and anticipation. Remember **the patient's expectations must not be at odds with the therapists**. Sometimes **just taking part is enough** to have a placebo effect. It depends on what kind of an experience the taking part was.

It has also been found that different responses to 'the same treatment' occur in different environments. The learning of expectation is closely linked **to experience and belief**. In other words the outcome can be determined by whether or not a person believes the treatment will have the desired effect based on their past experience. **The skill of the therapist is to satisfy this expectation or modify it**. Therefore **conditioning** can be involved, but by definition it is not a stimulus, as you do nothing. However, the patient must be verbally aware of what will happen. **If nothing is said, nothing will happen!** Yet again we emphasise the importance of **communication**.

Placebo response is not related to gullibility but to make it powerful the giver must make the receiver **trust** them and then convince them into believing the treatment is beneficial. **However, if this is overstated, or the therapist over promises too much, the effects can be negative**. These facts are not revolutionary as the advertising and pharmaceutical industry has been using them for years. **Linked** to this **expectation and anticipation is a belief and faith** that the treatment will work. This is linked to a person's **knowledge**.

On the other hand there are those people, referred to as **nocebos/non-responders** (*Wall, P., 1999*) who don't appear to respond, no matter what is done to them and who, in fact, expect to get worse. According to Professor Patrick Wall there are a lot of these people around and both nocebos and placebos are not related to personality, which the author finds hard to believe.

Adams, 1997, states there are gains to the patient in the presence of symptoms of chronicity – these are primary, secondary or tertiary. **Primary gain**, resulting from minor trauma, is the reduction of psychological conflict associated with such trauma. This leads to **secondary/illness gain**, where the person sees their illness situation or the injury as a way of 'getting something out of it', not only possible financial but also personal, e.g. sympathy, attention, abdication of responsibility, etc. The concept of 'illness or secondary gain' is well recognised in the medical profession and relates to not only litigation/financial compensation but can also relate to responsibility, sympathy, attention seeking, lack of autonomy and excessive pressures (*Tanner, J., 1998*). Clinicians and lately lawyers faced with a plethora of confusing symptoms and signs often point to three major findings to rationalise patient's complaints:

1. A high incidence of psychological dysfunction.
2. Long-term disability, secondary to spinal pain, is proportional to the level of disability payment.
3. In countries which had no facilities for compensation, a persons' perception of severity can be considerably affected, e.g. In Lithuania, road traffic accident patients showed little or no additional long-term disability and the 'patients returned to normality far more quickly' than in countries where it was an issue. No win, no fee, sometimes clouding the issue as to the severity of an injury. Schrader, H., et al., 1996, refers to whiplash as:

"A Western disease related to the high level of compensation available."

Fordyce, W. E., 1995, holds the view that by withdrawing disability benefit 'encourages' people to return to work. In the professional sporting context, some sports are now seen more as businesses and the employees/athletes, armed with agents, lawyers and financial advisors, see themselves going to work as opposed to going to play sport. This is something that sports therapists need to be aware of, especially if job satisfaction is poor, for whatever reason.

Injury/pain can sometimes be seen by some as a way of 'abdicating' responsibilities because they cannot cope with the pressures of having to decision make/perform:

- It may be just that it's raining outside and the athlete prefers to stay in with the physiotherapist rather than go out in the cold/damp weather training/playing.
- It may be that the athlete doesn't go along with the accepted, 'no pain no gain' mentality and so therefore exaggerates a problem to get help/attention.
- It may be that the injury causing the pain is the subject of a compensation claim and so financial consideration may start to cloud the issue. This could be confused with malingering which can be seen as a deliberate attempt to feign injury/illness. Do sports people feign illness/injury?

Tertiary gain, Dansak, *1973*, relates to the possible advantages, e.g. emotional, financial, or 'significant others' associated with the injured party.

So we ask the final question: 'Do we treat people or just see them?' There is going to be a significant mismatch of what the therapist expects to happen and what the patient expects, when the therapist does not address the fact that a sports person is an individual who has these traits/qualities related to what they expect. This is not only from the behaviour of the therapist but also in the treatment they give. This can manifest itself in a lack of progress in treatment and rehabilitation.

To reinforce what has previously been said, communication is vital and whilst outcomes are important, being the yardstick by which the therapist will be judged, clearly the success of these are directly related to the effectiveness of the process.

Clearly the issue of what is best for that person at that moment in time is not simply a recipe of doing x, y and z and the outcome being predictable. Success will always be determined not only by the generally accepted factors of intensity, duration, knowledge, commonsense, skill and expertise of the practitioner but also the personal interactive factors of the people involved and the power of placebo.

To achieve this, to be safe and effective in decision-making and to provide the best possible healthcare for any individual, a good practitioner must address not only the patient's needs and expectations but also should reflect on and be informed by all forms of evidence, including research. This will ensure that it's not what you do but the way that you do it and it's not what you say but the way that you say it, will definitely get results.

Part 3

The Pain Factor

Historical Perspectives and Definitions

"As an entity, pain can provoke a cascade of humoral and emotional responses designed to force the body to face its challenger. This mechanism is a twofold process and requires the chemistry of pain propagation combined with the direct responsiveness of nerve pathway conduction."
Tortora, 1998

Pain is a fascinating yet vast subject to cover and one that all sports therapists must study. After all, pain is usually the sole reason why athletes seek help and can be somewhat of a battle cry to display sporting prowess – no pain, no gain!

Acute pain is a protective mechanism as part of the body's response to injury and indicative of a problem, i.e. damaged tissue and indicates that the disease process has begun. So to encourage acquiring more of it in the pursuit of sporting excellence is a little strange. **Pain should be seen as a red flag/barrier only to be crossed, under certain circumstances, with extreme caution, as opposed to a red rag to a bull to be charged at**.

In simplicity pain is pressure/irritation and sensitisation on/of a nociceptor/free nerve ending which are found in all tissues in the body, apart from the brain and intestine. This pressure can be mechanical, thermal, electrical or chemical and finding the cause of the pressure or irritation and trying to relieve, release, reduce, or remove it is the secret to successful pain relief. 'Running it off' is usually the chosen course of action in sport, but when you run it off where does **IT** go? However, such is the multidimensional aspect of pain, this simplistic action plan will not always work and may cause further damage.

Descartes the 17th century philosopher postulated the view of pain as not the work of demons, as was first thought, but as a phenomenon related to a mechanism that relayed messages from the extremities of the body to the central mind. This was termed the **DUALISM PERSPECTIVE** and related to the pathway of a nerve from the periphery to the centre and back. This simplistic view of a mind-body connection has since been developed and refined. It shows pain to be a multidimensional, subjective phenomenon that cannot be measured objectively.

The sufferer has no direct control over it and involves the physiology of nerve impulse/transmission; tissue damage and resultant pathology; it is related to psychological, emotional qualities, thoughts, beliefs, anxiety, mood, states, sensations, feelings, sufferings of guilt and punishment. It can also be related to postural imbalance and compensations. Therefore its sources can be neurological, philosophical, psychiatric, behavioural, subjective, physiological, pathological, psychological, mechanical and postural.

> **"Pain is an abstract term which refers to many different phenomena from which one makes a selection, depending on whether one is giving a neurological, physiological, behavioural, subjective or psychiatric description."**
> *Sternbach, R. A., 1977*

One such perspective came from James Cyriax, 1985, who defined pain as:

> **"A highly subjective, personal, unpleasant, sensory, emotional, sensation, experience which is interpreted by the sufferer as being indicative of actual or impending tissue damage. It is a physiological rather than a pathological event involving peripherally and centrally acting mechanisms."**

Therefore because different people interpret and deal with pain in vastly different ways some research has highlighted a biophysio, psychosocial model to try and encapsulate this personal, multifaceted aspect.

> **"Psychosocial responses contribute to the experience of pain, which makes it difficult to assess pain, treat pain and study the effects of treatment upon pain."**
> *Degenaar, J. J., 1979*

Biopsychosocial Aspects

Three aspects of pain **NEED** to be considered in relation to the perception and response of pain as these help to unravel the complexity of chronicity. In other words why does pain persist long after the acute phase has passed?

1. Sensory/Descriptive

This is related to how people describe their pain in terms of emotion, sensation and/or what they feel, i.e. sharp, stabbing, prickly, burning, aching, terrible, dreadful, sickening, worst ever, etc.

Pain can be classified in different ways. Somatic pain is generally localised and originates from the skin. Deep somatic pain originates from muscles and joints, and is less well defined. Myotomes may help us in our diagnosis as to its origin. Visceral pain originates from internal organs, such as the gut, and is poorly localised. According to its duration, intensity and nature, differentiation can be made between phases of pain, i.e. acute and chronic (*Scott, Dr. J., 1998*).

Phase 1   'Ouch!' pain or acute pain – most commonly associated with the skin following injury. If there has been tissue damage, this may be followed by;

Phase 2   Variations on burning/aching/soreness etc. This can last for hours or days.

Phase 3   Pain lasting for months or years can be defined as chronic pain, and is classified under basic headings.

- Pain persisting beyond the normal healing time for a disease or injury.
- Pain related to chronic degenerative disease or persistent neurological condition.
- Pain that persists without identifiable cause. This can be related to abnormal illness behaviour.
- Cancer pain.

During the consultation/history-taking part of examination and assessment, open and probing questions can help to ascertain the cause and how best to treat it. **Don't forget, symptomatic treatment is ineffective**.

2. Cognitive/Evaluative/Relative

This is related not to emotion but to how people evaluate their pain based on previous, personal or related experience or knowledge. However, a person's emotions may start to enter their thought processes if their original evaluation isn't confirmed. Therefore, if an athlete has a pain in a particular place or has been given a diagnosis which they believe to be either the same as a similar, previous problem, or in the same place as someone else they know, they may consider their present pain to be equal to, more severe or less severe, than this pain. This then becomes subjective and emotional.

This is very much related to the re-occurring theme of perceptions, beliefs, awareness and expectations, etc. that are very important issues in injury/pain management (*see Chapter 5, Part 2*).

3. Affective/Motivational/Behavioural

This is related to what pain does to people and can become very individual. Does it motivate, demotivate, depress, make them anxious, etc. **SOMATOTYPE, PERSONALITY, PHYSICAL** as well as **BIOPSYCHO–SOCIOECONOMIC** factors start to become an issue. To re-iterate what the cognitive therapists tell us, it is not the problems themselves that distress us but the views we take of them.

Obviously if one is aware of a problem, via pain, then it follows that they have an idea of what they want to do about it and more significantly what they want the therapist to do about it. Therefore treatment needs to be directed towards:

Therefore it is important to address this issue of expectation in any verbal contract of agreement. Sometimes the expectations of the patient can be at odds with the therapists. The perception of pain is linked to a wide variety of physical, psychological and social factors. With severe pain, it can be easy for an athlete to slip into an all-embracing sense of helplessness, adopting what has been described as illness behaviour. Therefore treatment needs to be directed towards;

> **"Changing negative thoughts lowers pain arousal and lets the nerves settle down."**
> *McWilliams, Dr. A., 1998*

Others may reinforce the reporting of pain. Moving around on crutches may also gain sympathy from others. In the absence of training an athlete will have time to reflect on the pain, which does little to reduce it.

Many of the issues discussed in Chapter 5, Part 2, can enter the discussion. All of these issues and the psycho-social factors may lead to the treatment of pain being less effective and lack of, or poor recovery. The skill of the sports therapist is in knowing his/her charges. In order to gain a better understanding of how various theories, mechanisms and modalities suggested for the treatment of pain work, we **MUST** know some underlying neurophysiology.

'An Action Potential'/A Nerve Impulse

Neurons possess an axon, a nerve cell body and many dendrites. Axons behave like cells. Neurons can be irritated and conduct impulses. A nerve impulse is an all-or-nothing wave of fluctuating, electrical discharge that passes from one neuron to the next to an end organ, such as a muscle fibre, and is brought about by depolarisation. The cell membrane of a neuron is voltage sensitive; cations are ions that are positively (+) charged and electrons are ions that are negatively (-) charged. Outside the cell membrane there is a slight excess of high voltage, positive sodium ions, whilst inside there is a slight excess of negative, low voltage potassium ions (*Davis and Rawls, 1974, 1985*). Therefore, potentially high voltage, positive ions can be attracted into and low voltage, negative ions out of the cell. The difference between the two polarities is measured in millivolts (mV) in relation to the inside of the cell membrane. When not conducting impulses, the cell membrane is said to be resting and **polarised** and is known as the **resting membrane potential (RMP),** which is held at approximately -70mV. It is caused by a separation of charges across the membrane. This electrical charge difference is called a 'potential' because it is a type of potential stored energy. Opposite electrical charges having the potential to move toward one another if allowed to cross the membrane. For proper functioning, this differential must be at least -60mV (*Washnis and Hricak, 1993*). This resting potential is brought about by the membrane permeability and the difference between the intracellular and extracellular fluid which, as previously mentioned, contains electrolytes with an electrical charge (+ or -). The main electrolytes are potassium (K^+), sodium (Na^+) and chloride (Cl^-). Sodium is quite volatile and unstable. The difference in pH is 7.4 to 7.0 between extra and intracellular fluid.

What Controls the Movement of Ions In and Out of the Cell?

1. Membranes can be non-permeable, selective or semipermeable because they can possess specific membrane channels/gates that are open, non-existent or closed to certain ions. If a membrane doesn't possess gated channels for that particular ion then passage in and out of the cell is impossible. In neurons, plasma channels for transport of negative electrons are either non-existent or closed. Therefore negative chloride ions, the dominant extracellular ions, are trapped on one side. The positive potassium and sodium ions can move into and out of the cell.

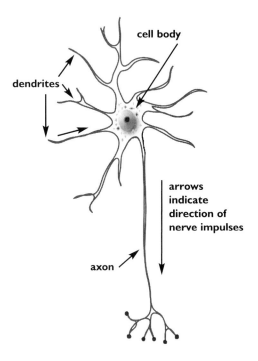

▲ *Figure 49. Individual nerve fibres (nerve cells) are called neurons.*

2. Diffusion through the membrane is either by:

- Simple diffusion, where ions move freely in and out of the cell along a concentration gradient, high to low. The rate depends on the number, the energy they've got, the size of the holes/gates, if those gates are open or closed, as well as the concentration and electrical gradient.
- Facilitated diffusion, which depends on the chemical bonding with protein molecules, i.e. in and out of the cell on the back of protein molecules.

What Maintains the Negative Potential?

A mechanism known as 'THE SODIUM POTASSIUM PUMP' actively pumps sodium ions out and potassium ions in at the ratio of 3:2. Also, more potassium gates are open than sodium, which ensures that when resting there is approximately 14 times as much sodium outside as in and 30 times as much potassium in as out. The negative chloride is trapped on the outside.

Depolarisation is the reduction of a membrane potential to a less negative value, and occurs when excitation by a stimulus/shock (chemical, electrical, thermal or mechanical) of the neuron triggers the opening of more sodium gates/channels. This allows more positive sodium ions into the cell, by overpowering the existing ions, thus reducing the degree of positive, high voltage ions outside the cell. This continues until the cell membrane inside possesses an action potential of +30 to +40mV at which point repolarisation occurs. During repolarisation, the sodium channels are closed and extra potassium channels opened to return the cell to negativity.

This polarisation, depolarisation, repolarisation fluctuation is what generates an action potential or nerve impulse and is local and isolated to one area of the membrane. However, as long as the stimulation is applied, a wave of electrical negativity, starting at the point of stimulus, affects the adjacent cells in a kind of domino effect by triggering voltage sensitive sodium channels to open in the next segment. As one becomes repolarised the other depolarises and so on. In neurons that are myelinated, action potential leaps from node to node (nodes of Ranvier) known as saltatory conduction, which accelerates conduction. Therefore the speed of conduction of a nerve impulse is dependent on the presence or absence of a myelin sheath and the size and diameter of the neuron. At the synapse, the action potential/impulse is carried by chemical neurotransmitters.

What is a Synapse and How Does the Synaptic Barrier Work?

This is the non-physical gap/barrier found periodically along the efferent and afferent neural pathways, where the sensory and motor impulses are interrupted. At its free end (no cell body/dendrites) the axon breaks up into minute branches called **pre-synaptic knobs**, the ends of which are **pre-synaptic vesicles** containing **neurotransmitters (chemical messengers)**. These are near to the dendrites and cell body of the next neuron. The space between the two, calculated as one millionth of an inch, is called the **synaptic cleft**. The neurotransmitters carry impulses/messages across the cleft, i.e. nociceptive (pain), thermal messages etc. and because there isn't any physical continuity at the junction/barrier it is said there is **contiguity** but not **continuity**. A synapse differs quantitatively and qualitatively from a nerve fibre in that:

- It offers more resistance to impulse hence the term barrier.
- It is susceptible to fatigue.
- Chemicals increase or reduce its continuity.
- It is affected by lack of oxygen.
- It emits only one way transmission.

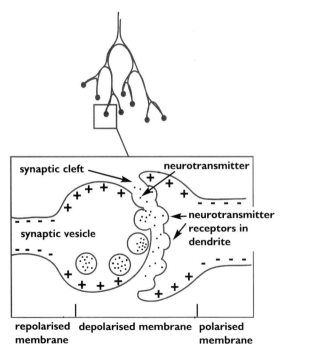

◀ *Figure 50. The junction between two neurons is known as the synapse.*

Therefore the function of the barrier is to:

1. **Prioritise** – allow priority of messages.
2. **Be selective/protective** – not all messages are conducted.
3. **Allow movement** – only one way.
4. **Conduct** the impulses.

As mentioned, the barrier is vulnerable to the action of the chemicals and neurotransmitters found in the area that can increase and decrease its conductivity as well as the intensity of the stimulus/impulse. A normal physiological action of the nervous system is the **law of facilitation/accommodation**, where similar, successive nervous impulses travelling along the same pathway to the exclusion of others, encounter less resistance each time it travels that way. This is because there is a cumulative breakdown of the barrier. This is how engrams/patterns of movement memory and habit are formed.

Unfortunately, if certain types of impulses (e.g. nociception pain) constantly bombard the barrier, eventually less stimulation will be required to trigger its function and more will be able to cross it and the easier it will be for the message to be received by the brain. Eventually even small stimulations are 'picked up'. When this happens the barrier is not doing its job and is said to be 'broken down'. Occasionally cellulomes are found in areas where the synapse has broken down.

Cellulomes are physiological phenomena found in connective tissue, which cause pain as they interfere with the neural pathways. According to Rola Pennell, an American chiropractor, cellulomes are one of six conditions that cause disease, i.e. the interference with normal nerve action. The others are trauma, diet, rest, exercise and poison. Cellulomes can be segmental-local, crossed-contralateral, intersegmental-remote. Once the barrier is broken down, the body perceives pain and healing needs to take place to re-establish the barrier. **Pain receptors do not adapt and so therefore the longer the nociceptor is irritated the more intense the pain gets. ANALGESIC DRUGS** work by inhibiting the opening of sodium channels therefore reducing or eliminating nociceptor impulses. When the action potential/nerve impulse reaches the synaptic knob this releases acetylcholine into the synaptic cleft. This is because the voltage sensitive sodium channels in the membrane open and allow sodium into the knob, increasing intracellular sodium that triggers release.

The neurotransmitter diffuses across the cleft and binds to protein molecules (facilitated diffusion) at the post-synaptic neuron/cytoplasmic membrane and creates an excitatory or inhibitory channel in the membrane through which sodium ions can diffuse into and potassium ions move out of the post-synaptic neuron. The sodium moves in faster than the potassium moves out. This can create depolarisation and an action potential that will transmit the nerve impulse. Alternatively, chemicals inhibit the impulse being generated. Excitatory channels are permeable to sodium and potassium, inhibitory channels are permeable to potassium or chloride but not sodium. If potassium channels open, potassium rushes out, otherwise chloride rushes in. Either causes the inside of the cell to be hyperpolarised (more negative and no action potential is set up). However, one dose of neurotransmitter from one synaptic knob is not enough to trigger an action potential. Its effect is cumulative, in that successive doses are needed to trigger an effect.

SUMMATION is the cumulative effect of the neurotransmitter to trigger an impulse. **Electrical, mechanical, thermal, chemical and nutritional/pharmacological stimuli** can affect either the release of chemicals, which irritate/stimulate the action potential, or the passage of the nerve impulse across the barrier.

A **NEUROTRANSMITTER** is a chemical substance that transmits impulses across a synaptic cleft. More than thirty compounds are known to be neurotransmitters and dozens more are suspected. They are specifically localised in discrete groups of neurons and are found all over the body, e.g. brain, spinal cord, autonomic nervous system, 'motor end plate'. They can be classified into:

Small-molecule, rapid-acting transmitters:

Class 1   ACETYLCHOLINE.
Class 2   AMINES, e.g. seratonin, histamine, dopamine, epinephrine and norepinephrine.
Class 3   AMINO ACIDS, e.g. glutamate, glycine and gamma-aminobutyric acid (GABA), or;

NEUROPEPTIDE, slow-acting transmitters, e.g. substance P, (excitatory), enkephalin, (inhibitory) and β-endorphins.

Their mode of action is fast and very specific and although not yet fully understood, is the way in which neurons talk to each other. Their action is determined by post-synaptic receptors. They are secreted by nerve cells, carried along axons, stored in vesicles within a synaptic knob and after they have carried out their action, by binding to post-synaptic receptors, they are either neutralised by enzymes, e.g. cholinesterase, or transported back and repacked in vesicles by mitochondrial energy to be re-used. If there is a lack or deficiency of neurotransmitters, the nerve cannot carry out its action, which can lead to problems, e.g. Parkinson's Disease, which is related to tremors and pin-rolling movements of the fingers/hand and is linked to the lack of the neurotransmitter Dopamine. LDopa introduced into the body makes Dopamine.

It has now been found that the types of pain signals are controlled by different neurotransmitters produced in the brain such as Factor P and Neurokinin A.

Nerve Fibres (Nociceptors) and Transmission

Nerve fibres (neurons) can simply be classified as:

1. TYPE A. ALPHA – which are myelinated and can be grouped as:

GROUP I. BETA.
GROUP II. GAMMA.
GROUP III. DELTA.

2. TYPE B.
3. TYPE C – which are unmyelinated.

The type A neurons are the largest, fastest conducting with type C neurons being the smallest, slowest conducting. Each fibre type has been identified with a particular afferent sensation, e.g. type A Beta fibres are associated with touch and proprioception. Sherrington coined the term **NOCICEPTORS**, to identify free nerve endings associated with pain transmission and these are identified as:

* Type A Delta, Group III, myelinated, which transmit impulses at 40 pulses per second/3–20 metres per second, which is more than 200 mph. Generally these nociceptors give a sharp, short-lived, localised, prickly type of pain. In sudden onset pain this is usually felt first for a few seconds.
* Type C, unmyelinated, which transmit impulses at 15 pulses per second/0.5–2 metres per second, approximately 20 mph. These nociceptors give a dull, diffuse, long lasting, burning type pain that follows the prickly pain.

The speed of their transmission is related to their myelination.

Both enter the central nervous system via the posterior, dorsal horn of the spinal cord synapses, decussate, enter the white matter (**SUBSTANTIA GELATINOSA**) and travel via tracts to the thalamus, the most important subcortical sensory centre, and the cortex for interpretation. There are six ascending/sensory/afferent and five descending/motor/efferent tracts.

Type A Delta nociceptors travel via the ascending **LATERAL SPINOTHALMIC TRACT (EPICRITIC PATHWAY)** together with the thermal and touch neurons straight to the **THALAMUS – CORTEX** whilst type C fibres travel via the **ANTERIOR, LATERAL SPINOTHALMIC TRACT (PROTOPATHIC PATHWAY)** to the thalamus, with only a few fibres going to the cortex. The rest enter a widespread area of interconnecting nuclei in the brainstem and are significant in the overall effect in arousing the whole nervous system, i.e. waking from sleep. Relatively recent research in Scandinavia has shown that there is not just one centre of the brain responsible for pain, as was once thought, but many.

Pain Generation

Pain will only be registered in the brain following a sequence of well-defined actions. The process is complex, intense, and not easily controlled (*Raj, 1995*). Part of this process results in the high stimulation/sensitisation (pressure or irritation) of nociceptors in the tissues. Up until then the nociceptor is a 'sleeping nerve'. This high stimulation can be as a result of chemical build-up at the time of the injury or metabolic waste products which are not 'flushed away'. When the body is injured and there is tissue destruction, the inflammatory response to this triggers the release of noxious metabolic substances, serotonin, bradykinin, histamine, prostaglandins, oxygen free radicals and leukotrienes, which assist the inflammatory response. Factor P (excitatory) and neurokinin A have been identified as significant neurotransmitters associated with pain transmission.

As well as chemical irritation, nociceptors can be affected electrically and mechanically, and by ischemia and temperature.

According to Munglani, 1999/2000, 'central sensitisation' is a process that can act to maintain the pain state whereby the spinal cord becomes increasingly sensitive (**ALLODYNIA**) to incoming stimuli and even ordinary movements and sensations. **HYPERALGESIA** is a heightened response to noxious stimuli.

Damage to the peripheral nerve, via prolapsed disc or peripheral tissue inflammation, may initiate a cascade of molecular events and neurobiological changes within the peripheral nerve and spinal cord, leading to chronic pain. Tissue inflammation can sensitise peripheral nerves so that they respond much more dramatically to stimulation. The release of neurotransmitters activates certain receptors, which in turn triggers a further cascade of events within the nerves. The nerves also start to alter their function and start to misinterpret stimuli with non-painful as painful.

Nerve injury reduces the effect of opioids and so therefore, according to Munglani, chronic pain after whiplash has to be managed differently than post-operative pain. Sympathetic nerve fibres may sprout in ordinary nerves within the dorsal ganglia, near to the cord, so that when the sympathetic system is activated so are these extra fibres.

Adrenergic receptor expression on peripheral nociceptors can cause sensitisation to circulatory noradrenalin, which is released into the blood in times of stress. Therefore in times of stress or changes in weather ordinary touch and pain fibres become activated as a result of the increased blood flow, due to the release of noradrenalin. **Because of all this sensory misinterpretation, pain can spread to previously uninvolved areas**.

Law of Facilitation

Nociceptors do not adapt and weak signals summate and become stronger over a period of time. If the pressure or irritation is not removed and there is constant bombardment/sensitisation, this summation can eventually cause **SYNAPTIC BREAKDOWN** with less stimuli needed to trigger the passage of signals. **HYPOSENSITIVITY** and **HYPERSENSITIVITY** are related to **PAIN THRESHOLD** and **PAIN TOLERANCE**. The former being related to the minimal stimulus needed for a person to perceive pain and the latter the maximum stimulus the athlete/patient can tolerate. With threshold there is no difference between males and females but with tolerance there are wide variations.

Law of Specificity

Discharge from the nervous system following stimulation continues long after the stimulus has been removed. This is why emotional responses are prolonged and far outlast the stimulus that provoked the response.

Pain Control Mechanisms, Modulation, Theories and Practicalities

A familiarity with the more pertinent theories of pain and sensation allied to an understanding of neuroanatomy and physiology may help in our work as sports therapists in the treatment of pain.

As suggested previously there appears to be two ways to remove, stimulate, modulate, block, utilise and interfere with the nociceptive pathways, both being very interrelated.

SHORT-TERM, via peripheral or centrally acting mechanisms to interrupt the impulses and can include oral, injected or implanted drugs. However, all drugs have side-effects. Non-steroidal anti-inflammatory drugs (**NSAIDS**) work by affecting the inflammatory response mechanism of the body (*see Chapter 3*).

A clinical review in the *British Medical Journal (BMJ)* in 1999, reported advances in the development of effective NSAIDS, with fewer side-effects, e.g. associated gastrointestinal problems. Analgesics (painkillers, e.g. aspirin) can work by inhibiting the opening of sodium (Na^+) channels therefore not allowing depolarisation. In other words the impulse is not transmitted but there is little research on their long-term effectiveness (*Smith, Hopton and Chambers, 1999*). There is strong evidence for the use of co-analgesics such as anti-depressants (*Smith, et al., 1999*). Certain foods also contain varying amounts of natural salicylates. Although the long held view that pain was a single phenomenon that can always be attacked by one type of drug is now not true and different drugs need to be targeted for specific neurotransmitters.

Recent research in the BMJ (2000), supports existing studies which have proven that women perceive pain more intensely than men, which has led to the suggestion that in future drug companies market gender, specific painkillers.

HEAT AND COLD can compete with nociceptive impulses in the spinal cord for transmission therefore overriding their effect. **MANUAL THERAPY**, involving physiotherapy, via massage, exercise, mobilisation, manipulation, hydrotherapy, electrical stimulation, acupuncture, posture training and ergonomic advice, etc. have been shown to have analgesic effects. Cutaneous stimulation (touch) can also compete with nociceptive impulses in the spinal cord. One reason for this can be attributed to **THE PAIN GATE THEORY**, postulated by R. Melzack and P. Wall in 1965. They suggested that all afferent impulses enter the spinal cord through the dorsal horn and all afferent nerves must pass impulses through an area there called **SUBSTANTIA GELATINOSA**. Researchers have postulated that all pain information must pass unopposed through this 'gate' area upwards for appreciation in the cortex. However, if the gate is also concurrently receiving other information produced by stimulation of thermoreceptors or mechanoreceptors, i.e. fast conducting sensory afferent pathways, then these impulses will take precedence and cause pre-synaptic inhibition of the slower conducting pain fibres. Therefore, if large diameter, fast conducting nerve fibre afferent impulses, e.g. type A are superimposed on small diameter slow conducting ones, the 'gate' is effectively closed to pain. If the brain is not made aware of the pain, no reactions can be initiated, e.g. muscle spasm or other reflexes.

Anxiety and excitement and anticipation can keep the gate open. All of which go hand in glove with sport. The most effective way to keep the pain gates closed and reduce the pain messages reaching the brain, is by:

- Avoiding stimulation of damaged nerves in the first place. This will involve pacing, which involves managing old physical activities in a new way to avoid over-exertion.
- Engaging in exercise and relaxation to keep natural painkiller levels stable.
- Using breathing and relaxation to manage pain when it does happen so that the pain does not increase further, or get out of control.
- Change our thinking, from frightening to less frightening thoughts, to manage pain when it does happen, so that the pain does not increase further, or get out of control. Obviously trained therapists need to be consulted.

LONG-TERM, via the removal of the perpetuating factors and can be considered as a development in dealing with acute pain.

However, as the causes of chronicity of pain are multi-factorial so should the treatment and this may be one reason why randomised controlled trials of a single therapy show poor results (*Munglani, 2000*). **MECHANICAL, CHEMICAL/NUTRITIONAL, PSYCHOLOGICAL** and **ELECTRICAL** methods have all been found to give pain relief.

MANUAL/MECHANICAL/PHYSICAL THERAPY, (via massage, mobilisation, manipulation, exercise, hydrotherapy, electrical stimulation, acupuncture, posture training and ergonomic advice, acupuncture/dry needling, etc.) and **ELECTRICAL** stimulation (**TENS, PULSED RADIO FREQUENCY, IMPLANTABLE DEVICES** etc.) can trigger the body's own pain control mechanisms, via spinal cord stimulation. **TENS** machines activate touch fibres.

Manual and exercise therapy can physically relieve the pressure or irritation on the nociceptor, via manipulation, mobilisation and massage, by improving circulatory flow which can remove the metabolic waste, reduce swelling, free restrictions, relieve tension etc. It can also enhance inhibitory control to reduce muscle spasm. However, research on massage for pain is disappointing (*Vickers, 2000*). There is some evidence to support the idea that regular exercise can induce physical fitness as well as mood elevation and potential pain reduction (*Murray and Pizzomo, 1998*). An active exercise programme with relaxation has shown significant improvement in self-reported function and pain (*Minor and Sandford*).

CHEMICAL AND NUTRITIONAL/DIETARY methods include **ANTI-INFLAMMATORY (NSAIDS)**, opiate drugs which will reduce the peripheral inflammation and block the effect of the prostaglandins. **NUTRITIONAL SUPPORT** can affect membrane permeability and mineral balance, as can nerve membrane stabilisers. Vitamins C, E, K, B1, B6, B12 have all been found to have anti-inflammatory effects. DLPA, essential fatty acids, magnesium and zinc have all been shown to modulate pain. Anti-depressants and oral opioids can enhance the spinal cords' own pain control mechanisms. Anti-convulsants can slow the firing rate of the damaged/injured nerves.

There are also a choice of foods that have implications for their ability to mediate pain, which contain varying amounts of natural salicylates, e.g. cherries, curry powder, almonds etc. (*Carper, 1994*). These are equivalent to aspirins and can produce the same effects, as well as side-effects. Therefore individuals suffering from asthma, hay fever or urticaria may be contra-indicative to the use of such foods. Conversely, consideration of the temporary elimination of such foods from a persons' diet, may help relieve tension headaches (*Carper, 1994*). Cloves, ginger and curcuma have been shown to have anti-inflammatory properties (*Lust, 1974, Carper, 1994*). Ginger is linked to reduction in the formation of prostaglandins and leukotrienes. Chilli pepper contains capsaicin, a known antagonist to the formation of Factor P (*Carper, 1994*).

However, it must be understood that the use of diet to control or reduce pain must be employed with the understanding that any foods consumed help to contribute to the stability of the blood sugar balance (*Duccini, 2000*). Dietary and nutritional intervention can also be used as part of the psychological strategy.

PSYCHOLOGICAL intervention can also be useful (counselling, imagery, biofeedback, hypnotism and nutritional intervention) can involve changing breathing rhythms which lowers arousal and tension; changing negative thoughts, relieve stress, anxiety and promote relaxation etc. (*Ogden, J., 2000*). Antidepressant drugs can also be used, reducing anxiety, excitement and anticipation with positive results (*Smith, et al., 1999*). Mood may be altered via exercise (*see Manual/Physical Therapy above, Chapter 2 and Chapter 5, Part 2*).

On the question of nutritional intervention, certain foods have been found to enhance serotonin levels, e.g. mashed potatoes, pasta and bread. This may help reduce stress and anxiety levels (*Yeager, 1998*). Bananas and prunes, which contain B6, a precursor in the formation of dopamine, a hormone known to be related to mood a sense of wellbeing, may prove useful in anxiety reduction (*Yeager, 1998*).

More radical approaches can include nerve blocks, via the injection of chemical cocktails to facet joints, discs, sympathetic nerves, epidura or even cutting the nerve supply. **Pain management programmes can involve a multidisciplinary approach addressing key issues related to the causes of chronicity of pain**.

The Body's Own Pain Control Mechanisms

Pain can be affected by the presence of certain substances in the brain which influence interpretation and reaction to pain signals (*Raj, 1995*). The Endogenous Opiate Theory, Werle, 1972, found that the body manufactures, stores and maintains its own opiate-like substances to react at receptor sites throughout the body to inactivate pain sensation (*Rang, D. R., 1999*). These chemicals owe their origins to dietary and biochemical sources and their role in analgesia is linked to their connections with other brain substances which control mood and blood sugar balance (*Des Maisons, 1998*). In simplicity these substances block or interfere with the impulses peripherally at the site of injury, or centrally, at the synapses in the spinal cord i.e. substantia gelatinosa, so that they either don't arrive at the thalamus/cortex or are considerably diminished if they do.

The injury/inflammatory response triggers the release of the noxious metabolic substances which irritate/activate type A Delta and type C nociceptors. In response to this, the thalamus triggers via descending fibres:

1. The periaquaductal grey, to release **ENKEPHALINS**, (grey matter around the cerebral aquaduct and 3rd ventricle) which are small peptide molecules found in the anterior hypothalamus and substantia gelatinosa. Once released they neutralise/inhibit the excitatory neurotransmitter, Substance P, found at the synapse. The enkephalin has only a rapid effect, approximately two minutes, and so therefore;
2. The pituitary is stimulated to release **DYNORPHINE CATECHOLAMINES** and β-**ENDORPHIN**. Endorphins have a longer effect on blocking the impulses. One trigger for endorphin release is exercise. In simplicity the effect of these neurotransmitters causes temporary hyperpolarisation at the synapse which means the post-synaptic membrane is less likely to reach the threshold potential and initiation of an action potential is thus inhibited.
3. The adrenals can also be stimulated to release **CORTISOL** from the cortex of the supradrenal gland. Cortisol is part of a group of hormones known as glucocorticoids that react to stress/injury and by stabilising the cell membrane (affect its permeability) it can have an anti-inflammatory effect. **ADRENALIN** released during high levels of stress has also been found to block pain transmission. Therefore if therapeutic techniques can be employed to produce stimuli along fast conducting fibres (type A fibres, touch, thermal) the same effects can be produced, i.e. intense cutaneous stimulation, both hot and cold.

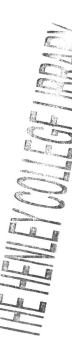

Let us also not forget the power of placebo and the mind–body connection (*see Chapter 5, Part 2*).

What Do We Need to Know?

(*see Chapter 4, Part 2*).

Regarding pain, during consultation/history-taking, we need to ascertain:

1. **DISTRIBUTION/RADIATION** – where is it/how far does it go? **DERMATOMES**, **SCLERATOMES** and **MYOTOMAL** distribution can be helpful. **CORD SIGNS** are indicative of an upper motor neuron (UMN) problem, the signs and symptoms of which are the 'D's, dizziness, diplopia – double vision, dysarthria – disturbed joint sensation, dysphagia – difficulty swallowing and drop attacks. Plus bilateral increased (clonus) reflexes, loss of pain, temperature, proprioception, vibration and simple touch. **ROOT SIGNS** are dermatomal, unilateral and give proximal pain.
2. **CHARACTER/DEGREE** – what is it like/sensation?

   - In the morning? – if it's worse it could be inflammatory.
   - On activity? – it could be mechanical.
   - At the end of the day? – it could be fatigue/stress.
   - Levels of pain can be measured on a 1–10 rating. McGill's Pain Questionnaire can also be used.

3. **LOCALITY** – is it local or referred? If the pain doesn't increase on palpation the problem is probably referred and/or the area is exquisitely sensitive to cotton wool. If the pain does increase on palpation the problem is probably local. Tender, palpable musculoskeletal points that are 'active' (referring) or 'sleeping' (local) have been identified as **TRIGGER POINTS** (*Travel and Simons, 1983*).
4. **PERSISTENCY** – what makes it worse/better?
5. **REGULARITY** – is it episodic/permanent/temporary?

Part 4

The Role of Soft Tissue Manipulation in the Care and Treatment of Sports People

Whilst for many people today, massage is considered 'new', 'alternative', 'complementary', it is certainly not new. Massage in general has had a roller coaster history, moving from medical orthodoxy to complementary, in the first part of the 20th century; declining to virtual extinction, post 1945; and back on the path returning to orthodoxy in the 80's and 90's (*Professor Goldstone, 1999*). However, the use of massage in sport has maintained a high profile.

"Manual therapy has long held pride of place amongst therapists and their grateful patients."
Sperryn, P., 1983

"A very useful but somewhat neglected form of therapy."
Colson, J. H. C., and Armour, W. J., 1986

"Massage treatment brings about sympathetic improvement when used in sports injury treatment and should be involved to a far greater extent."
Peterson, Dr. L., and Renstrom, Dr. P., 1986

In 1989, *Athletics Weekly* claimed that massage was a means of obtaining optimum athletic performance by:

- Allowing the athlete to compete with lower levels of stress on his/her body and at the same time perform more effectively and increase the workload of his/her muscles. It can also change moods or minimise pain.
- Improving the metabolic rate, i.e. improving cellular nutrition and toxic removal.
- Helping reduce pain and swelling after injury thus speeding up rehabilitation.
- Helping prevent injury, aiding recovery after training or competition and making the athlete less prone to stiffness. Enhance the cool down period, cutting down DOMS and fatigue.

Soft Tissue Injury – a Team Approach (6.7.90) emphasised the point:

"Employment of a masseur/masseuse specifically for a club, team, etc. may be worthwhile although VALIDATION OF STANDARDS was needed."

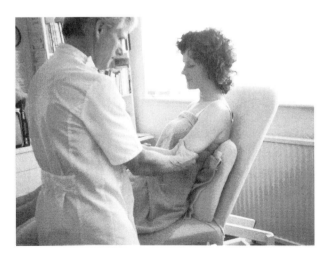

◄ *Figure 51. The role of soft tissue manipulation in the care and treatment of sports people. (model: Karen Probert).*

This was not at the expense of the physiotherapist whom is considered a very busy practitioner, but to work alongside, but doubted if there were enough qualified masseurs to go round! In 2001 much of what has been written previously holds true today especially in terms of validation of standards, although the profile of massage, especially sports massage, has risen dramatically, with the number of courses being offered also on the increase. Sports massage now has its own creams, lotions and oils!

In October 1998, the Sports Massage Advisory Group (SMAG) was set up under the auspices of the National Sports Medicine Institute in an attempt to standardise sports massage education in the UK. A core curriculum and course standards document has since been produced – sports massage can be considered as:

> **"The application of soft tissue manipulation techniques on an individual regardless of their stage of athletic development for the purpose of improving athletic performance."**
> *Lindsey Stiles, 2001*

Five areas can be identified for the involvement of soft tissue manipulation, especially remedial sports massage, in the care and treatment of sports type injuries, as part of the overall care and maintenance of athletes not as a substitute for anything, e.g. warm-up.

1. Pre-competition ('tuning-in' the athlete).
2. Post competition ('switching-off' the athlete).
3. As a modality in its own right in the treatment of sports type injuries.
4. In training and conditioning, i.e. restoration and rehabilitation for acute or chronic injuries.
5. Assisting in the psychological preparation of the sports person for competition.

Pre-competition

'Tuning-in' the athlete 15–45 minutes before competition is considered generally stimulatory. The body is a unique piece of mechanical poetry but like most machines cannot possibly be expected to perform at high levels of efficiency and effectiveness immediately it is switched on. If the body is not properly warmed-up or fatigued, its defence mechanism (muscle spindles etc.) cease to function effectively therefore increasing the risk of injury/re-injury.

The physiological and psychological value of a good warm-up is generally accepted by all who participate in sport. So as part of this warm-up schedule, which should be designed to raise temperature, stretch tissue, improve range of movement/ease of movement at joints and psychologically prepare the athlete for action, sports massage can be used to:

- **Improve circulation therefore raising muscle and body temperature**
  (*Ylinen, Y., and Cash, M., 1988*). Muscle contractions being affected by
  temperature. Nerve impulses travel faster in a warm muscle. In human beings
  lowering the muscle temperature below normal decreases muscle irritability
  and work capacity. A warm muscle is less viscous therefore contraction is
  easier and more efficient. A viscous muscle can cause irritation and rubbing of
  fibres. By improving circulation (venous and lymph flow) nutrients are
  brought to the area and toxic waste products are taken away. This can lead to
  an increase in the conversion of glycogen and its flow into the circulatory
  system. Glycogen is stored glucose and is vital for energy. There will be an
  increase in heart rate, stroke volume and respiratory rate (oxygen being vital
  for energy and top soccer players have oxygen absorption values of 6
  litres/min).
- **Loosen, soften and stretch connective and any residual immobile scar
  tissue** from an old injury that will remove stiffness (*Samples, P., 1987*),
  this will help the athlete to achieve full stretch and greater range of
  movement/ease of movement therefore reducing the risk of injury/re-injury.
  Stretching a muscle relaxes it and gives it greater potential (*Ryan, A., 1980;
  Stamford, B., 1985*). Passive stretching can be used initially but to maintain
  optimum temperature active stretching is called for. It also helps
  proprioception and co-ordination by allowing far freer and easier movement.
  Deep frictional massage assists the body in breaking down adhesions and
  fibrotic scar tissue aligning torn myofibrils by 'spinning the fibres' in a parallel
  fibrillary network helping to create soft, pliable, scar tissue. A strong,
  pre-stretched muscle resists better than a strong unstretched one.
- **Enhances muscular tone and flexibility to prepare for all out
  competition**.
- Tapotement techniques have been shown to cause reflex muscle contractions,
  therefore improving muscle tone.

Post Competition

'Switching off' the athlete with a cool down period is just as essential as a warm-
up period, if not as long (15 minutes–6 hours after exercise and is considered
generally sedentary). To this end, massage can assist by helping to:

- Clear away toxic waste materials that have built up during exercise (*Bonen, A.,
  et al., 1975; Dodd, S., et al., 1984; Gaeserr, G., 1984*).
- Re-distribute the blood and prevent pooling, therefore improving recovery
  time and decreasing the risk of injury.
- Relieve the muscle stiffness, pain and physical tension (*Ryan, A., 1980;
  Stamford, B., 1985*). Pain relief, via massage, is achieved by the removal of

noxious substances and via afferent input along larger diameter type A Beta fibres (Motor Gate Theory). Athletes generally report less muscle soreness on the day following competition if cool-down routines are practiced. Smith et al., 1994, found that massage reduced creatine kinase levels and elevated neutrophils.

- Identify areas of micro-trauma.
- Reduce psychological tension and upset in the event of loss.
- Helps return the body to homeostasis.

As a Modality in its Own Right in the Treatment of Sports Type Injuries

Masseurs/masseuses should carry out a detailed examination and assessment of the athlete, injured or otherwise. The purpose of this is to:

- Recognise and treat potential, minor, and more serious problems. The 'hands-on', sensitivity and touch become very powerful tools in diagnosis. This also helps maintain the physical condition of an athlete and improves time between treatment sessions.
- Recognise those conditions which may need referral to other practitioners, e.g. doctors, osteopaths, chiropractors, nutritionists, dietician, chiropodist etc. An expert is one who knows when to refer, **NOT** one who thinks they can treat everyone.
- Advise accordingly on training, rehabilitation, posture, diet, lifestyle, self-help exercise stretching etc.

In Training and Conditioning

Regular 'fine tuning' will help eliminate trigger points and biochemical stress, relieving the tender areas before they become problem areas (*see page 246*). This will help athletes perform more vigorously and consistently, lessening the chance of pain or injury.

Assist in the Psychological Preparation of the Sports Person For Competition

This is done by relaxing the mind and 'tuning in' to the job its about to do by reducing tension and anxiety (*Weinberg, R., 1988; Drew, T., 1991*). Tension and anxiety can lead to skill breakdown. This 'tuning in' can lead to an increase in motivation. Warm-up can set off chemical reactions (e.g. adrenaline) which prepare the body for action.

Where's The Evidence To Show That Massage Actually Does What it Claims To Do?

Over the years the value of soft and bony tissue manipulation (manual therapy) has been under scrutiny and any research to prove the efficacy of such treatments has proven difficult, for various reasons, to come to any definite conclusions. Much of the research to date has proven equivocal certainly on the physiological benefits of massage and less so on the psychological.

> **"Massage is commonly seen as a therapeutic art without scientific foundation."**
> *Goats, 1994*

However, as pointed out in Chapter 1:

> **"No scientific study can ever 'prove' anything; scientific research merely provides evidence to support or reject various hypothesis."**
> *Bledsoe, J., 1999*

Anderson, G., et al., (1999), demonstrated similar clinical outcomes when osteopathic spinal manipulation was compared to standard care for patients with low back pain. Returning to the topic of research, which was discussed in Chapter 1, and again emphasised in Chapter 5, Part 2, according to the ACPSM, it can be based upon:

1. **BIOLOGICAL EVIDENCE**, providing a rationale based on an identification of a symptom and the application of a therapy which is known to reverse that mechanism.
2. **EMPIRICAL EVIDENCE**, relating to the valid, clinical evidence of the efficacy of such treatment based on randomised, controlled trials.
3. **CONVENTION** (*see page 62*).
4. **CONSENSUS** is agreement by experts, in the absence of scientific evidence in the literature, based on experience and/or assumptions in such literature. Into the arena we can also include **anecdotal evidence, 'unverified methods'** (*Macdonald, 2000*), based on subjectivity and justified/unjustified opinion.

However, with so much positive, anecdotal evidence and with the sophistication of modern research methodology it is surprising that no such research has been undertaken that unequivocally gives us more answers than questions.

Much of the case for massage having a positive effect on the physiology and psychology of the athlete has tended to fall into this anecdotal category. However, as more and more research has been carried out into the efficacy of massage its use has tended to coincide with the positives and negatives of such findings. Kamanetz, 1985, proposed three reasons for the decline in the use of massage over the greater part of the twentieth century:

- The development of the pharmaceutical industry.
- New machines supporting older forms of physical therapy.
- De-humanisation in the patient-therapist relationship. To this we could add;
- Traditional image, with massage being thought of as a luxury not a necessity and considered a beauty treatment and far too effeminate for sport.
- Its labour intensity, which in the world of team sports makes it hard work if all the team want 'hands-on'.

In 1993, Michael J. Callaghan looked at much of the research into massage in the sporting context to date and its contents make interesting reading. Some issues raised in the article were:

- There is little scientific evidence to support the hypothesis that pre-event sports massage will enhance athletic performance.
- There is no definite or consistent evidence that massage enhances body physiology apart from muscle tone.
- Studies which show a reduction in fatigue and increase in performance are few in number and contradictory mainly because all were in a laboratory setting.

He concluded: **"Lack of comparable instrumentation and different research designs have led to little agreement amongst researchers over the type of massage to be employed or the length of time needed to be effective. Indeed the length of time and degree of use are often based solely on the athletes preference and not on scientific data. It is clear that the role of massage in the athlete needs to be evaluated further in an attempt to resolve some of these points and in an attempt to justify the requests from athletes for a time-consuming technique."**

Professor Goldstone, 1999/2000, looking at the history of massage from medical orthodoxy to complementary, concluded that in any comparable studies into massage, its effects and efficacy now and then, should not overlook the fact that frequency, strokes, speed and lubricants were considerably different then. When it was accepted as orthodoxy, to now, with modern techniques, oils and creams.

Van Wyk's, 1992 compilation, traced the history and research into massage and for students of massage is a good reference source to chart its roller coaster history. However, more recently two papers, by Professor Len Goldstone, 1999/2000, in relation to orthodoxy, nursing, orthopaedics and rheumatology provides excellent literature reviews for massage past and present. In relation to past and present in 1984, J. M. Walker stated that there is:

"No support for the hypothesis that frictions promote the repair of sprained ligaments."

However, Hunter, G., 1997, informs us:

"Much deep friction, by a qualified, experienced therapist, is necessary to reduce the adhesion so that it can be absorbed. The aim is to break down its mechanical properties."

Cafarelli and Flint, 1992, also looked at the last 40 years of scientific data related to the physiological and psychological responses to exercise and recovery. They conclude that although massage is generally recommended as an aid to speeding recovery, preparing for exercise and enhancing performance there was little data in the literature to support these claims. Although it could be shown that massage had some modest effects on local blood flow this was not directly related to improved performance. As for improved blood flow, research varies from; "no effect of massage to as much as 50% increase." (*Hemmings, B. J., 1999*). Shoemaker, 1997, showed no effect of massage on blood flow irrespective of the techniques used. However, Lederman, 1997, concluded that kneading was insignificant on fluid dynamics but that vigorous hacking increased blood flow lasting ten minutes after its cessation.

Cafferelli and Flint did not rule out the effect of massage to the feeling of well-being and euphoria and how this related to exercise performance and recovery, but their judgement was reserved, because of lack of evidence-based research, rather than the considerable body of anecdotal reports.

Hemmings also showed that the physiological effects in terms of blood lactate removal do not point to massage being beneficial and athletes were better served doing active exercise. This tends to confirm findings by Dr. Lederman who advocates the use of active/dynamic techniques to assist fluid dynamics (blood/lymph flow) as opposed to passive/static ones. He also seriously questions some of the long held beliefs as to what manual therapy does especially with its supposed effects on the motor system. With particular reference to peripheral and reflex mechanism, he quotes:

"Controlling the motor system via activation of peripheral mechanisms and segmental reflexes is equal to attempting to stop the flow of a river by throwing a pebble into it."

Hemmings also found that with the use of passive techniques, where there is no patient involvement, patient compliance is essential for relaxation. However, he found that active techniques, where there is direct involvement by the patient, affect the processes of the body far better.

> **"Controlling the motor system via activation of peripheral mechanisms and segmental reflexes is equal to attempting to stop the flow of a river by throwing a pebble into it."**

Hemmings also found that with the use of passive techniques, where there is no patient involvement, patient compliance is essential for relaxation however; he found that active techniques, where there is direct involvement by the patient, affect the processes of the body far better.

The power of **PLACEBO** must also be considered. In fact sceptics of the benefits of massage often claim it is the only reason people respond to a 'quick rub' (*see page 235*). The therapist patient relationship is very important in this respect with a person's knowledge, expectations, anticipation, perceptions, faith, beliefs and needs all playing an important role in the success of any modality. To this end communication, with a positive attitude, is vital for the therapist. Just taking part can have a placebo (*see Chapter 5, Part 2*). Finally:

> **"Massage seems to be a popular technique to aid recovery for athletes. Its use for physiological recovery and improved performance appears to be in doubt: however, its potential to bring about psychological benefits should not be overlooked."**
> *Hemmings, B., 1999*

In conclusion, constant appraisal of why we do what we do by keeping abreast of the latest research/studies should be part of our continuing, professional development. Also all evidence should be viewed in totality not isolation.

Contra-indications To Soft Tissue Manipulation: Sports Massage

> **"Any condition that renders a particular treatment improper or undesirable."**
> *Sandy Fritz, 1995*

No treatment is entirely risk free and it is essential that every effort is made to minimise the risk to the patient. Risks should be put at an absolute minimum by ensuring that a precise history of the patient is taken and of course a thorough examination is conducted. Remember to adopt **P PRINCIPLES. By pursuing** and promoting proper procedures and following established principles, peak performance may be produced without problems. However, puffed up personalities and politics may prevent and prohibit this.

During history-taking and examination clues should be searched for likely causes to reveal problems contra-indicating certain treatments. Sometimes these contra-indications are classed as regional/general/systemic, treatment not appropriate; absolute and relative may also be considered. The treatment may be considered as general or specific. However, the fact that we are treating people must never be forgotten and commonsense, allied to knowledge, skill and expertise should always be used. No list is ever definitive or exhaustive and shouldn't be solely relied upon but adherence to principles and guidelines help to make the right decisions.

When considering and learning contra-indications to soft tissue work it is a good idea to try to classify under headings, e.g.

1. **BONES**. Where an underlying condition may have weakened the bone. Consideration here can be made to osteo…spondy…and artho…conditions.
2. **CIRCULATORY**. Where there is disruption to normal supply, i.e. peripheral vascular disease, phlebitis etc.
3. **NERVOUS**. When there exists a disturbance and altered sensation, e.g. numbness down both legs and into the groin or symptoms that suggest severe nerve pressure, e.g. disc prolapse.
4. **PATHOLOGY**. When it is suspected there is an underlying problem that needs further investigation, e.g. the person is in constant, unremitting pain that is not altered by sleep, rest, etc.
5. **DIAGNOSIS**. When this is uncertain.
6. **PSYCHOLOGICAL**. Where psychological reasons exist, e.g. hysteria or the patient just doesn't like massage.

The immune system in sports people can be compromised if the athletes are constantly over-training and they are therefore more prone to coughs, colds, etc. **Certain conditions that raise suspicion and doubts will always exist,** such as those previously mentioned. It should always be part of a masseuse/masseur's ongoing education to make themselves aware of all medical and non-medical conditions they might encounter so that referral can be made to the relevant professional.

There are very few absolute contra-indications to the use of massage where a masseuse/masseur can never do any soft tissue work e.g. obvious infections, Hodgkin's disease, malignancy. However, massage can be performed around the problem areas as well as the whole body. Local massage is contra-indicated in the conditions listed but general massage may be required for surrounding tissues to improve circulation and the conditions for healing. If massage is indicated, care must be taken. **Remember one of the aims of treatment is to effect the environment in which healing/repair takes place.** Without unduly alarming the patient, referral to a medical practitioner should always be made with any condition the sports therapist is unsure of. **If in doubt, leave it out!**

ACUTE TRAUMAS – open wounds – open lesions – muscle ruptures – tendon ruptures – contusions – burns – unstable fractures. Massage should not be performed during the acute stages of an injury for fear of exacerbating the problem. With open wounds, wait until the scar has formed (1–2 weeks) and, if considered for massage, work around but not over the wound. In connective tissue damage it is necessary to massage as soon as practically possible to prevent scar tissue formation, etc. and restore normal function. It is safe when there is no risk of inducing fresh bleeding. In the case of fractures, limbs will be immobilised and therefore inaccessible until healing has taken place but massage may be essential after removal of the plaster to combat swelling etc.

Acute Inflammatory Conditions

Massage is contra-indicated in the acute stages of inflammatory disorders but can safely be used on the soft tissues in sub-acute and chronic stages, e.g. rheumatoid arthritis, in flare-up, gout, periostitis.

Myositis Ossificans

This is a rare process of ossification in the traumatised area of muscle following haematoma. The quadriceps muscles in the thigh, following a blow, are commonly affected. Massage will aggravate the symptoms of swelling and pain, and will lengthen the period of calcification. It can be 12–21 days before this is evident on X-ray!

Infections/Skin Conditions

Two main reasons for care by the sports therapist are the possibility of spreading infection to other areas of the patient's body and, if transmittable, to her/himself. If in doubt, seek a medical opinion. The common infections are:

a) **Bacterial folliculitis** caused by skin friction. Lymphangitis from abrasions or small cuts in hand or feet. A red line up the limb with tenderness is often the first sign. Cellulitis – in subcutaneous fat layers. Erysipelas (acute streptococcal infection of the skin).

b) **Viral**. Influenza is most common. Toxins are already released into the system and therefore massage is contra-indicative. In childhood, measles, chicken pox and rubella may be encountered. Herpes cannot be transmitted by massage but blisters on the skin that contain clear liquid should be avoided. Warts and verruccae should also be left undisturbed.

c) **Fungal**. Ringworm is common as a result of poor personal and communal hygiene. It is not contagious during massage, as long as a high standard of hygiene is maintained by the therapist.

Thrombosis, Varicosity, Peripheral Vascular Disease, Phlebitis

A thrombus is a blood clot. If this occurs in veins, it can stop the circulation. This is mainly a problem of immobilisation or relative inactivity, e.g. post-fracture or surgery. **Phlebitis** is inflammation of the veins, often started by local trauma, which can also lead to thrombosis. Both require immediate medical attention and massage is prohibited because of the danger of dislodging the clot and releasing it into the general circulation. This is dangerous if it re-lodges into the heart, lungs or brain.

Any condition being treated by a medical practitioner is contra-indicative to massage unless he/she agrees.

Tumours/Swellings/Lumps and Bumps of Unknown Origin

Swellings caused by infection, obstruction and neoplasm (tumour) are contra-indicative. Intensive massage to malignant tissue risks irritation that can spread the growth and even spread the malignancy. Most lumps in the subcutaneous layers are fat tissue. Typically, these nodules are soft, freely moveable against the deeper tissues and surrounded by a smooth capsule. In muscle, lumps are usually contracted muscle fibres. These nodules are hard and feel striated. If a lump is noticed during massage and is not typical from the therapist's experience, medical advice should be sought. The subject of lumps, bumps, swellings and oedema is a vast subject and cuts into many areas of medicine but it is impossible to totally isolate one area of health care from another (*see Chapter 3, Part 6*). A quick rub is not always a good idea! **If in doubt, leave it out!**

Part 5

Mechanical Massagers

Although the thought of using machinery, other than the mechanics of the human body, might be tantamount to heresy for a 'hands-on' therapist, mechanical massagers do exist and can have their uses. Various companies supply branded named products that will fall under one of the following categories. They can be considered as:

1. **Percussors/vibrators**. Percussors come in a variety of forms, e.g. cushions, chairs, belts and sonic units, designed primarily for the home market. It is suggested that they operate in a vertical plane and in physiological terms their effect is equivalent to tapotements. The earliest form of 'percussing' was to send the patient horse riding!

2. **Gyrators/vibrators**. Gyrators operate in a horizontal plane and can be used to stimulate the movements of effleurage and petrissage. They come in hand held or pedestal form.

Both percussors and gyrators can be used with talcum powder. Whilst no machine can do the jobs that the human body can the use of mechanical massagers can be justified on the grounds of:

- A labour saving device for the masseur/masseuse – a smaller output of energy is required.
- Being more profitable as less time is spent with the patient.
- In a sporting scenario the problem of massaging many in a short time can be overcome using a machine.
- They are convenient and impressive and will have some **PLACEBO** effect. Remember placebo works on anticipation and involvement, related to experience and belief (*See Chapter 5, Part 2*).

However, it is a question of personal choice as to whether the masseur/masseuse wants to incorporate one into their treatment after considering the pros and cons of using such equipment.

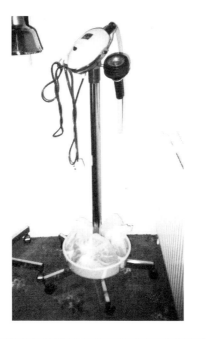

◀ *Figure 52.*
Mechanical
massagers.

Part 6

Bandaging, Strapping and Taping

Bandaging, strapping and taping techniques are widely used in the prevention, treatment and rehabilitation of sports-type injuries and therefore they do have a valid place in the work of the sports therapist working in the sports medicine arena.

Methods were initiated more than fifty years ago by coaches and trainers and developments are still being pursued.'The spray-on bandage that heals in an instant', is one such development.

> **"Scientists and doctors at the American Red Cross laboratories in Maryland, working with the US army on battlefield wounds have now made the breakthrough with a material that closes wounds in seconds."**
> *Daily Mail 13.4.99*

Bandaging and taping can be considered as the application of non-adhesive bandages and/or adhesive, elastic/stretch or non-elastic tape, in order to control bleeding and swelling, provide support and protection to soft tissues and weakened joints with minimal limitation of function. Dressings are used to maintain hygiene and are applied to cover and protect wounds, cuts and abrasions, therefore preventing or reducing the risk of infection.

The application of bandages, dressings and tape is relatively easy but if not carried out correctly is of little value and may be harmful. It is an area of skill and expertise that requires a knowledge of basic principles and procedures which initially is gained by instruction and then by practise and experience. It is, however, a contentious and at times confusing issue with certain commentators and authors.

> **"A good tape job can make almost any joint more stable and less likely to sprain."**
> *Southmayd and Hoffmann, 1981*

> **"It is never a good idea to strap up an ankle in order to do activities which would otherwise cause pain as the pain is a warning sign the ankle is not ready yet."**
> *Grisogono, V., 1984*

> **"Joints and structures that are recovering from injury may derive some benefits from taping."**
> *Dornan, P., and Dunn, R., 1987*

There has also been a long held belief that strapping if used indiscriminately and often would weaken the musculature around the joint but in recent reviews of the literature in the last thirty years there is no evidence to support this (*Minter, N, 1999*). In Australia the use of strapping for support is advocated from a young age. It must also be appreciated that **the psychology of strapping** for some sports people is important and could be very much linked to the power of **PLACEBO** (*see Chapter 5, Part 2*).

What is not in dispute is the fact that it is important that an understanding of the pathophysiology of response to injury, fluid dynamics, biomechanics and relevant underlying theory is undertaken. This will help the sports therapist to appreciate why bandaging strapping and/or taping is being contemplated (*see Chapter 1, Part 4; Chapter 3 and Chapter 4, Part 2*).

Indications – The Case For/What Can it Do/Does it Do?

Injury and re-injury may be avoided and so therefore its uses can be considered twofold:

1. For injury care and protection during the treatment and rehabilitation phases.
2. For injury prevention on return to activity (*Hodson, A., 1996*).

The following reasons being given:

- To protect a wound by covering it with a sterilised non-fluffy piece of gauze/dressing to maintain hygiene.
- To hold/support dressings, pads and protective devices over vulnerable areas, e.g. chiropody felt, second skin etc. to prevent blisters.
- To prevent injury by using it to protect limbs and structures from external forces related to particular activities, e.g. a gymnast using bars.
- To protect from further injury by supporting weakened or damaged structures and placing the part in a comfortable position, e.g. arm sling, elevation slings etc. However, Peterson and Renstrom, 1996, claimed that the latest research showed that taping doesn't prevent re-injury.
- To restrict unwanted joint movement such as immobilising a suspected fracture/torn ligament.
- To compress recent injury, thus reducing and limiting bleeding and swelling (oedema) and therefore improving the chances of good repair and recovery. This is one area where the use of compression bandaging is not disputed.
- To allow healing without stressing the injured structures.
- Provide reassurance – a psychological crutch some would say and the power of placebo must not be overlooked.

- To protect and support the injured structure, within safe limits, in a functional position, e.g. early weight-bearing during the rehabilitation programme. How long the effect of such support lasts is open to conjecture, with some commentators claiming 15–20 minutes maximum.
- To aid the muscle pump to effect circulation in the affected area.
- As an adjunct to the total health care programme.
- To improve the body's positional awareness of the ankle (proprioception).
- To improve the muscular response around the ankle via cutaneous stimulation.

Types of Taping, Bandaging, Strapping and Dressings

For Compression

1. Non-elastic cotton/crepe.
2. Cohesive, elasticated adhesive, 2.5cm, 5cm, 7.5cm, 10cm, and 15cm.
3. Tubular tubigrip.
4. Adjustable neoprene supports.
5. Inflatable pressure devices/splints – no good for more vigorous rehabilitation and training.

NOTE: Elastic bandages and tubigrip appear to be the most effective.

For Dressing

1. Cotton buds/wool eye pads.
2. Gamgee absorbent dressings.
3. Orthopaedic foam melonin.
4. Sterilised gauze reflex – sports dressing.

For Support and Rehabilitation

1. Triangular slings.
2. Plaster casts/waterproof casts provide a rigid support.
3. Braces and orthotics need to be fitted by specialists.
4. Walking sticks and crutches will provide additional support.
5. Bandages can be used to hold dressings in place as part of wound management.
6. Non-elastic.
7. Non-stretch adhesives 35mm and 12mm.
8. Stretch adhesives 2.5cm and 7cm.
9. Zinc oxide rigid adhesive.
10. Self-adhesive/cohesive – re-usable!

11. Adhesive – bulky and can't be re-used.
12. Commercial – *Vulcan*, *Pro sport* etc. can be used for expediency.
13. Hypo allergenic.
14. Water repellent.

Contra-indications/the Case Against/Drawbacks/Side-effects

The possible side-effects of every strapping and taping should be weighed against the desired effects and the following reasons have been given against its use:

- It can affect the body's internal pressures therefore creating homeostatic imbalance, affects the lymphatics and encourages the formation of adhesions.
- It can be self-defeating causing more problems than it was designed to eliminate, especially in the hands of the inexperienced, over exuberant therapist/trainer.
- It is neither a substitute for an anatomical structure nor is it a substitute for treatment and rehabilitation because it will not totally prevent unwanted movement.
- It can encourage further activity without seeking to eliminate the cause.
- Warning signs of a more serious impending injury can be ignored or other compensatory injuries develop.
- On the field of play it can act as a red rag to a bull. A motivator/confidence builder to the opposition.
- A variable amount of adipose and connective tissue exists between the skin and underlying structures allowing the skin a considerable amount of mobility that varies from site to site. This mobility can make the value of the strapping doubtful in certain situations, e.g. an injured thigh muscle.
- Most joints require additional support for physiological and functional protection.
- The priority therefore is to actively build up these functions.

Taping should not be used:

- If the injury has not been fully examined and assessed.
- To routinely strap an otherwise normal joint/limb thinking it provides something extra.
- If the patient is allergic to tape, plaster etc. Skin irritation may also occur by mechanical or chemical means if it is left on for long periods (maximum 2–3 days). Zinc oxide tape can reduce the risk of this.
- As a first aid measure before examination and assessment, i.e. strap it up and run it off!
- If the joint is swollen, irritable and painful.

- If there is diminished or abnormal skin sensation.
- Over an area that has recently been treated using hot or cold preparations.
- Where there is severe damage.
- To mask an injury to allow further use.
- If the operator is not familiar with the taping technique for the specific injury.

When in doubt, leave it out!

There is a school of thought that if people have to have their limbs in elaborately placed strips of tape then exercise of any description shouldn't be contemplated.

> **"If athletes cannot compete without metres of strapping to support a damaged structure they should not participate in sport until, through active rehabilitation, they are able to play without tape."**
> *Dornan, P., and Dunn, R., 1987*

Taping Terminology

1. **ANCHORS**. The first strips of tape to be applied and to which subsequent strips are attached. Anchors minimise traction on the skin.
2. **SUPPORT STRIPS/STIRRUPS**. Restrict unwanted sideways movement.
3. **GIBNEY HORIZONTAL STRIPS**. Add stability to the joint. **NOTE:** When stirrups and Gibney strips are used alternately they form a basket weave.
4. **REINFORCING STRIPS**. Adhesive tape strips to restrict movement and add tensile strength to strategic areas when applied over stretch tape.
5. **CHECK REINS**. Restricts range of motion during activity.
6. **LOCK STRIPS**. Secures the cut end of stretch tape that tends to roll back on itself. To secure check reins in place. To neatly finish the tape job when applied over anchors.
7. **HEEL LOCKS**. Gives additional support to the subtalar and ankle joints.

Accessories

1. Underwrap.
2. Vaseline.
3. Tape remover: *ElastoZoff*.
4. Leukospray – prior to application.
5. Ether.
6. Articare.
7. Astringent – *Friar's Balsam* applied prior to tape application.
8. Scissors.
9. Padding, gauze, felt.
10. Second skin.
11. Tweezers.

Taping/Bandaging Techniques

The number and variety of tapings that could be applied to the body is nearly infinite and so therefore the following represent the more familiar ones.

1. **CIRCULAR OR SIMPLE SPIRAL** – forearm.
2. **REVERSE SPIRAL** – calf.
3. **FIGURE 8** – knee, ankle.
4. **SPIRAL BASKET WEAVE** – medial and lateral ligament sprain.
5. **DIAMOND WRAP** – heavy activity.
6. **SPICA** – shoulder.
7. **CRYSTAL PALACE WRAP** – knee support.
8. **DOUBLE LOUISIANA** – heel lock.

The Application

Purpose

Are the aims of treatment to compress or support? Are all the required materials at hand? What is required: a bandage or a tape, stretch or non-stretch, cotton, cloth, gauze, elastic, crepe? What width is required: 2.5cm, 5cm, 15cm? The following guidelines may help. 2cm – wrist, thumb and hand; 3cm – ankle, elbow; 6cm – knee, shoulder; 10cm – thigh, trunk.

What pattern/type is the most suitable, spiral, basket weave etc? Narrow strips of adhesive tend to be easiest to apply and have greater combined strength. It is suggested that the use of adhesive strapping on skin for acute injuries should be avoided, as removal for medical examination would be too painful.

Position

The limb should be supported, elevated and be in a comfortable position with minimal fatigue or stress on the injured structure and at the appropriate height to ensure an even application of bandage or strapping. Leverage is required in most applications but unwanted or excessive leverage may not only be uncomfortable but detrimental. Cliniband/theraband or crepe bandage can be used to hold the limb in position. Always strap in a direction that will shorten injured structures/tissues, i.e. ligaments in a shortened position. Position the bandage/tape with the unrolled portion uppermost and the sticky side uppermost.

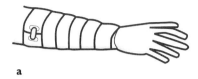

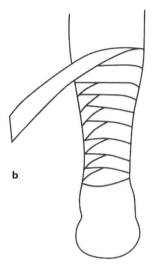

a

b

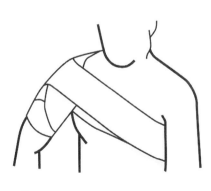

c

▲ Figure 53. Examples of types of bandaging, a. Circular or Simple Spiral, b. Reverse Spiral, c. Spica.

Principles and Procedures (Guidelines, Precautions and Rules)

Before commencing, the following should be considered:

- Knowledge of taping is gained initially by information and then by practise and experience.
- Think before you begin.

Can the following questions be answered:

- Has the injury been fully examined and assessed?
- How did the injury occur?
- Are you familiar with the anatomy and movement of the parts involved? i.e. surface anatomy, joint structure, biomechanics.
- Are you familiar with the physiology and pathophysiology of what has happened? i.e. inflammatory response, stages of repair and healing, types of oedema etc.
- What structures were damaged?
- What tissues need protection and support?
- What movements must be restricted?
- Is complete immobilisation necessary at this stage?
- Are you familiar with the technique?
- Are you competent?
- Do you have suitable materials for the taping technique?

Preparation For Taping

- Using soap and water, wash, dry and shave skin in a downward direction, as tape will not stick to oily skin. Shaving will prevent hair follicle inflammation and unnecessary pain when the strapping is removed. Conversely hair removal cream can be used.
- Cover broken lesions before taping.
- Check if allergic to tape or spray.
- Apply protective padding to friction and pressure areas.
- With sensitive skin or when strapping has to be repeated frequently, an under-wrap may be used.
- A mild astringent such as *Friar's Balsam* can be painted over the skin to help prevent a rash and ensuring better tape adhesion and to facilitate its removal.
- Pre-cut lengths of strapping from the roll.
- Cover the area to be taped with pre-wrap.

Pressure/Tension

- **Tension is one of the specific skills that differentiates a good strapper from someone who just knows how to put on a bandage.**
- Strapping that is too slack will be ineffective and uncomfortable.
- The strapping should be firm but not too tight in case the circulation and nerve pathways are compromised. There should be even, uniform, overall pressure.
- The pressure should not be greater proximally than distally (*Brodell, J. D., et al., 1986*).
- **Avoid** gaps, wrinkles, too many folds, layers and concertinas.
- **Avoid** excessive traction over the skin, e.g. nipping, blisters.
- **Never** use a patient's limb as an anchor to pull bandaging or strapping off the roll.
- **Allow** for expansion, i.e. foot when weight bearing and normal muscle function when running, jumping etc.
- **Never** completely encircle a limb with non-elastic tape.

Direction

- The bandage/strapping should go from within, to out/medial to lateral.
- Distal to proximal – far to near.
- With compression, spiral never circumferential.
- Overlapping should be a $^1/_2$–$^2/_3$.
- The application should be 15cm above and below the site of injury but consideration must be given to lymphatic drainage.
- The bandage should be smoothed as it follows the contours of the skin.

Finishing

- The application can be finished by pinning, taping or tucking.
- The application should be checked to see that it is functional and comfortable.

After Care/Advice

- Talk to the patient throughout informing them as to what and why the taping is being applied. **This is important for informed consent**. Also listen to the patient – they will inform you if all is not well.
- Advise your patient, e.g. Alcohol! Colour sensation – pink healthy; blue/black! numb, tingling!
- **Compression is removed when the limb is elevated but applied when it is in the dependent position** (*Murthy, G., et al., 1994; Rucinski, et al., 1991*).
- Any **home exercise** that is given **should not be considered as home treatment**.

Inform the patient about:

- If the circulation becomes compromised and what to do if it does.
- Weight/non weight-bearing (NWB).
- Rest.
- Elevation.
- Walking devices, sticks and crutches.
- For hygienic and allergenic reasons, tape shouldn't be left on too long (maximum 2–3 days) or after training and playing.

Don't forget – if in doubt, leave it out!

Strapping/Tape Removal

- Taping should only be kept on a maximum of 2–3 days.
- Remove the strapping immediately after training or match play, then wash the area with neutral soap and water.
- To remove encircling bandaging, use special strapping scissors with a snubbed nose that can slide under, lift and cut the strapping without piercing the skin. Keep the lower blade of the scissors parallel to the skin surface.
- When removing strips of strapping do not pull at right angles to the skin, or rip off violently, as this may lift and tear the skin. Support the limb with one hand whilst removing the tape with the other. This avoids disrupting any healing that has taking place. Pull the strapping back on itself keeping the removed strapping parallel to the skin surface. Where skin is very loose, use

the other hand to apply counter pressure, and try to push the skin away as opposed to trying to pull or tear the tape away from the skin. The easiest and least painful method is to use adhesive plaster/tape remover. Lift the end of the strapping and, while pulling parallel to the skin, rub the contact line between the skin and the strapping with a wad of cotton wool soaked in tape remover.

Part 7

Electrotherapy and Thermal Treatment

BEFORE considering the use of any modality for treatment purposes, therapists need to be **TRAINED** in its use as well as possess a sound theoretical knowledge to complement and underpin such practice. These matters can be dealt with by reference to the many excellent texts on the subject. These facts also have implications relating to insurance, compensation and litigation.

Electrotherapy

The use of electrotherapy equipment has many implications and should only be used after an acceptable course of study has been followed. The issue that is always raised is what constitutes acceptable? A quick demonstration by a salesperson is **not** acceptable.

Electrotherapy is a general term applied to treatment in which sound, heat, light and other forms of electromagnetic energy, which is the simplest form of energy, are applied to the body, e.g. ultrasound, diathermy, short wave, microwave, laser etc. to assist the healing process. Whilst the mechanisms of such are not fully understood the evidence points to a multiple response. Apart from the fact that in order for such energy to have an effect it must be absorbed the effects of such electrotherapeutic intervention can be considered as physical, physiological and therapeutic and the interrelationship of such. In other words any energy delivered to the tissues has the potential to produce a physical effect. This in turn alters the physiology, bringing about changes in the body to the structures and tissues (reduced viscosity, increased metabolic activity, increased blood flow etc.) and this in turn can achieve the required therapeutic outcome by affecting changes to the body, (pain relief, relaxation). The interaction is that a physical effect such as increasing blood flow can bring about a therapeutic one by raising temperature. Because of the potential effect of certain rays in the electromagnetic spectrum, eye protection (blue bottle sunglasses) should be worn when using lasers. The following responses to electrotherapy have been documented:

- There is an increase in collagen synthesis when direct current is used.
- An analgesic effect is noted.
- Lymphatic drainage is stimulated.
- There is an increase in the capacity of the blood capillary system.
- Cell realignment occurs so that current flow passes easily through tissues.
- Fibroblastic activity and function is influenced.
- There is a significant increase in cell ATP production (*Chandler, Dr. M., 1998*).

Electrotherapy can therefore have both a definite potential benefit, as well as a detrimental effect in relation to soft tissue healing and repair. As with all other modalities its success is dependant on many variables, not least the professionalism, commonsense, knowledge, skill and expertise of the therapist, allied to what is best for that particular person at that time (*see Chapter 3, Part 4*). In order to evaluate what is best, information needs to be assessed to know what equipment is available and the pros and cons of using such equipment. This can then be related to the knowledge of tissue healing and repair in order to arrive at a good clinical decision as to what piece of equipment would give the best clinical outcome.

Which Approach/Which Modality?

"**The secret of any electrotherapy treatment is to select the modality, dose and application method which is most likely to achieve the effects required.**"
Watson, T., 1997

The theme of: 'It's not what you do but the way that you do it', holds true for electrotherapy. The skill and expertise is not in the delivery but in the thinking behind it (*see Chapter 5, Part 2*).

Is the required outcome selected first and then the most suitable piece of equipment to bring about such success chosen next, or is the piece of equipment chosen first and then utilised to achieve the desired outcome? Obviously professional people will have their own particular process for arriving at such a decision that may vary slightly from another. The main criteria, is such a choice safe and effective?

Although many modern electrotherapy machines claim to be, 'all singing, all dancing' they are, on the whole, with the odd exceptions, nothing more than sophisticated variations on a theme, which have been used for many years. However, the range and availability of such equipment and the variety of treatment approaches ensures that in essence there is no one right way of doing things.

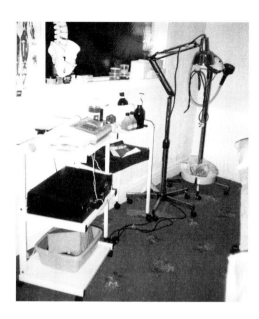

◄ *Figure 54.*
Electrotherapy
equipment.

According to Dr. Tim Watson, 1997, there appears to be several theoretical approaches to assist the body in its healing and repair that utilise electrotherapy.

1. **CHEMICALLY** which interferes or modifies the chemistry of the problem during the inflammatory stage. An example of this could be **ULTRASOUND**, which causes cellular excitation, via mechanical disturbance by oscillation, at three million times a second, which in turn affects the cell membrane potential and the cell transport mechanism. In other words: "a blinking Geoffrey Maitland." (*Tim Watson, 1997*).
2. **BIOMECHANICALLY**. This approach electrically stimulates the muscle activity that in turn activates the muscle pump that helps in the removal of oedema. An example of this could be **FARADISM**. Another benefit of this approach might be to improve muscle tone and strength to restore homeostatic balance around the joint.
3. **NEUROLOGICALLY** to stimulate the nerves to bring about a secondary pain relief, e.g. **TENS**. It has also recently been established that peripheral sensory nerve stimulation can be used to modify a peripheral inflammatory process, 'neurogenic inflammation'.

"In considering normal body response to injury or the repeated insults to soft and bony tissue there is considerable evidence in the literature that the healing process is mediated by the flow of endogenous electrical current (referred to as: 'the current of injury'). However, when the body is injured or damaged there develops a high resistance to current flow."
Chandler, Dr. M., 1998

Various opinions have been postulated as to why this occurs, but whatever the mechanism the body's own natural electrical energy is unable to enter the damaged site and assist repair. It is therefore hypothesised that outside electrical forces are required to assist the healing repair process.

Clearly the sports therapist is no different to other therapists in that clinical decisions must be made as to the choice of equipment and how best to utilise such equipment during the treatment of the athlete. A quick demonstration by the sales representative showing how to switch the machine on and where to put the pads is clearly not sufficient knowledge to satisfy the criteria of being safe and effective. Long before the sales representative is sent for the therapist must embark on a course of study to acquire the underpinning theoretical knowledge that would complement such tuition.

Thermal Treatment

The aim of this section is to provide the sports therapist with enough theoretical knowledge about hot and cold therapy so that he/she will be familiar with its role in the treatment of many musculoskeletal problems. It is not intended to present a treatise on the subject. The benefits of hot, cold and contrast treatment physiologically, psychologically and in particular their effectiveness in terms of pain relief is well documented, and therefore, for the inexperienced sports therapist, it may appear that either will do in the treatment of inflammatory conditions.

By looking at some of the biological, empirical, consensual and conventional perspectives this approach can be questioned. The aim should be to initially address the signs and symptoms presented to assist and control the natural responses of the body, which may then bring about a return to homeostasis. The evidence initially calls for the use of cold. Once the repair process is under way we should gradually start to introduce heat to the tissue, initially via contrast bathing, to improve the circulation (nutrients in – waste out) after any damaged vessels have been repaired. Therefore as an introduction to hot, cold and contrast therapy the sports therapist should note:

1. **ACUTE CONDITIONS** are the first 24–48 hours of an injury, but always remember this can last up to 6 days and the chosen modality should be **COLD**.
2. The **SUB-ACUTE CONDITION** lasts from acute up to resolution, which can be from 6–21 days and the choice of treatment here should be to **USE CONTRAST BATHING (HOT AND COLD)**.
3. **CHRONIC CONDITIONS** are non-resolved acute and sub-acute conditions, and here the choice should be to use **HEAT**.

Let us now consider these guidelines in greater detail. The **INTENSITY AND DURATION** of any treatment allied to the knowledge, skill, commonsense and expertise of the therapist will always determine its success or failure (*see Chapter 3, Part 4; Chapter 5, Part 2*).

Ice/Cold Therapy (Cryotherapy)

Types

Treatment can be by:

1. **EVAPORATION**.
2. **COMPRESSION**.
3. **IMMERSION**, and can be via sprays, which have a temporary/masking effect and arguably only 'numb' the superficial (31mm–62.5mm) of tissue. Ethyl chloride evaporates on the skin 'removing' the heat. The cold being absorbed into the tissues via conduction, with heat being transferred the other way. Cold water can be applied by putting the limb under cold running water, if possible. This is considered less traumatic than ice therapy.

COLD WATER AND ICE (33% water and 67% crushed ice). Here the affected part is immersed. 'Cold water, can be applied by, if possible, putting the limb under cold running water'.

FLOWTRON/CRYOCUFF is considered highly effective as it compresses and cools, studies indicating less pain than with other methods of applying compression and cooling (*Shelbourne and Rask, 1998; Zaffagnini, et al., 1998; Whitelaw, et al., 1995 and Scheffler, et al., 1992*).

ICE PACKS can be in the form of:

- Disposable cryogel/cold pads but these can lose their effectiveness after approximately 40 minutes.
- Re-usable, which need to be changed 45–60 minutes after dulling.
- Frozen packs, e.g. vegetables, etc are effective if nothing else is available. However, it has been found that leaving such packs on for longer than 30 minutes can cause frostbite (*BJSM, 2000*).

Ice is not to be used directly onto skin as it will cause ice burns and so cubes can be wrapped in a damp cloth and applied to the area or a layer of oil on the skin surface will allow water to drain away. If melted ice water collects under a tight pack it becomes super cool and drains salts from the skin that can cause blisters.

Chipped/crushed ice in a damp cloth appears to be the most effective application of cold, followed by ice in a plastic bag and then frozen gel (*McMaster, et al., 1978; Belitzky, et al., 1987*). Most guidelines advocate the use of ice packs for periods of 10–20 minutes depending on the volume of soft tissue around the injury.

Effects

These can be considered as:

1. **THERAPEUTIC** changes to the body, i.e. how the person responds and reacts.
2. **PHYSICAL/PHYSIOLOGICAL** changes in the body, i.e. the structures and what it does to tissues. These can be:

- **DIRECT**, with an immediate response, or;
- **INDIRECT**, i.e. reflex, periphery and deep and which include, circulatory, neural and excitatory mechanisms.
- There can be a **REDUCTION IN SWELLING/OEDEMA**, which seems to be dependent on the type of cold used and contrary to belief can actually increase swelling (*Kowal, 1983; Farry and Prentice, 1980*). It has been suggested the increase could be attributed to increased permeability of the lymph vessels, extra vascular protein accumulation and extravasated fluid, with temperatures below 15°C increasing blood flow (*Meeusen, and Lievens, 1986*).
- There can be a **REDUCTION IN MUSCLE SPASM** due to an increased activity of the motor neurone.
- There is a **REDUCTION IN BLOOD FLOW**, with an initial vasoconstriction and temperature change. However, there appears to be disagreement as to the exact response, known as, '*Lewis's Hunting Response*'. It appears that reactive vasodilation and increased blood flow occurs with skin temperatures below 14°C, whereas between 14–42°C vasoconstriction and reduced blood flow occurs. In the presence of exercise it is the exercise that increases blood flow and not cold (*Knight, and Londeree, 1980*). Intra muscular temperatures not being affected until after 10 minutes.
- There is **AFFECTATION OF TISSUE METABOLISM** with a reduction considered to be more important than the reduction in blood supply because if the inflammatory response is reduced secondary cell death is minimised (*Rivenburgh, 1992*). Hypothermia reduces cellular energy needs therefore reducing oxygen demands and usage (*Knight, 1989*). Metabolism can take up to 8–10 hours before it is truly affected and this can lead to **INCREASED TISSUE FLUID VISCOSITY**.

- There is an **ANALGESIC EFFECT** brought about because temperature and pain nociceptors travel in the same Lateral Spinothalmic Tract to the brain (*see Chapter 5, Part 3*). Some studies however, demonstrate an initial increase in pain upon the application of ice followed by a decrease in pain and numbness (*Knight, 1989*). Pain reduction does appear to occur after cooling to temperatures around 10–15°C.

Timings

Cold should only be used for as long as it takes to have an effect. To be effective the cold must be penetrative. Cold is transferred through conduction with heat travelling 'the other way'. The larger the area the longer the treatment, e.g. ankle/knee – 30 minutes, thigh – 45 minutes. Areas with more than 2cm of subcutaneous fat will need longer and areas with less, no more than 10 minutes. A 20–30-minute application every two hours for the first twenty-four hours (*McMaster, et al., 1978 and Knight, 1989*) appears the most effective. One application of 20–30 minutes will cause muscle temperature to remain below normal for two hours then cold needs to be applied again.

For the first 2–3 hours check the skin pallor after each change because the cooling needs to be constant. Once the application is not cold enough there may be a reflex action which can cause vasodilation.

Let us not forget the importance of compression bandaging and the reservations outlined previously as to whether the limb is elevated above the heart or in the dependency position. Evidence suggests (*Rucinski, 1991*) that when elevation can be maintained above the heart level, compression should not be applied at the same time as elevation. This is because it compromises lymphatic and venous return and produces a possible 'rebound phenomenon' caused by a sudden shift of vascular or lymphatic fluid. This phenomenon only occurs when compression and elevation are done together and not when elevation is carried out alone. It has been found that ice has little effect on joint swelling once intra articular effusion has formed, therefore ice treatments are of most value when used **IMMEDIATELY** after injury (*McLean, B. A., 1989*). Also, remember the **importance of placebo** that is 30–35% successful in all medicine and that **a person's needs and expectations can greatly influence its effect** (*see Chapter 5, Part 2*).

Contra-indications and Dangers

As with all contra-indications and dangers there are absolute, obvious and potential classifications and so the following list serves to remind the reader as to the more obvious:

- **WARN/INFORM PATIENTS** what is being done to them. This has significant implications for **INFORMED CONSENT**.
- **TEST PATIENTS** as to the effects of applying cold as skin character varies.
- **DANGERS** can be considered as – **BURNS – FAT NECROSIS – FAINTING – OVER SUPERFICIAL NERVES** (*Basset, et al., 1992*). Athletes with little subcutaneous fat are particularly vulnerable.
- **CARDIAC PATIENTS**. Don't apply cold to left shoulder, back or neck as this stimulates the autonomic ganglion to the vital organs. It is suggested that cold is not applied within six months after a heart attack as this affects the blood pressure and increases the heart rate.
- **ALLERGY TO COLD**, i.e. Reynaud's disease, arteriosclerosis, peripheral vascular disease, sickle cell anaemia, urticaria.
- **CIRCULATORY PROBLEMS**, i.e. atherosclerosis.
- **DIABETICS – EPILEPTICS** are particularly sensitive to thermal treatment.
- **DEFECTIVE NERVE/SKIN SENSATION**. If there is a history of or if suspected the treatment should not exceed twenty minutes and the patient should be checked every five minutes.
- Application over superficial nerves if too prolonged can cause nerve damage (*Covington and Basset, 1993*). It is suggested no more than ten minutes.
- **MENTALLY RETARDED**.
- **VERY OLD/YOUNG**. Some people are just adverse to it! The power of the mind-body connection has been highlighted many times during this book.
- **AFTER STEROID INJECTION** (for at least 24–48 hours because of deep vasodilation).
- Athletes should not return to activity immediately after the application of cold as nerve conduction and velocity, sensation and connective tissue flexibility could be reduced.

Contrast Bathing (Hot and Cold)

Contrast bathing is considered best after the first 48–72 hours or sub-acute phase. As it combines cold and heat, its effects, dangers and contra-indications are similar to those of the other two modalities. It must be remembered:

- Heat can cause vasodilation.
- Cold can cause initial vasodilation and then vasoconstriction.

Contrast bathing is useful because it helps:

- Aid oedema absorption, therefore reducing swelling.
- Stimulate circulation.
- Can have an analgesic effect.

The effects of the application of heat and then cold produce a pumping action via vasodilation and vasoconstriction. In many quarters it is considered a highly effective but somewhat neglected form of therapy. As with all modalities there are many variations on the theme all professing to be effective. It is very much a case of if it works then use it. However, for initial guidance here are two suggestions.

72 Hours–1 Week Post Injury

DAYS	4–5	6–7	8–9
TIME (Cold)	4 minutes	2 minutes	1 minute
TIME (Hot)	1 minute	2 minutes	4 minutes
	x 4 every hour	x 5 every hour	x 4 every hour

Another method is to immerse the limb in hot until it no longer feels hot and then in cold until it no longer feels cold. This can take 3 minutes and 1 minute respectively, with the cycle being repeated 5 times every hour, i.e. hot – 3 minutes, cold – 1 minute x 5 every hour until the desired effect is achieved.

Heat

> **"Now King David was old and stricken in years; and they covered him with clothes, but he could get no heat. Whereafter his servants said unto him: Let there be sought for my Lord the King a young virgin, and let her stand before the King, and be a companion unto him; and let her lie in thy bosom, that my Lord the King may get heat."**
> *Kings 1:1-2*

Since ancient times heat has been used as a form of treatment in one way or another. Today's technological advances may have refined certain apparatus and equipment but the basic objective remains the same, i.e. to raise the temperature. Is the above placebo, anecdotal and/or scientific? I'm also sure many sports people today would prefer the biblical approach rather than the more advanced forms of heating.

Types

Treatment can be by:

1. **IMMERSION**.
2. **IRRITATION**.
3. **CHEMICALS/LOTIONS**.
4. **ELECTROTHERAPY**.

- **SPRAYS, CREAMS, RUBS** can cause a superficial warming effect which temporarily mask any problems. In essence they can increase the reddish colouration of the skin surface and are known as rubefacients.
- **HOT WATER** can either be by immersion or via hot water bottles.
- **HEAT PACKS** (hydrocollator packs, chemical and commercial), these can take many forms from simple 'boil-in-the-bag' types to expensive hydrocollator pads which are applied after immersion in a heated tank.
- **PARAFFIN WAX** can be either by immersion or by coating the limb in the wax, which hardens and then covers to keep in the heat.
- **MASSAGE**. The effects have been previously discussed (*see Chapter 5, Part 4*). Other forms of heat prior to massage can act as an adjunct to treatment.
- **HEAT LAMPS**, ('**DIRECT HEAT**') infrared and ultra violet (UV) rays are; **REFLECTED, ABSORBED, REFRACTED** or **TRANSMITTED**. Any hot body will emit infrared rays e.g. sun, gas, coal, electric, radiator etc. Infrared can be considered as:

1. Type 1 – non-luminous (infrared only) or;
2. Type 2 – luminous (infrared + UV) – '**RADIANT HEAT**'.

Effects

These can be considered as:

1. **CIRCULATORY**.
2. **NEURAL**.
3. **EXCITORY**.

- **INCREASING METABOLIC ACTIVITY**.
- **INCREASING BLOOD FLOW** via **VASODILATION** and **RAISING TEMPERATURE**. The chemical irritants released at the site of injury are 'washed away' as a result of the increased blood flow. Repair cells i.e. white blood cells are brought into the area which increases oxygen and foodstuff demand.
- **REDUCING TISSUE VISCOSITY** therefore encouraging new healthy cell growth.

Heat also has:

- An **ANALGESIC EFFECT**, by stimulation of the neural receptors in the skin. The body's own opiate-like substances are released, e.g. endorphins and enkephalins (*see Chapter 5, Part 3*).
- **PSYCHOLOGICALLY** it feels good for most people.

- **LOOSENING SKIN** and **SOFTENING SUBCUTANEOUS TISSUE,** which aids stretching.
- **PROMOTING MUSCLE RELAXATION** which is considered a good adjunct to massage therapy.
- **DECREASING STIFFNESS IN JOINTS.**
- **HELPS PREVENT INJURY** and **IMPROVE PERFORMANCE** if used as part of a warm-up procedure but this will depend upon:

1. The method/modality used.
2. The size and type of tissue.
3. The depth of absorption of the specific radiation.
4. The duration of heating.
5. The intensity of the treatment.
6. The 'human factor'.

Contra-indications and Dangers

- **WARN/INFORM PATIENTS** as to what is being done to them. This has significant implications for **INFORMED CONSENT.**
- **TEST PATIENTS** as to the effects of applying heat as skin character varies.
- **SHOCKS.**
- **BURNS.**
- **HEADACHE.**
- **FAINTNESS.**
- **DIZZINESS – AFFECTING THE EYES.**
- **OVERDOSE.**

Goggles may be worn during the use of applying heat that is transmitted via rays. The following must be considered before applying heat:

- Oils or linament on the skin.
- The patient is under the influence of drugs or alcohol.
- The patient is an epileptic and/or diabetic.
- Skin diseases.
- Respiratory conditions.
- The patient has either a heart condition and/or blood pressure problems.
- The patient is in the late stages of pregnancy.
- Menstruation.
- Defective nervous system/blood supply, within a few hours of a heavy meal or conversely the patient has not eaten for a long time.
- Very old/young people are very wary of thermal treatment.
- Psychologically some people are just adverse to it.
- Recent injury with haemorrhage.

Don't forget that we are dealing with a person with a particular condition. Commonsense must be used allied to the skill and expertise of the therapist at that particular moment.

References

1.   Adams, N.: 1997. The psychophysiology of low back pain. Churchill Livingstone.
2.   Anderson, G. B. J., et al.: 1999. A comparison of spinal manipulation with standard health care for patients with low back pain. *New England Journal of Medicine*, 341, (19), 1426–31.
3.   Basset, F. H., et al.: 1993. Cryotherapy induced nerve injury. *The American Journal of Sports Medicine*, 20, 5, 516–518.
4.   Belitzky, R. B. et al.: 1987. Evaluation of the effectiveness of wet ice, dry ice and cryogen packs in reducing skin temperature. *Physical Therapy*, 67, 7, 1080–1084.
5.   Benjamin, H.: 1986. Everybody's guide to natural care. Health For All.
6.   Bogduk and Mercer: 1995. The selection and application of treatment, musculoskeletal physiotherapy. *Clinical Science and Practice*.
7.   Bonen, A., et al.: 1975. Lactic acid removal rates in controlled and uncontrolled recovery exercise. *Journal of Applied Physiology*, 39: 932–936.
8.   British Journal of Sports Medicine. 2000. The use of makeshift ice packs, 34:382–384 and reported in *SportEx*, 7, December/January 2001.
9   British Medical Journal: 2000. Sex specific painkillers. Found in *SportEX*, 5, April, 2000.
10. British Medical Journal: 1999. Chronic pain. Vol. 317.
11. Brodell, J. D., et al.: 1986. The Robert Jones bandage. *Journal of Bone and Joint Surgery*, 68–B, 5, 776–779.
12. Callaghan, M. J.: 1993. The role of massage in the management of the athlete: a review. *British Journal of Sports Medicine*, 27, 28–33.
13. Carper, J.: 1994. Food your miracle medicine. Rodale Press.
14. Chandler, Dr. M.: 1998. Healing arthritis the drug free way. Microleve International Ltd., Medical Researcher.
15. Covington, D. B. and Basset, F. H.: 1993. When cryotherapy injures. *The Physician and Sports Medicine*, 21, 3, 78, 82, 84, 93.
16. Dansak, D.: 1973. On the tertiary gain of illness. *Comp. Psychiatry*, 14, 523.
17. Davis, A. R., Rawls: 1974. Magnetism and its effects on the living system. Exposition Press, New York.
18. Davis, A. R., Rawls: 1985. The magnetic effect 4th Ed., Exposition Press.
19. Degenaar, J. J.: 1979. Some philosophical considerations of pain. *Pain*, 7: 281–304.
20. Des Maisons, K.: 1998. Potatoes not Prozac. Simon and Schuster.
21. Dodd, S., et al.: 1984. Blood lactate disappearance at various intensities of recovery exercise. *Journal of Applied Physiology*, 57: 1462–5.
22. Dornan, P. and Dunn, R: 1987. Sporting injuries. Chapter 3, 70–73.
23. Drew, T., Kreider, R., Drinkcord, B., et al.: 1991. Effects of post-event massage therapy on psychological profiles of exertion, feelings and mood during a four-day ultra endurance cycling event. *Medicine, Science, Sport and Exercise*, 23:97.
24. Duccini, K.: 2000. The natural medicine chest. Nurse, 1:4, *Pain Management*, 26–27 August.
25. Farry, P. J., and Prentice, N. G.: 1980. Ice treatment of injured ligaments: an experimental model. *New Zealand Medical Journal*, 91, 12–14.
26. Fordyce, W. E.: 1995. Back pain in the workplace. International Association in the Study of Pain Press, Seattle.
27. Fourcault, M.: 1973. The birth of the clinic. New York, Routledge.
28. Furnham, A., Forey, J.: 1994. The attitudes, behaviours and beliefs of patients of conventional v complementary/alternative medicine!
29. Gaeser, G.: 1984. Metabolic bases of post exercise oxygen consumption. *Medicine Science, Sport and Exercise*, 16, 29–43.
30. Goats, G. C.: 1994. Massage – the scientific basis of an ancient art: Part 1, Techniques. *BJSM*, 28(3) 149–152.

31. Goldstone, Professor, L.: 1999. From orthodox to complementary: the fall and rise of massage, with specific reference to orthopaedic and rheumatology nursing. *Journal of Orthopaedic Nursing*, (3) 152–159.

32. Goldstone, Professor, L.: 2000. Massage as an orthodox treatment past and present. *Journal Complementary Therapy in Nursing and Midwifery*, November.

33. Green, J.: 2000. Evidence-based medicine or evidence-informed osteopathy. *Osteopathy Today*, 6:04, 21–22, April.

34. Greenwood, H.: 2000. An investigation into the congruency of health beliefs between selected osteopaths and patients who visit them. *Bri. Ost. J.* XXII.

35. Hammond, Dr. P. L: 2000. 'Mind over matter.' ITV, February.

36. Hemmings, B. J., et al.: 1999. Effects of massage on physiological restoration, perceived recovery and repeated sports performance. *British Journal of Sports Medicine*, 34 (2): 109–115.

37. Holden, C.: 1978. Cancer and the mind: how are they connected? *Science 2000*: 1363.

38. Hopwood, A. L.: The social construction of illness and its implications for alternative and complementary medicine. *Complementary Therapies in Medicine*, 5, 152–155.

39. Hunter, G.: 1997. The timetable of soft tissue healing, OCPPP Seminar, Dynamic Tissue Healing and The Effects of Physiotherapy, Manchester.

40. Jenkins, Dr. S.: 2000. Demystifying the penalty kick. Found in *Sportscare Journal*, 20, Autumn, 2000.

41. Kamenetz, H. L.: 1985. History of massage. In Basmajian, J. V., ed.: Manipulation, Traction and Massage, 211–249.

42. Kane, M.: 1995. Measuring success: what of the patient's perspective. *British Osteopathic Journal*, XV1: 14–15.

43. Kirk, R.: 2000. Health promotion, part 5. *Osteopathy Today*, October, 2000.

44. Knight, K., and Londeree, B. R.: 1980. Comparison of blood flow in the ankle of the uninjured subjects during therapeutic application of heat, cold and exercise. *Medicine and Science in Sport and Exercise*, 12, 1, 76–80.

45. Knight, K. L.: 1989. Cryotherapy in sports injury management. *International Perspectives in Physiotherapy*, 4, 163–185.

46. Kowal, M. A.: 1983. Review of physiological effects of cryotherapy. *The Journal of Orthopaedics and Sports Physical Therapy*, 5:2, 66–73.

47. Lederman, Dr. E.: 1997. Fundamentals of manual therapy. 101, 218.

48. Macdonald.: 2000. Evidence-based osteopathy. *Osteopathy Today*. Vol 6:2, 6.

49. McLean, B. A.: 1989. The use of cold and superficial heat in the treatment of soft tissue injuries. *British Journal of Sports Medicine*, 23:1.

50. McMaster, W. C., et al.: 1978. Laboratory evaluation of various cold therapy modalities. *The American Journal of Sports Medicine*, 6:5, 291–294.

51. McWilliams, Dr. A.: 1998. Talkback. *Journal of The Backcare Association*, Winter.

52. Melzack, R., and Wall, P.: 1965. Pain mechanisms: a new theory. Science 150: 971–979.

53. Minor, M. A., and Sandford, M. K.: The role of physical therapy and physical modalities in pain management (review). Rheumatic Diseases Clinics of North America 0 AD/9, 25 (1): 233–248.

54. Minter, N.: 1999. To strap or not to strap – that is the question. Hockey Sport, March.

55. Munglani, R., Hunt, S., Jones, J. G.: 1996. Spinal cord and chronic pain. In *Anaesthesia Review*, Kaufman, L.: (ed.), 53–76, Churchill Livingstone.

56. Munglani, R.: 1997. Advances in chronic pain therapy with special reference to back pain. In *Anaesthesia Review*: Kaufman, G.: (ed), Churchill Livingstone.

57. Murray, M., and Pizzono, J.: 1998. Encyclopaedia of natural medicine. Churchill Livingstone.

58. Murthy, G., et al.: 1994. Intramuscular pressures beneath elastic and inelastic leggings. *Annals of Vascular Surgery*, 8:6, 543–548.

59. Ogden, J.: 2000. Health psychology: a textbook, 2nd ed. OUP.

60. Peterson, Dr. L., and Renstrom, Dr. P.: 1998. BASM Conference.

61. Peterson, Dr. L., and Renstrom, Dr. P.: 1986. Sports injuries. In Chapter 5, 156–164.

62. Quigley, T. B.: 1981. In *Sports Health*. Southmayd, and Hoffman.

63. Rang, D. R.: 1999. Pharmacology. Churchill Livingstone.

64. Raj, P.: 1995. Pain medicine. Mosby.

65. Rivenburgh, D. W.: 1992. Physical modalities in the treatment of tendon injuries. *Clinics in Sports Medicine*, 11:3, 645–649.

66. Roberts, J.: 1996. 'It's not what you do but the way that you do it.' *Inter Medica*, *Journal of the Guild of Osteopaths*, (Now the BOA).

67. Rodgers, W. S.: 1991. Explaining health and illness. Harvester Wheatsheaf.

68. Rucinski, T. J.: 1991. The effects of intermittent compression on oedema in post-acute ankle sprains. *The Journal of Orthopaedic Sports Physical Therapy*, 14:2, 65–69.

69. Ryan, A.: 1980. The neglected art of massage. *Physician and Sports Medicine*, 8:25.

70. Samples, P.: 1987. Does massage have a role in sports medicine? *Physician and Sports Medicine*, 15, 177–183.

71. Schrader, H., et al.: 1996. Natural evolution of late whiplash syndrome outside the medicolegal context. *Lancet 347*, 1207–1211.

72. Scott, Dr. J.: 1998. Pain explained. *Talkback, Journal of The Backcare Association*, Summer.

73. Shoemaker, J., et al.: 1997. Failure of massage to alter limb blood flow. *Medicine, Science, Sport and Exercise*, 29, 610–614.

74. Smith, B. H., Hopton, J. L., Chambers, W. A.: 1999. Chronic pain in primary care (review). *Family Practice*, 16 (5) 475–482.

75. Smith, L. L., Keating, M. N., Holbert, D., et al.: 1994. The effects of athletic massage on DOMS, creatine kinase and neutrophil count: a preliminary report. *JOSPT*, 93–99.

76. Stamford, B.: 1985. Massage for athletes. *Phy. and Sports Med.* 8:25.

77. Stapleton, C.: 1997. Multidimensional health focus of control and the osteopathic patient. A study to assess the difference between long and short term patients at the British School Of Osteopathy clinic. BSO student dissertation no. 53, 32–33.

78. Sternbach, R. A., et al.: 1977. On the sensitivity of the tourniquet pain test. *Pain, 3*, 105–110.

79. Stiles, L.: 2001. The right course, sports massage. *SportEx*, 7, 17–19, December/January 2001.

80. Tanner, J.: 1998. Illness gain and whiplash. Speaker's Corner, *Talkback, The Journal of The Backcare Association*.

81. Tortora, G.: 1998. Principles of anatomy and physiology. Wiley.

82. Van Wyk, R.: 1992. The bodywork knowledge base.

83. Vickers. 2000. Found in Touch Therapy by T. Field, Churchill Livingstone.

84. Walker, J. M.: 1984. *JOSPT*, 6:2, 89–94.

85. Wall, Professor, P.: 1999. Pain relief by manual therapy. London lecture, organised by the Centre for Professional Development in Osteopathy and Manual Therapy, 11.2.

86. Washnis, G. J., Hricak, R. Z.: 1993. Discovery of magnetic health, Nova.

87. Watson, T.: 1997. Electrotherapy for the promotion of healing – what to use and when. Dynamics of tissue healing and the effects of physiotherapy seminar, Manchester.

88. Wenberg, R., Jackson, A., Kolodny, K.: 1988. The relationship of massage to mood enhancement. *The Sports Psychologist*, 2: 202–211.

89. Werle, E.: 1972. On endogenous producing substances with particular reference to plasmakinins. In *Pain*, Williams and Wilkins, Baltimore.

90. Yeager, S., (ed.): 1998. New foods for healing, Rodale Press.

Bibliography

1. ACPSM: 1998. Guidelines for the management of soft tissue injury, September.

2. Athletics Weekly, 1989. Summer.

3. Austin, K., Gwynn-Bretton, K., and Marshall, S.: 1994. Illustrated guide to taping techniques.

4. Beiersdorf: Taping and strapping – a practical guide, 2nd ed.

5. Calliet, R.: 1984. Pain mechanisms and management. Running Magazine, August.

6. Colson, J. H. C., and Armour, W. J.: 1986. Sports injuries and their treatment.

7. Dornan, P., and Dunn, R.: 1987. Sporting injuries.

8. Electrotherapy explained, principles and practice.

9. FA basic and intermediate treatment and management of injury course notes.

10. Foster, A., and Palastanga, N.: 1985. Clayton's electrotherapy, theory and practice, 9th ed.

11. Fritz, S.: 1995. Fundamental of therapeutic massage, 1st ed. Mosby.

12. Grisogono, V.: 1984. Sport injuries, a self-help guide.

13. Hoskins, T. Michel, ed.: 1985. International perspectives in physical therapy. Pain, Churchill Livingstone.

14. Kennedy, R.: 1995. Mosby's sports therapy taping guide.

15. Kitchen, S., and Bazin, S.: Clayton's electrotherapy.

16. Macdonald, R.: 1994. Taping techniques – principles and practice.
17. Montag and Asmussen: 1986. Taping seminar, Beriersdorf
18. Peterson, Dr. L.: and Renstrom, Dr. P.: Sports injuries.
19. Southmayd, W., and Hoffman, M.: 1981. Sports health.
20. Sperryn, Dr. P.: 1983. Sport and medicine. Butterworth.
21. Textbook of orthopaedic medicine, 8th ed., 1, Diagnosis of soft tissue lesions.
22. Therapeutic modalities in sports medicine, 3rd ed.
23. Woodham, A., and Peters, Dr. D.: 1997. Encyclopaedia of complementary medicine. Dorling Kindersley.
24. Ylinen, Y., and Cash, M.: 1988. Sports massage.

Chapter 6
Rehabilitation

What could you achieve and what could you attempt to do if you knew you could not fail?

Part 1

Aims, Objectives, Principles and Practicalities

Chapter 2, Part 4, looked at exercise and some of its uses in treatment, training and rehabilitation. The following continues to develop the theme of rehabilitation, the aim of which should be:

> "To restore full functional fitness in the safest, shortest, time."
> *Smith, G. N., 1990*

The differences between rehabilitation of the non-sports person and the sports person are those of **DEGREE** and **SPECIFICITY**. With sports people, treatment must continue to a much greater degree or advanced level of activity and must be designed to meet the specific demands of the sport. An office worker with a hamstring strain needs rehabilitation that will probably cease when he/she can walk without a limp and manage stairs. Much more will be required for a county high hurdler or a hockey player with this condition.

The Rehabilitation Process

The process should begin at the moment of injury. It is particularly frustrating for a therapist to be faced with 'late' referrals where either nothing or the wrong things have been done over a period of time since the injury occurred. The programme should have the optimum balance of exercises to promote strength, endurance, flexibility, speed, co-ordination and proprioception, etc. Not only should the programme fit the sport, but for team games it should be tailored to the various positions. For example:

- Forwards in hockey or soccer will need running speed and endurance/stamina.
- Goalkeepers will need to be able to fall and recover quickly.
- Weightlifters may be aiming for power.
- Sprinters will require explosive speed.
- Marathon runners will want to rebuild stamina/endurance.

The Patient

Home advice is not home treatment. It is essential that the patient must be absolutely clear about:

- What to do.
- How to do it.
- When to do it.
- How many repetitions etc.

This avoids re-injury and a breakdown in communication between the therapist and athlete. The whole programme should be carefully progressed and altered on a **DAILY FEEDBACK** basis if necessary so that the injury is permitted to take a little more strain at each stage without being suddenly overloaded. For example, 70% of good limb – 75% of good limb – 80% of good limb, etc. until both limbs are equal, then both limbs are worked.

At each stage can the athlete produce the previous days work without any adverse reaction? Self-help rehabilitation programmes are based on stopping the programme at the first sign of pain. During rehabilitation the patient should be working in the **PAIN FREE** and **STIFFNESS AND MINIMAL DISCOMFORT** range.

The Rest of the Body

Part of any rehabilitation programme for any sports injury is to provide exercise to all the unaffected parts of the body, to maintain cardiovascular fitness, to keep the patient active and involved in his recovery. You can't tell a sports person to totally rest – they need active rest.

Rehabilitation Schemes

These can be used in conjunction with the different stages of rehabilitation which are to be discussed next. Many excellent texts can be referred to for advice on what types of exercises to include in the rehabilitation.

Stages of Rehabilitation

As previously discussed, injury is usually the result of abnormal movement patterns imposed on the musculoskeletal system and in treatment/rehabilitation we are looking to re-educate these patterns, to eliminate compensations, whilst considering what physiological movement patterns may be going on inside the body. **Every injury should be progressed through these stages** and they can be considered as progressions of treatment. There is a need to look at:

- Functional patterns of movement (active – dynamic) v physiological processes.
- Progressive overload.
- Sports specificity.

Early Rehabilitation – Working the Injury – 'The Clinical Stage'

This stage includes the period of time **when the limb is immobilised or the patient is non-weight bearing (NWB) or partial weight bearing (PWB) on crutches**. It is usually characterised by loss of normal movement, swelling, pain and a reduction in tensile, muscle strength. During this stage the rest of the body can be worked provided no adverse stresses or strains are placed on the injury site. Meanwhile specific local treatments are applied to the injury itself. **The starting point for treatment are the signs and symptoms of the lag phase.**

All activities should be done so that **full weight is not taken through any part of the injured limb at any time. At no time** during this stage **should competitive elements be introduced** that might involve physical contact. It is, however, possible to play games whilst sitting such as sit down volleyball, sit down cricket etc. It is the therapist's responsibility to ensure that no 'risk' situations arise. Although the least active stage, it is often the hardest to control as both the injured sportsman and the therapist must be constantly aware of risk situations and the possibility of accidents occurring from sporting mentality. At this stage, open chain, non-weight bearing, non-functional exercises can be used.

Intermediate Rehabilitation – 'The Conditioning Stage'

This **is the stage from PWB/FWB walking to the commencement of running**.

It begins when joints can pass through at least 2/3 full range, e.g. 90 degrees of flexion in the case of knee injuries, with no swelling or pain and the movement is smooth and co-ordinated without muscular judder.

This stage is complete when all swelling/effusions have receded, the full range of movement (ROM) has returned and co-ordinated muscle activities are possible including the beginning of running. Ease of movement (EOM) is improving in line with range of movement. Re-education in gait patterns and later running should be included during this period.

At the start of this period there should be no rotational work (twisting, turning), no single leg, weight-bearing movements (hopping) and no weights used on the injured limb but as this stage progresses, proprioceptive loss must be addressed. Multi-gym circuits are possible and hydrotherapy work is permissible as is cycling. **This is often the longest stage** and must be progressed through completely. **At this stage we are aiming for quality of work.**

NOTE: FWB in lower limb fractures is the stage of callus formation.

Late Stage Rehabilitation – 'The Fitness Stage'

This is the most dynamic stage so far, when the patient will have all activities increased, for example running, hopping and jumping for lower limb injuries and resisted progressive strengthening programmes for the upper limb. Muscles need strength, power, endurance and extensibility. There is more emphasis placed upon general fitness and such work is combined to include the injured limb with the rest of the body. **As an athlete becomes fitter and more confident, the degree of complexity and difficulty of specific exercises can be increased and the injured part is exercised without protection or limitation. It is at this stage that more functional work is introduced** that is related to the demands of the sport. **At first this functional work will be as closely controlled as possible.** However, relatively uncontrolled situations will eventually have to be used to ensure complete rehabilitation. Don't forget that fit to train is very different from fit to play (*see Chapter 1, Part 5*). Where sport specific, functional deficiencies are present, correction may be achieved by breaking down the movement pattern concerned into sub-components which are practised, improved and finally reconstructed, although **complete movement patterns are best to re-educate the motor system. REPETITION** is vital for skilled activity and is necessary to achieve skilled performance.

> **"A single motor event or manipulation will be lost very rapidly if not repeated over and over again."**
> *Schmidt, R. A., 1991*

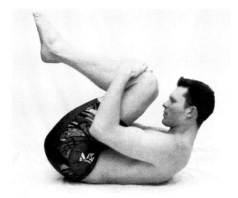

a

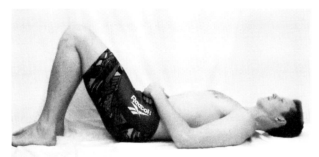

b

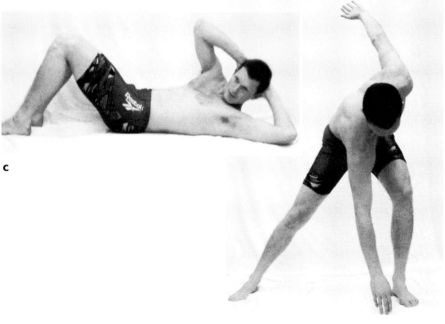

c

d

▲ *Figure 55a, b, c and d. Late stage rehabilitation.*

Also a single episode does not allow for tissue adaptation. Research into stretching **suggests four cycles** obtain the best results; the first four cycles will improve elongation by 80% at the musculo-tendon junction. **A cycle can involve 15 seconds stretch/15 seconds contraction**.

The transfer principles of learning any new skill or movement are not only very much related to repetition but also to the fact that the activity needs to be closely matched to the intended skill. In other words **goal orientated. This is a basic principle of rehabilitation**. An injury can be caused by **ABNORMAL MOVEMENT PATTERNS** on the musculoskeletal system (*Lederman, E., 1997*). This is because the afferent signalling discharge, signalling input is not totally synchronised with the efferent discharge response and the reactions and responses in certain situations are not fast enough. Therefore **NORMAL MOVEMENT PATTERNS** must be introduced to avoid re-injury. Final performance will be diminished if functional discrepancies are not identified and corrected. Therefore skill, hand and eye co-ordination is vital.

Progress to this stage too early is often a major cause for re-injury or regression. It is, therefore, important that patients do not tackle this stage too quickly. It is far better to spend longer in the intermediate stage ensuring that the quality of work is good, rather than to rush through to the late stage before the sports person is able to cope with the increased demands. It must be stressed once again that unless the walking pattern is correct, it will be impossible to run properly. Similarly, with all joint activities and gross movements (either lower or upper limb) the quality and co-ordination of the movements must be mechanically sound before the increased stresses and strains of the late stage are placed upon them. **In many cases, this stage should be one of the shortest and should be a stepping stone to the final stage to come, rather than a high hurdle that is not cleared comfortably, with failure resulting in a fall back to an earlier level**. Therefore careful assessment and realistic, unemotional decisions must be made before the sports person embarks on late rehabilitation. If in doubt, leave it out!

Circuits at this stage can be:

- Injury specific or cardiovascular fitness.
- Against the clock – speed.
- Fixed time – number of repetitions.
- One against one – competitive!

Remember that the guiding principles will be **DEGREE – INTENSITY – SPECIFICITY – OVERLOAD**.

Pre-discharge Rehabilitation – 'The Fitness Testing Stage'

This stage is arguably the most important as the aim should be to expose any weaknesses so that there is no breakdown in the skill factor. There is no treatment as such at this stage. This stage should be aggressive!

Some rehabilitation programmes stop when the patient can run but in sports rehabilitation the demands of the sport will dictate to what physical level of fitness the patient needs to be taken. Also it is important that besides being physically fit he/she is also mentally prepared. The psychology of sport is now a course of study in its own right. Therefore, **the aim of this stage is to include everything that the athlete's sport demands so that on his/her return to full, unrestricted training there is no breakdown. They must also be able to recover and reproduce similar activities on consecutive days. Then and only then can they be passed 'fit' to return to unrestricted training with confidence**.

It is important that the sports therapist is familiar with the demands that are likely to be placed upon the athlete when he/she returns to their particular sport so that cumulative stress is placed on the injured limb. The therapist should be optimistic, positive and encouraging during this stage as it is more than likely that the patient will be apprehensive and reluctant, to say the least. Quite often the patient will be asked to do activities which originally caused the initial injury and so it is vital that he/she is encouraged and helped over these hurdles and not pushed. If the rehabilitation process is 'rushed' then the athlete will arrive at this stage too soon and breakdown is inevitable which may lead to the therapist's credibility being lost. If short cuts are taken then injuries will re-occur and become chronic and then the athlete may suffer not only physically but also psychologically. Pre-discharge rehabilitation should aim to find an athlete's weakness.

Part 2

The Role of Proprioception in Treatment and Rehabilitation

The literature related to joint sensation can be found to be confusing in its definition of proprioception, the relationship of proprioception to and with kinaesthesia and both their physiological functions. Discovered in the 1890's proprioception is not one of the special senses of sight, smell, hearing, taste, touch or vestibular equilibrium but 'a secret/sixth sense' that collects information from the body, related to position tone and motion and automatically and unconsciously monitors and adjusts (*Montague-Cook, 2000*). The somatic senses usually described in the literature involve nociceptors, thermoreceptors and mechanoreceptors, which includes tactile and 'positional sense'.

Positional sense can be **STATIC**, which is conscious orientation of one part to another, or **DYNAMIC**, which is related to rate and direction of movement and which can be further sub-divided into **CONSCIOUS** (voluntary) and **UNCONSCIOUS** (involuntary/reflex). Lephart, S. M., 1995, talks about **CONSCIOUS PROPRIOCEPTION**, which is considered essential for proper joint function in sports, activities of daily living and occupational tasks, and **UNCONSCIOUS PROPRIOCEPTION**, which modulates muscle function and initiates reflex stabilisation. Returning to Lederman's thoughts on the cause of injury being abnormal movement patterns imposed on the musculoskeletal system he re-emphasises this fact by saying that sometimes non-productive motor activity produce abnormal postural or movement patterns. These patterns, with repetition, are stored and become part of that functional activity but are of no functional use, e.g. tensioning the neck and shoulder muscles when typing. This leads to fatigue and discomfort, affects skill and can eventually lead to structural damage. Therefore proprioception can be considered as:

> **"A complex neuromuscular process that involves both afferent input and efferent signals and allows the body to maintain stability and orientation during both static and dynamic activities. In general it is the process by which the body can vary muscle contraction in immediate response to incoming information regarding external forces."**
> *Hoffman, M., and Payne, V. G., 1995*

What are the **mechanisms** of proprioception and which **'reporting stations/receptors'** are involved in them? Classification of their exact locations and precise functions involves a certain degree of overlap and debate. What is not in dispute is that there are countless thousands of reporting stations in myofascial and articular components entering the spinal cord via the dorsal roots.

Mechanoreceptors/Proprioceptors

These represent:

> **"The complex, harmonious, delicately balanced orchestration of the contraction and relaxation of many muscles."**
> *Korr, Professor, I., 1976*

They form part of the balance/movement mechanisms of the internal environment. There are a variety of such receptors found in the skin, joints, tendons, ligaments and muscles that respond to internal, mechanical stresses and movement. The main categories of proprioception relate to joint position and motion, tendon tension and muscle length.

Proprioceptors in simplicity provide information on the position of the tissues, acting only in feedback but do not directly control motor centres. Instead they provide information so that the system can choose/decide on an appropriate response (*Lederman, E., 1997*).

EXTEROCEPTORS play an important part in motor activity and these receptors respond to external stimuli and physical movement in the environment, i.e. sound waves. **Vision and hearing,** balance and equilibrium sensors, found in the ear (i.e. perilymph, endolymph in the semicircular canals – the vestibular apparatus), are very much involved in the 'righting reflex' and balance – 60% of the balance mechanism coming from the eyes. **Balance** also relates to growth, the centre of gravity, size of the base and the relationship/interaction between the point of contact with the ground.

All this sensory information is added to by changes in the internal and external environment, i.e. conscious and unconscious thought, blood chemistry, carbon dioxide and certain ions, all of which the sympathetic nervous system is sensitive to.

Receptors Found in the Skin

These are activated by the skin being stretched and are either fast adapting or slow adapting. Their role is primarily one of proprioception to provide information in sensory events, e.g. contact, texture, slippage, fast gripping etc.

1. **FREE NERVE ENDINGS** are simple or complex, relate to the senses and are found in the dermis or epidermis.
2. **MEISSNER'S CORPUSCLES and MERKEL'S DISCS** are complex and relate to touch.
3. **END BULBS OF KRAUSE** respond to mechanical stimulation.
4. **HAIR FOLLICLES** respond to afferent stimulation.

Receptors Found in and Around the Joint

These detect mechanical changes in and around the joint itself and convey information about range, speed, pressure, position and pain.

1. **FREE NERVE ENDINGS** found inside the joint, are stimulated by excessive movement and pressure causing pain. **NOCICEPTOR** is the name given to free nerve endings that convey pain impulses.
2. **PACINIFORM ENDINGS** mediate pain and are non-adapting.
3. **RUFFINI'S CORPUSCLES** and **PACINI'S CORPUSCLES** are most complex and are found subcutaneously in the superficial fascia and respond to pressure.

Pacini's corpuscles are also found in periarticular connective tissue and are sometimes referred to as '**accelerator receptors**' as they report the rate of accelerated movement taking place. **Ruffini's corpuscles** are found strategically placed within the joint capsule and report direction and velocity of motion and position accurately. They also respond to muscular contraction, stretch and pressure, which alter joint capsule tension. Each is responsible for a 15–20 degree angle with an overlap. They are not easily fatigued and facilitate smooth as opposed to jerky movement. Their prime concern is a steady position and directional movement.

Receptors Found in the Ligaments

GOLGI END ORGANS help to let the body know where a joint is at any given moment, irrespective of any muscle contraction or activity. In simplicity they report position.

Receptors Found in Tendons and Muscles

1. **FLOWER SPRAY FIBRE** compensates for over reaction at primary receptors and also relates to conscious mind.
2. **ANNULOSPIRAL FIBRES** detect small changes in muscle length.
3. **GOLGI TENDON BODY/ORGANS/RECEPTORS** are found in the tendon, close to the musculo-tendon junction. They are connected to 10–20 muscle fibres and are not affected by mechanical events in other fibres. They reflect how hard a muscle is working via tension, force of contraction and load (*Houk, J., and Henneman, E., 1974*). It is not a stretch receptor as was once thought and they are stimulated better by active-dynamic more than active-static techniques (*Lederman, E., 1997*).
4. **MUSCLE SPINDLES** lie in parallel to muscle fibres, and are much more complex than the tendon receptors, sensitive, non-adapting receptors which will sustain a stream of influences on the motor system as long as they are stimulated. This influence is highly specific. The greater the spindle density, the finer the control. They detect, evaluate, report and adjust to the lengthening of the muscle in series, therefore setting tone. In other words they respond to lengthening and shortening, (*Houk, J., and Henneman, E., 1974*). **Stretch in series refers to the stiff elastic component. Stretch in parallel refers to soft elastic spring.**

There are two types of muscle spindle:

1. **PRIMARY NERVE ENDINGS** are **found in the central core of the spindle, which is non-contractile**. When a muscle is stretched the central non-contractile core is also stretched. They are dynamic, fast adapting and respond to deceleration, acceleration, length and velocity (rate of stretch).
2. **SECONDARY NERVE ENDINGS** are found in the **outer portion of the spindle, which is contractile**. They are located either side of the primary nerve endings but on average there is only one primary to one secondary. They are static, slow adapting receptors, which detect displacement of how much the spindle stretches in series, i.e. instantaneous muscle length.

Both joint and muscle receptors contribute to the sensory appreciation of joint position by modifying the function of each other (*Grigg, P., 1976; Baxendale, R. A., 1988*). **The muscle spindles and Golgi tendon organs are the two receptors that have most significance with regards manual therapy and proprioception.**

The motor system and its control is far more complex than was first imagined with the afferent receptors providing information but the control coming from the centre. Lederman, Dr. E., 1997 emphasises this by stating:

"Controlling the motor system via activation of peripheral mechanisms and segmental reflexes is equal to attempting to stop the flow of a river by throwing a pebble into it."

We are also told that descending motor drives can override or totally eliminate peripherally mediated activity.

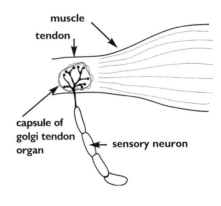

▲ *Figure 56. Golgi tendon organ.*

Joint afferents contribute to central nervous system function at three levels of motor control (*Lephart, S. M., 1995; Atter, T., 1997*):

1. **SPINAL LEVEL**, i.e. reflex muscle splinting for 'protection', with the muscle spindle playing a major role here. This is achieved by a sudden alteration in the joint position.
2. **BRAIN STEM**, to maintain posture and body balance. Input here is from the joint proprioceptors, vestibular centres in the ears and the eyes. Stimulation may be achieved via balance and postural acts, both with and without visual input.

3. **MOTOR CORTEX**, basal ganglia and cerebellum. Here motor commands for voluntary movement and actions are initiated, modified and programmed. The cerebellum modifying the intended movement initiated by the cortex and basal ganglia. This is known as the difference between actual and intended movement. These levels can be stimulated via conscious performance of joint position activity, especially at the end of the joint range.

It has also been found that relevant portions of the reporting station also reach and are utilised by the autonomic nervous system in tuning of visceral, circulatory and metabolic activity related to the musculoskeletal demands.

Affectation of Proprioceptive Mechanisms via Injury

Injury can directly, via direct trauma disrupting the soft tissues, or indirectly, via pressure from effusion or haemarthrosis, disrupt the sensory information provided by the mechanoreceptors, the 'positional sense', leading to; "deafferentiation, proprioceptive loss/deficit", (*Schutte, M. J., 1990; DeCarlo, M. S., 1986; Freeman, M. A., 1965*). Injuries to muscles and joints may lead to loss of proprioception leading to functional rather than structural instability (*Barrett, D. S., Cobb, A. G., Bentley, 1991*). An example of this is when the ankle keeps giving way but upon examination there is no structural damage to account for this.

With regards to pressure disruption, the receptors are intact but provide incorrect information, leading to inhibited function. The function of the vastus medialis muscle has been found to be inhibited by up to 60% by even a small knee infusion (*Young, 1987*). Also the affects of this proprioceptive defect on motor activity may take time to develop and isn't always readily apparent. If this disruption is not addressed during the rehabilitation process it can prove to be a major risk factor for re-injury (*Bunton, F. E., Pitney, W. A., Kane, A. W., et al., 1993*). It has been shown that proprioception can be improved through training.

The longer an athlete is unable to compete the greater the loss of proprioception (*Beard, D. J., 1994; Thara, H., 1986*). It is also expected that disturbance to sensory input from the muscoloskeletal system, whether local or general, will not only impair motor but other systems. Proprioceptive loss in the long-term is believed to contribute to progressive joint disease and muscle atrophy (*Skinner, H. B., et al., 1984*). Therefore proprioceptive training and rehabilitation should be an integral part of any rehabilitation programme.

The Practicalities

Proprioceptive rehabilitation programmes need to:

- Challenge, enhance, and improve the system (*Laskowski, E. R., 1997*).
- Stimulate the joint and muscle receptors in order to encourage maximum efferent discharge to the respective CNS level; **spinal level, brain stem level and motor cortex, basal ganglia and cerebellum levels** (*Lephart, S. M., 1995; Atter, T., 1997*).
- Be tailored to suit the individual.
- Be sport specific, thereby utilising the transfer principle of skill acquisition, i.e. adopting a downhill, crouched, skiing stance and doing lateral jumps, from one leg to the other as quickly as possible.
- Promote normal function of abnormal movement patterns and posture via visualisation, cognition, volition and repetition of the correct movement (*Lederman, E., 1997*). **Guided motor imagery** is to do with facilitating motor learning, relaxation, introspection and awareness. The patient is asked to visualise the movement pattern, with closed eyes, focusing on a point slightly beyond what is at present possible at the end range. After visualising this for several minutes the person physically goes through the movement. This can be used with active and passive techniques to try and improve **ROM** and **EOM**. **Mental imaging is an exception to the rule regarding repetition. Introspection and awareness** is related to the inability to relax and feel movement which will impede progress.
- Challenge dynamic joint stability by stork standing with and without the eyes open, using balance boards, Profitter etc.
- Include balance training, closed kinetic chain exercises (movement at one joint producing predictable movement at other joints usually involving axial forces), open and closed chain movements with manual resistance. For example, leg presses, double or single leg hops, bunny hops, bounding, stretch/shortening exercises, plyometrics, trampette work, ball throwing, squats, circle running, foot drill passes, figure of eight running, lateral bounds, single leg, balance board, Profitter, long jumps, vertical jumps, carioca/cross over walking etc.

Part 3

The Psychology of Injury and Rehabilitation

> **If you think you're beaten, you are,**
> **If you think you dare not, you don't,**
> **If you like to win but think you can't, you won't,**
> **If you think you'll lose, you've lost.**
> **Success begins with a person's will**
> **It's all in the state of mind.**
> *Unknown*

Whilst athletes can obtain a wealth of guidance regarding physical repair, they may receive little or no guidance at all regarding the psychological impact their injury may have on their emotions and behaviour. As recovery rates are very much dependent on the combined effects of these stressors it is important that both the therapist and athlete are aware of such. Response to injury can be considered in terms of:

1. Emotions and behaviour – how the 'athlete' reacts to the injury and this is related to the stress response.
2. Mediating factors – social and physical.

Emotions and Behaviour

Injury can have both positive and negative consequences. On the positive side it may provide 'time-out' from a physically demanding schedule and/or provide an opportunity for the individual to pursue other interests whilst recovering. However, there is ample evidence to show that injury can be accompanied by immediate increases in negative mood, depression, anxiety, irrational beliefs, loss of self esteem, feelings of isolation, sleep disturbance, lowered vigour and feelings of loss of control (*Lucas, T., 1998.*) These responses can be considered in stages or phases and are highly individualised but with little evidence to suggest athletes follow these reactions in a wholly sequential manner:

- Initially there is **SHOCK/DISBELIEF** especially if the athlete is not injury prone and this may lead to **DENIAL** that the injury exists and if it does it is not serious.
- Then there can be **ANGER**, either directed at anyone within their 'ring of influence', or at themselves for allowing it to happen.
- There follows a **BARGAINING MENTALITY**, where the injured party will try to establish control over the injury. If at this stage 'the athlete' doesn't believe in the treatment, rehabilitation or prognosis offered, he/she will lose interest and **NOT COMPLY** with what is asked of them. This is related to their perceptions, beliefs, expectations, anticipations and awareness.
- The longer the player is injured and not part of the team the greater the potential for them to become **ANXIOUS, DEPRESSED, TENSE** and **HELPLESS**, and at this point they may seek solace in alcohol/drugs to mask the problem.
- Finally, there is an **ACCEPTANCE** and **RESIGNATION** of what has happened to them and an **ADAPTATION** and **REORGANISATION**, in terms of what they need to do to overcome and recover from it.

Mediating Factors – Social and Physical

Factors Affecting Recovery

Apart from the physical pain of the injury and the physical rigours of the treatment/rehabilitation these specifically relate to the psyche and can be considered along with the complications of healing.

Somatotypes and Personality

Endomorphs, mesomorphs, ectomorphs, hypochondriacs, positives, negatives, placebos, nocebos, extroverts and introverts. Extroverts tend to be impatient whilst introverts indecisive, guarded and apprehensive. Placebos are positive, whilst nocebos negative, but there is no evidence to date that this is related to personality type.

Overuse injuries are most frequent in people with high levels of abdication of responsibility. Personality is very much involved with 'the athletes' perceptions, beliefs, expectations, anticipations and awareness of their injury. In much the same way as with pain they will have their own ideas as to its severity and this in turn will either motivate or demotivate them (*see Chapter 1, Part 5*).

Self-motivation/Self-esteem/Concept (Body Concept)

Again the opinions/views the athlete has of themselves and the threat to their life/sports goals and self-esteem will affect their attitude and approach/involvement to the treatment and rehabilitation programme. To deal with these factors the sports therapist needs to:

- Be **POSITIVE** and have **EFFECTIVE COMMUNICATION** skills. The sports therapist may have a constant battle against negativity.
- Be able to '**TRAIN THE BRAIN**', which will involve referral to specialist help.
- Put **EFFECTIVE SUPPORT SYSTEMS** in place – the better the support systems, the better the recovery.

The road to recovery is not straight,
Inch by inch is such a sinch,
Yard by yard is too hard,
There is no quick fix and short cuts should not be taken!

Strategies to Control the Stressors

How can we train the brain? The help of a sports psychologist can be of tremendous benefit, and they will use motivational and relaxation techniques involving:

- Imaging.
- Relaxation.
- Visualisation.
- Goal setting.
- Positive self-talking.
- Social support – vital as the injured athlete in professional sport can be somewhat of 'a leper' and a network of support people who have gone through similar experiences can help.

Psychological Readiness to Return to Competition

Here the sports therapist must be able to identify whether the athlete is in fact ready or just full of false optimism. Is the athlete:

- **CONFIDENT?** Both of the injury 'to stand up' and themselves. Fear of re-injury is a great psychological barrier and fear of failure or not being accepted 'back' especially after a time out of the game.
- **ANXIOUS?** Whilst a little apprehension is normal the 'athlete' must not have any negativity upon his return to competition.

The final decision is with the player, as long as they are not minors, but the therapist must know his/her charges to advise the athlete. We must also not forget that the return to competition is both physiological and psychological.

Part 4

The Role of Nutrition in Rehabilitation

Finally, if the role of the sports therapist is to restore full functional fitness in the safest and shortest time then the role that nutrition can play must not be forgotten in this restoration process. As Professor C. Williams, 2000, states:

"The role of sports nutrition in rehabilitation is another area of study that will require a multi-disciplinary approach in order to develop effective strategies for the benefit of injured athletes."
See Chapter 1, Part 5; Chapter 2, Parts 3 and 8; Chapter 3, Part 4; Chapter 8, Part 1.

References

1. Atter, T.: 1997. The importance of proprioception. OCPPP Seminar, Dynamic Tissue Healing and The Effects of Physiotherapy. Manchester, 15.11.97.
2. Barrett, D. S., Cobb, A. G., Bentley, G.: 1991. Joint proprioception in normal osteosynthetic and replaced knees. *Journal of Joint and Bone Surgery* (Br), 73 (1), 53–56.
3. Baxendale, R. A., Ferrell, W. R., Wood, L.: 1988. Responses of quadricep motor units to mechanical stimulation of knee joint receptors in the decerebrate coat. *Brain Res*, 453: 150–156.
4. Beard, D. J., Dodd, C. A., Trundle, H. R., et al.: 1994. Proprioception enhancement for ACL deficiency: a prospective randomised trial of two physiotherapy regimes. *Journal of Joint and Bone Surgery* (Br), 76(4): 654–659.
5. Bunton, E. E., Pitney, W. A., Kane, A. W., et al.: 1993. The role of limb torque, muscle action and proprioception during closed kinetic chain rehabilitation of the lower extremities. *Journal of Athletic Training*, 28(1):10:20.
6. De Carlo, M. S., Talbot, R. W.: 1986. Evaluation of ankle joint proprioception following injection of the anterior talofibular ligament. *Journal of Orthopaedic Sports Physical Therapy*, 8(2): 70–75.
7. Freeman, M. A., Dean, M. R., Hanham, R. W.: 1965. The etiology and prevention of functional instability of the foot. *Journal of Joint and Bone Surgery* (Br), 47: 678–685.
8. Griggs, P.: 1976. Response of joint afferent neurons in cat medial articular nerve to active and passive movements of the knee. *Brain Res*, 118: 482–485.
9. Henneman, E.: 1974. Peripheral mechanisms involved in the control of muscle. In *Medical Physiology*, edited by Mountcastle, V., Mosby.
10. Hoffman, M., Payne, V. G.: 1995. The effects of proprioceptive ankle disc training on healthy subjects. *Journal of Orthopaedic Sports Physical Therapy*, 21 (2): 90–93.
11. Houk, J., Henneman, E.: 1974. Feedback control of muscle. In *Medical Physiology*, 13th ed., edited by Mountcastle, V., Mosby.
12. Ihara, H., Nakayama, A.: 1986. Dynamic joint control training for knee ligament joint injuries. *Am. Journal of Sports Medicine*, 14(4): 309–315.
13. Korr, I.: 1976. The spinal cord as organiser of the disease process. Osteopathy 2000 Conference, London.
14. Laskowski, E. R.: 1997. Refining rehabilitation with proprioceptive training. *The Physician and Sports Medicine*, 25, 10, October, 1997.
15. Leach, R. E.: 1982. Overall view of rehabilitation of the leg for running. In Mack, R. P., (ed.) Symposium of the foot and leg in running sports, Mosby.
16. Lederman, Dr. E.: 1997. Fundamentals of manual therapy. 101.
17. Lephart, S. M., Fu, F. H.: 1995. The role of proprioception in the treatment of sports injuries. *Sports Exercise and Injury*, 1, 96–102.
18. Levin, S.: 1993. Early mobilisation speeds recovery. *The Physician and Sports Medicine*, 21, 8, 70–75.
19. Lucas, T.: 1999. The psychology of injury. Society of Sports Therapist Annual Conference, Wycombe Wanderers FC, May.
20. Montague-Cooke, B.: 2000. Osteopaths = conscious manipulators of the unconscious. *The Osteopath*, April.
21. Read, Dr. M., and Wade, P.: 1998. Sports injuries.
22. Schmidt, R. A.: 1991. Motor learning and control: a behavioural emphasis.
23. Schutte, M. J., Happel, L. T.: 1990. Joint innervation in joint injury. *Clinical Sports Medicine*, (2): 511–517.
24. Skinner, H. B., et al.: 1984. Joint positional sense in total knee arthroplasty. *Journal of Orthopaedic Research*, 1, 276–283.
25. Smith, G. N.: 1990. Sports therapy diploma course notes. Society of Sports Therapy.
26. Tyldesley, B., Grieve, G. R.: 1989. Muscles, nerves and movement: kinesiology in daily living. Blackwell Scientific, 268–284.
27. Williams, Professor, C.: 2000. Sport and exercise nutrition – sports nutrition – what will the future bring? *SportsCare News*, 18, Spring.
28. Young, A., Stokes, M., Iles, J. F.: 1987. Effects of joint pathology on muscle. *Clinical Orthopaedics*, 219 (June) 21–27.

Chapter 7
Legal, Professional, Ethical, Moral and Practice Management Issues

"None of us is perfect,
I for myself am peculiarly susceptible to draughts."

"I can resist anything but temptation."
Oscar Wilde

Part I

The Compensation Culture

In 1986, the Central Council for Physical Recreation estimated that in the UK alone, 22 million people participated in sport/exercise on at least one occasion per month, embracing all generations and for various reasons. Whilst this had, and still has, significant social and health implications for society, it is now seen, with an even greater emphasis on participation, as a growing source of income and increased workload for the legal profession. At present, the practice of sports therapy is not regulated by Statute, therefore anyone can call themselves a sports therapist! But like other professional groups seeking registration, this state of affairs will not be allowed to continue. At present, common laws affect the right of an individual to participate and practice and therefore a sports therapist must abide by the laws of the town/country in which he/she legally performs, practices or resides.

"Neither does the law of the land stop at the touch-line."
Payne, S. D. W., 1995

The legalities of sports therapy are no different to other professions. The therapist must be guided by his/her professional association with regards to a code of conduct, professional practice, discipline, advertising, insurance, ethics, morals, and patient care, as well as the common, civil and criminal laws of the land. The various ramifications of the legal system with all its technical jargon may seem of little relevance/significance to a person running onto a field of play. However, to ignore the law in today's compensation culture/climate would seem ill-advised.

"The great tragedy of science – the slaying of a beautiful hypothesis by an ugly fact."
Ologenesis and Abiogenesis, 1834/5

The legal system with regards to young children/minors must definitely not be overlooked; *loco parentis*, in place of the parent, applying to anyone accepting responsibility for the training, coaching and treating of youngsters in the absence of their parents/legal guardians. It is also true to say that the more successful or highly qualified a person becomes the higher the risks and responsibilities. Sportsmen and women are now being paid weekly wages, plus fringe benefits, which the rest of the population would gladly accept as their annual salary. The cost of financial compensation if a sports therapist was found negligent in their duty of care in looking after such sports people and their treatment led to career threatening

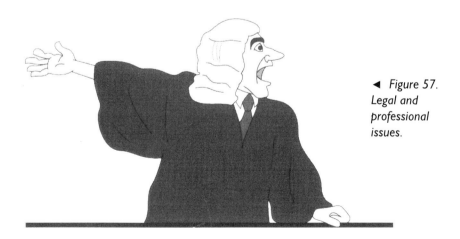

◀ *Figure 57. Legal and professional issues.*

injuries then the professional, personal and financial loss to the therapist would be highly damaging. Damages can come out of bodily injuries and mental/emotional, injury, illness, disease or death.

> **"Liability issues have dramatically changed the focus of the sports industry. Liability for a sports-related injury can extend far beyond the school or team to reach individuals such as players, coaches, and even officials. Claims often are not limited to only medical or property damages but include claims for pain and suffering, loss of society and companionship, wage loss, loss of earning capacity, and possibly punitive damages. Claims can be made by others besides the injured party, such as the injured party's spouse and children, or even the injured party's own insurance company. The old saying 'win at all costs' has new meaning when liability issues are considered. Perhaps the saying should be 'win if you can avoid all costs' in today's litigious society."**
>
> *Green, J. C., 1998*

Whilst all along this text has stated that it is not and does not purport to be a medical document it nevertheless is virtually impossible to isolate any health related course from its medical implications. In fact during the planning, preparation and writing of it no attempt has been made to do this and reference to medical matters, where appropriate, have been included. Neither is it the intention of this chapter to consider every conceivable permutation of what might happen in the life of a sports therapist that has legal implications. However, hopefully it offers help, advice and guidance to make the therapist more aware and strongly emphasises the importance of many of the issues discussed. Don't forget though that if people go looking for problems they will always find one! It is true that although risks for complementary practitioners are much less than for the medical practitioner they still, apart from drugs and surgery, fall into the same categories.

In these days of accountability, registration, protected titles, NVQ's and the standardisation of many competencies required to carry out 'a job' it is important that the sports therapist is aware of not only these risks but also his/her responsibilities and duties.

Part 2

Terminology and Practical Issues

Here it is intended to consider in general, various issues pertaining to sports therapy, keeping, wherever possible, jargon and terminology in layperson terms. It is relevant to consider not only the difference between the meanings of certain terminology, words and titles, but also to highlight the fact that some words are deemed 'protected titles'. Only those qualified to do so or belonging to a professional body can use them, i.e. doctors, chartered physiotherapists and osteopaths (*May 2000*).

A PROFESSION is a body of specialised knowledge directed towards an individual problem whose function it is to take over and share such a problem. A sports therapist in practice will in fact be two persons, a private and a professional person, the two being indivisible. Professionalism is something that is acquired during long periods of training and development and there are no short cuts to acquiring it.

ETHICS AND MORALITY are issues that are concerned with right and wrong conduct. The boundaries are difficult to define because they are related to individual value concepts. They are difficult to deal with as they involve some perplexing questions that ultimately relate to why people do what they do. They become even more important when discussing the standards of behaviour expected from qualified members of a profession.

> **"Because sport is competitive it is full of opportunities to bend or break the rules in order to gain an advantage. This means the coach, athlete, official and administrator is constantly faced with moral questions; should I do this or that?"**
> *Butcher, Dr. R., 1999*

A sports therapist working in such an environment will be aware of such conflicts and will be, at some stage, subjected to the issues involved. For example, Should I cut corners to get this athlete fit? Should I let him/her compete knowing that he/she may breakdown?

Dr. Robert Butcher identifies certain morally sensitive issues that although related to coaching can also be considered in therapy. These issues concern making decisions in relation to; fairness, respect for yourself, other people's interests/autonomy and competition. Or issues that could result in harm which could be physical, mental, emotional and financial. An athlete's experience and enjoyment of sport and self-esteem/life can be greatly enhanced or destroyed by his/her relationship with 'significant others'. These experiences being:

> **"Characterised by close physical and emotional relationships and distinct power dynamics."**
> *Antonia, K., 1999*

This is particularly important when working with children (*see Chapter 1, Parts 5 and 6*). It is therefore essential that all working as part of a team do so by supporting the concepts/values/ideals of responsibility, integrity, trust, competence, effectiveness, efficiency, equality of opportunity, fair play, professionalism, equity, sportsmanship, safety, encouragement, respect, effective communication, positivism, etc. This should be through a code of conduct/ethics, to which all members are legally duty bound to respect and uphold. We all have/owe a **DUTY OF CARE** to anyone, which means that we are responsible to anyone who we can reasonably foresee may be affected by our actions. There is no room for the assumption that allegations can be swept aside or that they will go away. Tort, or civil wrong doing, can easily become an issue when dealing with minors as well as adults. As previously mentioned in sport such a duty of care applies to participants, referees, competitors, organisers etc. In treatment the question that arises is do we have a duty of care to the person who pays or the beneficiary of the treatment? Injury arising from a violent act executed deliberately and/or recklessly is actionable in both civil and criminal codes.

> **"The skills in treating, alleviating, counselling and mentoring can be learnt, developed and certificated by a training body and enshrined in a code of ethics and conduct. But an inability to carry such principles out – or an allegation by someone else that they were not – puts the issue squarely into a legal arena, where a different set of ground rules can operate."**
> *Balen, D., 1995*

NEGLIGENCE is where a person sues for a breach of a legal duty of care, although three points need to be proven:

1. The defendant (the perpetrator of the act) was under a duty of care to the plaintiff (the person who was acted upon).
2. There has been a breach of that duty.
3. That as a result the plaintiff suffered damage.

With regards to football and 'The Common Law of Negligence,' which was established over a hundred years ago, one of the first recorded cases happened in the mid-1990's. Gordon Watson of Bradford City, sued Kevin Gray of Huddersfield Town for a tackle which Watson claimed could have ended his career.

Damages can be recovered for playing field injuries caused by participants via:

- Trespass to a person.
- Negligence.

- Nuisance, which can be public or private. Public nuisance referring to an unlawful act or omission that endangers or interferes with the lives, safety or comfort of the public in general.

TRESPASS is related to the invasion of a person's personal boundary. Such a **BOUNDARY** can be related to a person's space approximately one arms length away. Problems associated with invasion into this space are related to the **REASONS AND INTENT**. Three possible forms can be considered:

1. **ASSAULT** is an act that causes another person to apprehend immediate and unlawful personal violence. Doing something physical to someone without consent is assault.
2. **BATTERY** is when force is applied, however slight, to a person in a hostile manner or against his/her will.
3. **FALSE IMPRISONMENT** is holding a person against their will and/or making them do actions they don't wish to do. When someone makes an appointment to see a sports therapist in his/her practice are they doing so under their own free will or are they being co-erced? (e.g. someone made it for them).

Within the context of contact sports, the defences against action for trespass are:

1. Self-defence, where a person can defend themselves against assault and battery provided the defence is reasonable, proportionate and commensurate to the attack.
2. Consent, where no legal wrong can be done to a willing person. However, whilst participants may be aware of the risks and dangers of participation they can not be expected to consent to wrong doings outside the accepted rules and standards of behaviour.

   "There is a legal concept of implicit acceptance of risk of injury, provided the risk is a known one and occurs within the rules and practices of the sport concerned. Spectators, competitors and organisers of sporting events have legal duties towards one another and consent to risk of injury is implied only if these duties are fulfilled."
   Smith, G. N., 1990/97

Unfortunately the practicalities of this are that in today's society everyone feels they have a right to do what they want, to whom they want, with scant regard to the consequences. Statements of what constitutes fair play and what is and what is not acceptable behaviour/conduct are pointless if those subscribing to them only pay 'lip service' to their significance. Sport is a reflection of society and sadly, not only in the past but also the present, has been seen by the general public to condone unacceptable standards of behaviour justifying it as part and parcel of the game.

> **"Normal codes of behaviour do not apply to footballers so why should they apply to fans? Footballers can beat their wives, get coked up in night clubs, behave like animals and drive as fast as they like, and nothing is done. Fans can be stabbed or beaten to death and still the game must go on............it is a cynical business from top down. It is about what goes on in peoples' bank accounts, not their hearts. It is not about the playing of the game but about winning. These are the values that it now encapsulates, let's not fool ourselves any longer."**
> *The Mail on Sunday, 2000*

Is this sensational journalism, more fuel for the discussion on sporting mentality or the realities of certain sports going into the new millennium?

A CODE OF ETHICS/CONDUCT is designed to ensure that members maintain the highest levels of responsibility in their everyday lives and avoid litigation. This code is not only useful in clarifying goals and ideals of acceptable behaviour/conduct but also ensures that benefits to the participants are maximised and the risks/injuries are minimised. Remembering that harassment and abuse in sport can be physical, mental, emotional/psychological and sexual. A code of conduct/ethics allows any problem to be integrated without surprise. How best can a therapist perform their duty of care and how can this be achieved?

A code of ethics/conduct can include the following, where the term athlete is used to infer all people involved in sporting activity who comes into contact with the sports therapist. This list is not definitive:

- Athletes should take precedence whilst considering all other considerations.
- Make the care, protection and health of the athlete priority one.
- Act with the athletes' welfare at heart.
- Treat every athlete politely and considerately and don't abuse your authority to jeopardise the therapist/athlete relationship.
- Don't do anything to make the athlete feel threatened.
- Respect an athlete's dignity, privacy, needs and personal persuasions. A sports therapist is responsible for finding not only the '**COMFORT ZONE**' of their athletes/patients but also themselves. This requires self-analysis and introspection.
- Be yourself whilst appreciating you are a private and professional person. There is a need to be honest in appreciating personal prejudices, fears, behaviours, likes/dislikes etc. Only then can the individual needs of others be respected.

- Only provide treatment for which you are trained and qualified to give.
- Never take unnecessary risks in the treatment of an injury.
- Inform, advise and take preventative measures if necessary on potential dangers to all involved in the sporting experience.
- Give the patient adequate information in order for him/her to make an informed decision about subsequent future actions.
- Communicate regularly with the club, team, medical officer and the player's own GP regarding injuries and treatment.
- Maintain good medical records.
- Exercise clinical judgements to the highest standards of which the therapist is capable.
- Insist on high standards of personal and communal hygiene.
- Be constantly aware of the dangers facing children and adolescents in combat/contact sports and try to minimise such risks.
- Avoid any emotional involvement with the athlete. In the past, those involved with sport running off with other people's wives has been shown to be a bad career move! This statement has wide and deep implications of problems relating from sexual misdemeanours to taking on board a person's personal problems. Unless qualified to do so, advice and help should only be offered but emotional involvement should be avoided. Referral to a psychiatrist, social worker and/or counsellor would appear to be much more appropriate. There are well publicised accounts of athletes needing help for marital problems and from drug and alcohol abuse. In order to fulfil such duties the therapist should ensure they possess the necessary knowledge, skills and expertise of the particular physical and mental demands/risks required in sport.

Sport needs to be seen to severely deal with breaches of such codes, whether perpetrated by irresponsibility, arrogance, ignorance or just illegally, via an effective complaints procedure in accordance with the principles of natural justice, the laws of the land and which deals with the rights of all parties concerned.

How Should One Behave and Present Oneself?

Following on from the issues related to ethics and morality this question relates to acting in accordance with a practice accepted as proper by a responsible body of opinion skilled in that particular art. The issue is what constitutes proper in terms of usual and normal practice. Also a practitioner has to demonstrate acting with reasonable care and skill and taking whatever reasonable precautions where appropriate in the situation. Again the issues here are what constitutes reasonable. If a person is going to gain respect there is a need to consider various social skills, which in the clinical situation, has much to do with **BODY LANGUAGE, via the choice of words and tone of the voice:**

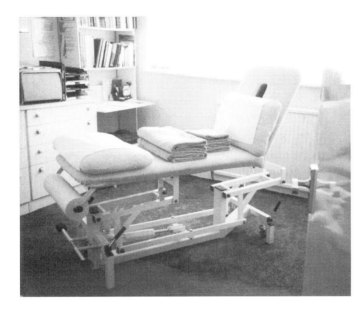

◀ *Figure 58.*
Creating the right
impression is vital.

- By using simple/plain words and by not trying to impress! The patient may not have studied anatomy and physiology.
- By actively listening to what the athlete says – all the clues are then available to solve the problem.
- By asking the right kind of questions and then actively listening – the skill is when to interrupt without being rude (*see Chapter 4, Part 2*).
- By talking to a patient not gossiping.
- Always seek permission, **NEVER ASSUME**. It makes an ass of you and me! A patient upon presentation has only consented to a consultation; if you wish to examine and treat you must seek **INFORMED CONSENT**, i.e. I would like to examine you. Would you take your clothing off? etc. **GIVE OPPORTUNITY TO CONSENT**. The Patient's Charter states:

  "you have the right to any proposed treatment, including risks and alternatives, clearly explained before you decide whether to agree."

- Be positive but never make sweeping statements, e.g. "we'll soon have you right in a few days. Hip replacements are wonderful, I think you should have one."
- By explaining to the patient what it is that is being done or would like to be done. **TRUST AND CONFIDENTIALITY ARE VITAL**.

Your **facial expressions** should be largely reflex and your **manner, gesture and movement** should be unthreatening and non-suggestive. This will help to relax and put the patient at ease. Professional distance is important without creating a barrier. Each patient should be given individual attention. Be confident and in control.

Your **dress and appearance** should reflect a professional image although there are those who feel it is not what people wear but how they behave that really matters. **FIRST IMPRESSIONS ARE VITAL – YOU DON'T GET A SECOND CHANCE TO MAKE A FIRST IMPRESSION**. Personal hygiene is, without question, of utmost importance, hair, nails, facial hair etc. Creating the right impression is vital. **Your job title should reflect the nature of your work, and your training/qualifications for that particular work. For example:**

PHYSIOTHERAPY in simplicity means treatment by physical means and, as such embraces treatment by massage, exercise, light, heat, cryotherapy, electrotherapy, hydrotherapy etc.

MASSAGE is a definite art/science involving skilful management by the masseurs'/masseuses' hands. It also involves more than just massage movements.

Practitioners/therapists are quite rightly proud of their roots, knowledge, skills and expertise **but must only call themselves what they are trained and qualified in**. This also applies to the name you give to your premises and the inferences this gives in relation to what knowledge, skills and expertise you are offering, e.g. sports injury clinic (*see Chapter 8, Part 2*).

This brief explanation is not included to denigrate or promote one therapy more than another, but to keep in mind **THE NEED TO EARN THE RESPECT AND CO-OPERATION OF FELLOW PRACTITIONERS AND PROFESSIONALS**. Respect, however, has to be earned and is not achieved by waving diplomas around, wearing a white jacket/tunic/tracksuit or by telling everyone how good we are and how poor someone else is. Is that arrogance, ignorance or is it both?

FULL DISCLOSURE is the provision by the therapist of the complete picture of the known facts so that 'the athlete' can give their consent or refusal to treatment. This must not be confused with disclosure to third parties relating to record keeping (*see Chapter 7, Part 3*). Refusal can also apply to the sports therapist if the athlete is not honest.

INFORMED CONSENT is giving permission for treatment to start or continue after being furnished with all the known relevant facts and infers respect for that person.

MALPRACTICE is acting in a manner that is not in accordance with a professional code of ethics and conduct.

SLANDER refers to maliciously spoken defamation of a person's character/reputation in front of a third party.

LIBEL refers to maliciously written defamation of a person's character/reputation.

What Are the Needs of a Sports Therapist?

Whilst considering some of the duties expected of a sports therapist and in the absence of guidelines from any one specific governing body it is intended to use a modification of the advice given by the General Medical Council in November 1995 to doctors. Much of this is relevant to complementary practitioners.

When discussing needs we must consider these also as potential risks, as failure to carry them out can lead to problems and possible litigation. All of the needs become relevant in **LITIGATION** cases where there has been injury and questions raised related to:

- Was the injury due to someone's actions or lack of care etc?
- Was someone negligent in carrying out their duty of care etc?
- Is compensation relevant?

There is a Need to Examine Properly

There is a need to follow principles and a set procedure and to use these as a matter of routine, even if this differs from fellow practitioners. It is the procedure that is relevant not the variation (*see Chapter 4*). The details/results of such should be fully documented (*see Chapter 7, Part 3*).

There is a Need to Diagnose

Sports therapists are not and will not be qualified to medically diagnose but the fact remains that correct diagnosis is the key to successful treatment. However, sports therapists are entitled to an informed opinion/hypothesis and working diagnosis based on the information obtained during the examination and assessment.

There is a Need to Treat

Legally a therapist is obliged to give the best treatment of which they are trained, qualified and capable of giving, irrespective of race, creed, colour or social status. The athlete/patient should never be allowed to dictate the treatment. It should never be agreed and/or accepted to treat a patient that is being treated by a fellow professional/colleague unless referred by them or without their permission. The treatment should be considered reasonable and appear reasonable and the patient should benefit from it. A cure should never be promised.

RIGHT OF REFUSAL – a person has a right to stop treatment at any time. Conversely a sports therapist may refuse to accept a person for treatment if there is **JUST AND REASONABLE CAUSE**. However, failure to treat a condition that may benefit from a therapy could lead to legal or disciplinary measures.

There is a Need to Obtain Consent/Permission to Examine and Treat

A person who makes an appointment has only consented to a consultation. Permission must be sought to examine and treat. However, there is an **IMPLIED CONSENT** if a person makes an appointment with a sports therapist that they know what type of therapy is on offer.

There is a Need to Warn of Risks

Outrageous claims should not be made but the patient should be informed of the possible side-effects/benefits of the therapy. A therapist is not negligent if they act in accordance with a practice accepted as proper by a responsible, professional body, even though other therapists may adopt a different practice.

There is a Need to Communicate Properly

- By talking to athletes/patients about findings, problems, treatments and techniques – **INFORMED CONSENT**.
- By actively listening to patients and respecting their views. After all without them there is no one to manage/treat/advise/rehabilitate/coach/train etc.
- Avoid innuendo and suggestions.
- Give patients information in a way they can understand.
- Respect the rights of patients to be fully involved in decisions about their care.
- Be prepared to justify your actions to them.
- Recognise the limits of professional competence.
- Keep professional knowledge and skills up-to-date. Remember expertise is not a static quality but a never-ending process of learning, modification and change.
- Maintain the standard of performance by taking part regularly in educational activities which relate to work and by keeping knowledge, skills and expertise up-to-date throughout your working life via continuing professional development.

- Be honest and trustworthy.
- Respect and protect confidential information.

There is a Need to Consider/Respect Confidentiality

In England, the law courts usually respect the confidentiality of communication between a client and his/her lawyer but not necessarily between a patient and his/her therapist. Sports therapists have a duty to keep confidential all information about a patient given to them in good faith:

- Make sure personal beliefs do not prejudice patient care.
- Act quickly to protect patients from risk if there is good reason to believe that you or a colleague may not be fit to practice.
- Avoid personal relationships with patients – keep a professional distance.
- Avoid abusing a professional position.
- Be willing to consult fellow practitioners.
- Work with fellow practitioners in ways that best serve patient's interests by arranging investigations or treatment where necessary.
- Serve patient's interests.
- Keep fellow practitioners informed when sharing the care of patients.
- Do not be critical of other practitioners.

There is a Need to Keep Full Medical Records

The quality of kept records can make the difference between being found negligent or not.

There is a Need to Refer Patients

A sports therapist must have the professional integrity and honesty to recognise when he/she should refer the patient to another practitioner. Sometimes the failure of all therapists is to believe their therapies are always beneficial for everyone. Remember that expertise is a never-ending process of learning, modification and change. **Success in practice is dependent not only on who and how you treat but also on those you don't.**

- Do not entice patients away from other practitioners.
- Do not treat a patient being treated by a fellow practitioner unless asked to do so.
- Carry out an adequate examination and assessment of the patient's state of health.

Part 3

The Importance of Record Keeping

Therapists are required to record their activities:

- For personal use; especially for personal protection in the event of litigation.
- For legal requirements.
- For statistical records.
- For educational purposes.
- For insurance purposes.
- For professional requirements.
- For ethical requirements.
- For research purposes.
- As information for further planning, treatment, rehabilitation and training.
- To assist other practitioners taking over/involved in treatment, i.e. a multidisciplinary approach.
- To critically assess techniques and standards involved in treatment/rehabilitation.

Adequate records are important as they can provide for a logical approach to patient care and improve quality of practice.

> **"Case notes are intended to prevent problems rather than cause them."**
> *Medical Defence Union, 1996*

What Records/Documents Should Be Kept at the Office/Clinic

The taking of, keeping of and storage of written records are essential in running a business. Today many sports are considered a business and many sports people consider training as going to work! Depending on what type of record is kept will be determined by the kind of business. In physical therapy, medical records must be kept regarding the patient (**THE CLINICAL SIDE**) and non-medical records must be kept regarding the financial aspects (**THE OFFICE SIDE**). In sports therapy records must also be kept relevant to that sports governing body.

The Clinic

Medical records and documents need to be kept to record:

1. Personal data.
2. Medical history.

3. Primary complaint.
4. Secondary complaint.
5. Examination and assessment details/decisions made.
6. Treatment record/information given to the patient.

They must possess:

- Subjective information.
- Objective information.
- Positive as well as negative findings.
- Routines and procedures.
- No judgements of a personal nature (*see Appendix 4*).

They must:

- Be confidential – **CONFIDENTIALITY** is **VITAL**.
- Be clear, understandable, contemporaneous, relevant, concise, comprehensive and accurate.
- Follow a standard format, demonstrate key points, record relevant information and retain meaning.
- Satisfy legal requirements. Remember everything that is written down has legal implications. If it is not written down it is presumed that it has not been done.
- Be securely stored in accordance with existing policies and current legislation. If stored on computer the data must be registered under the 1984/98 Data Protection Act. A one key locked storage system is advised, written up within 24 hours of an examination/assessment and kept for a minimum of 5 years to 8 years, as are X-rays, after the conclusion of treatment. Records relating to children and the young must be kept until their 25th birthday or 8 years after the last entry if longer.
- Obstetric records (the care of women during pregnancy) should be held for 25 years. A person can sue for negligence even after 10 years and with regards a minor there is no time limit.
- The records can only be released with a patients' permission although the patient has not got an automatic right to see the notes if the practitioner thinks it may be detrimental for them to see them, i.e. physical or mental distress.

"There is no place for humour in medical records."
Medical Defence Union, 1996

NOTE: Ownership of information is a tricky issue with various agencies having claim to it, e.g. courts and/or lawyers.

The following circumstances permit **DISCLOSURE**:

1. Patient consent. However, when disclosure is required by either the law or the order of the court this is not required.
2. In the patient's interest or if it is impossible to obtain consent.
3. The law requires, e.g. certain diseases.
4. When there is a duty to society, e.g. a serious crime has been committed. **Interest to the public and in the public interest, are not the same thing. Also, in the public interest does not require patient consent**.
5. To prevent serious risk to public health.
6. For research if appropriate and approved by an ethics committee. It must be appreciated that if information is shared it may be passed on.

Medical Records and the Law

There are three Acts of Parliament which give patients certain rights with regard to any medical notes, records or information which has been written about them or which is held on computer. However, at this moment in writing, these rights are balanced against the therapist's right to only allow the seeing of such information at their discretion.

The Medical Records Act 1988

- The patient must give consent for a **MEDICAL REPORT** to be given to a third party (e.g. a solicitor).
- The patient must have access to any **MEDICAL REPORT** written on their behalf by a practitioner.
- The patient has the right to request any alterations to the report before it is sent off.
- If the practitioner refuses, the patient may add to the report his own statement regarding her/his disagreement.
- The patient may request a copy of the report for which a fee may be charged (i.e. £10).
- Access to the report may be denied by the practitioner on health grounds, i.e. physical or mental distress.

Access to Health Records 1990

- The patient has the right to see his written health records – but only back to November 1991.
- Application should be in writing. Parents may apply for access to their child's records provided the child has consented or is incapable of understanding. Application by minors under 16 years of age will be considered.

- A fee of up to £10 may be charged.
- Access should be granted within 40 days or 21 days for information recorded within the last 40 days.
- Information may be withheld if it is felt that to include it would be harmful. Also there is no legal duty to inform the patient that information has been withheld.

The Data Protection Act 1984 (Updated in 1998 and implemented on 1.3.00)

The Act refers to not only personal data held on equipment operating automatically but also manual files, e.g. clinical and hand written notes. Personal data is information about living, identifiable individuals, and can be as little as just a name and address. (This Act is not specific to medical records). The Act is administered by the Data Protection Registrar which is an independent officer who reports directly to Parliament. It gives the 'data subject' rights and ensures that proper practices are followed by the 'data user'.

A sports therapist holding any personal data (even just a list of names and addresses of patients) with or without medical notes must register. The registration fee is currently £75 for a 3-year period. It is a criminal offence not to register. The Registrar regularly prosecutes, with fines of up to £5,000. Using a computer only for text processing (writing letters to doctors or patients), keeping your business accounts, or calculating wages for your staff need not be registered.

Once registered, a person must comply with the eight data protection principles of good practice. Failure to comply is a criminal offence. The eight original data protection principles state that data must be:

1. Obtained and processed fairly and lawfully.
2. Held only for the lawful purposes described in the data user's register entry.
3. Used only for those purposes, and disclosed only to those people, described in the register entry.
4. Adequate, relevant and not excessive in relation to the purpose for which they are held.
5. Accurate and where necessary, kept up-to-date.
6. Held no longer than is necessary for the registered purpose.
7. Accessible to the individual concerned who, where appropriate, has the right to have information about themselves corrected or erased. Patients may apply in writing for access to all data held on them so they may have it corrected or deleted where appropriate (subject access) if it is causing, or is likely to cause damage, physical or mental distress to them or another or is unwarranted. This

does not apply if a person has consented to the processing of such information; the processing is necessary for entering information; the performance of a contract or compliance with legal obligations or to protect the therapist's vital interests. Response to such a request must be within 40 days. A fee of up to £10 may be charged by the 'data user'.

8. Surrounded by proper security.

The increased patient's rights afforded by the 1998 updated Act extends the definition of processing to include obtaining, recording, holding, carrying out any operations or set of operations on the information or data. This includes the organisation, altering, blocking, erasure, obstruction, retrieval of information or data, as well as simply storing or retrieving it. As a result, greater obligations are now imposed on the 'data controllers' when processing or authorising processing.

Referral to the relevant professional association is recommended for a more detailed analysis of the Act. There is only one Registrar for England and one data protection office, but they will answer any personal queries, and send registration forms on request. The address is:

The Office of the Data Protection Registrar
Wycliffe House
Water Lane
WILMSLOW
Cheshire
SK9 5AF
Tel: 01625 524510
www.dataprotection.gov.uk

Part 4

Referrals and Reports

As a member of a professional body there may be occasions when a sports therapist needs to refer a patient to a fellow practitioner or to write a report for insurance/litigation purposes and whilst referrals and reports are different they contain roughly the same kind of information.

A referral is when you want a fellow practitioner's help, advice and/or opinion, whilst a report is more related to an account of what you have done and is usually part of an insurance claim or litigation or both. **Initially in the case of reports, it is vital to seek help and advice from a professional body. Whereas with referrals initially it may be a good idea to seek the help and advice from a** more experienced colleague without direct recourse to the professional body, who will probably furnish you with guidelines anyhow. In the absence of such here are a few guidelines:

REFERRALS should be typed on headed notepaper, be approximately two hundred words and consist of three paragraphs. For example, the patient's personal history/data; what has been done/found and what is being requested.

THE CONTENT should include:

- The patient's name, address and date of birth.
- The referral's address.
- What has been done, i.e. history, examination and treatment, if any, and its effectiveness.
- What conclusions have been made.
- The reason for the referral, requesting what is required and may include an opinion based on the known facts to date (*see Appendix 4*).

REPORTS need a lot more time and preparation but remember that whatever information is disclosed, it will be closely scrutinised, possibly in a court of law.

To re-iterate, everything written down about a patient has legal implications. If it is not written down it is assumed it has not been done and so it is important to write down all the relevant information.

It is important that the therapist's professional association is contacted for help and advice on these matters, as is the insurance/legal profession as to what information is and what is not required. It is also important that the patient's records are kept fully up to date. Things should be kept simple when replying to requests. Nothing should be done until two things have been achieved:

1. The written consent of the patient to write the report is received.
2. The fee for services is received. This may seem a little mercenary and materialistic but in the world of litigation, payment can be a longtime coming.

Characteristics to avoid in writing reports are flippancy, levity and jocularity. Expressing an opinion without sufficient reflection on how that opinion will be justified, expressing a view glibly and lengthy jargon should all be avoided.

Part 5

Advertising and Attracting Patients

By treating one sports person successfully, 'word of mouth' will ensure that at least another is informed. But how are people initially attracted to a practice? This is via education by:

- Letting people know who you are.
- Letting people know where you are.
- Letting people known what you have to offer.

This can be one of the most challenging roles a sports therapist has to perform. These things can be done in a variety of ways:

1. Advertising in relevant journals, magazines and directories, e.g. yellow pages, professional registers/directories.
2. Giving talks to local groups, etc.
3. Using professional and informative stationery.
4. Using mail shots to target groups, e.g. sports clubs, health centres etc.
5. Via direct introductions by personally visiting places that may find a use for your knowledge, skills and expertise, e.g. health centres, fitness clubs.
6. By working in an environment that promotes your knowledge, skills and expertise.

There are many innovative ways that can attract patients but don't get carried away and sacrifice professional quality for quantity. It is important that a strategy is planned involving thoughts on the kind of clientele you envisage treating. Advertising must pay for itself but must be considered a legitimate expense. Also remember you are treating people and it is these people who will bring other patients. **Advertising is important but not half as important as looking after existing patients**. When deciding on an advertisement, bear the following in mind:

1. Who is it aimed at? This will decide where the advertisement is to be placed, e.g. a box advertisement under a professional directory in the yellow pages or a postcard in the window of a local public house? **NOTE**: 95% of a therapists' patients should give them 5% of their problems, **NOT** 5% giving 95%. The advertising will decide who is attracted.
2. What is included in the advert? The advertisement is not only advertising services but representing a professional body who may have some definite ideas on how its members advertise their services. Don't forget that every word that is used will be carefully scrutinised by someone. Don't make false statements.

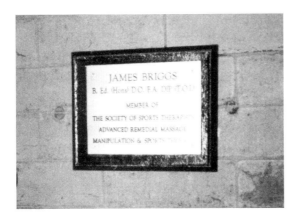

◄ *Figure 59. Door Plaque advertising.*

3. How often is advertising necessary? An advert will need to run long enough for the public to become familiar and comfortable with it, i.e. 4–6 times.
4. The office stationery and business card will say a lot about the therapist and his/her practice other than what is blatantly obvious.
5. Time should be taken and a lot of thought put into the kind of image that you wish to portray on paper.

Part 6

Insurance and Sport

> **"Even with the best training available, and a conscientious, experienced therapist, it must be admitted that none of us is perfect or infallible."**
> *Balen, D., 1995*

The cost of insuring oneself against public, employer, professional and product liability and possible loss of earnings, as a result of malpractice, may appear relatively expensive but false economies should not be made. The potential legal risks faced by those who participate in what they may regard as a harmless leisure activity should not be trivialised. In the world of professional sport the rewards paid to certain sports people are astronomical and if, heaven forbid, a person's actions prevent a sports person from earning such sums then this compensation culture will come crashing down upon their head.

PUBLIC LIABILITY refers to liability in law for causing injury to other people, or damage to their property, whether they are your patient or not, providing no treatment or advice is involved.

PROFESSIONAL INDEMNITY. Inherent in such insurance is the principle of accountability and responsibility.

EMPLOYER LIABILITY refers to injury to staff following alleged negligence of the employer.

PRODUCT LIABILITY refers to the supply or sale of goods to patients, causing injury or damage.

CLAIMS MADE/CLAIMS OCCURRING are such that they need expert clarification from a more knowledgeable source but are nevertheless included here to emphasise their importance when choosing insurance.

The subject of sport, insurance, litigation and the law is a fascinating, yet frightening one, so be warned that studying the subject may lead to a person not wanting to get out of bed in the morning, never mind putting on their trainers!

In summary, a practitioner must plan, organise, implement and manage the delivery of the effective and efficient operation of their professional life by identifying and defining the needs and requirements for a fully operational practice.

References

1. Balen, D.: 1995. Insurance for complementary health professionals, making sense of the jargon. *Inter Medica*.
2. Balen, D.: 1995. Professionalism in practice insurance. *The Therapist*, Summer, 1995.
3. Butcher, Dr. R.: 1999. Moral decision-making in sport – a guide to practice. *Faster, Higher, Stronger*, 6, December, 1999.
4. Green, J., C.: 1998. Insurance and sports. *Sport and Law Journal*.
5. Huxley, T. J.: 1834/5. Olegenesis and abiogenesis. Collected essays.
6. Keiran, A.: 1999. Ethical issues in coaching. *Sports Coach*, Winter, 1999.
7. Mail on Sunday: 2000. Now let's ban this greedy, yobbish game. 25.6.2000.
8. Medical Defence Union: 1996. Patient records and case notes. In *Touch*, 79, Spring, 1996.
9. Payne, S. D. W.: 1995. Sports medicine and the law. From *Sports Exercise and Injury*, 1, 70–75.

Bibliography

1. Artfile Sport, Phaidon Press, Oxford, ISBN 0–7148–2667–7.
2. Ethics who cares? 1999. *Faster, Higher, Stronger*, 6. N.C.F. Publication.
3. Gardiner, T.: Coaching and the law – An NCF Workshop.
4. Grayson, E.: 1998. Ethics injuries and the law in sports medicine. ISBN 0 7506 15761.
5. McLatchie, G.: Essentials of sports medicine, Chapter 1, 1993.
6. Payne, S. D. W. (ed.): 1990. Medicine, sport and the law.
7. Stone and Matthews: 1996. Complementary medicine and the law.
8. Swisher, D., Krueger-Brophy, C.: 1998. Legal and ethical issues in physical therapy. ISBN 0 7506 97881.

Chapter 8
Final Thoughts and Considerations

"Come to the edge," he said.
They said, "we are afraid."
"Come to the edge," he said.
They came,
He pushed them..........
And they flew.
Guillaume Apollinaire

Part I

The Drugs/Cheating Issue – Sports Nutrition, Supplementation, Performance Enhancement, Alcohol, Smoking and Caffeine

The Drugs/Cheating Issue

Competitive sports people have always and will always use any means to try and gain an advantage over their rivals. That is inherent in their competitive nature (*see Chapter 1, Part 2*). In today's sporting world, such advantages range from highly sophisticated to down right blatant methods. An 'athlete' will employ:

- The best coach/trainer using the most up-to-date training, tactical coaching methods to gain, **'a tactical/physiological edge'**.
- The best psychologist to improve/focus the mind and 'psyche out the opponent' to gain, **'a psychological edge'**.

- The best nutritionist to improve the fuelling of the machine, which can assist/optimise healing, repair and performance to gain, **'a nutritional edge'**.
- The best sports scientist using advances in sports science to 'fine tune' the machine to gain, **'a scientific edge'**.
- The most up-to-date equipment supplying not only data feedback but also protection to gain, **'a technical edge'**.
- On a more cynical level, a player may consider, 'taking players out,' to 'negate their effectiveness'.

This may be done under instruction, "let him/her know you are there", or under the player's own volition. **Can we call this a physical edge?** Is this justification for 'the professional foul'? To this we can add being encouraged, or under a person's own volition, to bend and manipulate the rules before, during and after the competition. Sometimes this will involve quite blatant intimidation of the referee. Such practices are rarely condoned/admitted to unless a TV and/publishing company offers an astronomical sum of money to, 'come clean and tell-all'. Sometimes videos are made to record such misdemeanours. Such practices may at times be explained, rather patronisingly to the uninitiated, as being, 'part and parcel of the game'.

A recent newspaper article reported that cheating was even evident in the recent Paralympic Games in Sydney, where the category of 'intellectual handicap' was open to abuse (*Slot, 2001*).

In such a climate it is understandable why some athletes may try to gain, **'a pharmaceutical or nutritional edge'**. In the words of Oscar Wilde: **"I can resist anything but temptation."**

Are athletes competing on a level playing field? If they feel they aren't, or the goalposts keep being moved, then they may either take a few risks or give up in frustration. Whilst not condoning cheating or the use of drugs, the author does feel that certain sports are highly hypocritical when it doesn't suit. Here we are re-entering the realms of sporting mentality, ethics, morals and what constitutes fairness, cheating and an unfair advantage. In other words can drugs ever be justified in sport?

> **"...there can be no justification for athletes to cheat in order to win....the pressures and temptations are the same for all athletes, yet most show great character and do not succumb.....The problem is not educational, economic or social but, essentially, a moral problem.......the use of doping substances or methods to enhance performance is cheating. It undermines the foundation of fair competition and can be illegal and/or dangerous, putting the performer at risk."**
> *Faster Higher Stronger, 2000*

What Constitutes a Drug?

According to the Association of Chief Police Officers:

> "A drug is any substance which may affect a person's emotional state, body function or behaviour. Alcohol, tobacco, caffeine and over-the-counter medicines in this sense are drugs. The effect of a drug may be harmful or beneficial."

Another definition widens the scope as to their use:

> "Any substance that affects the structure or functioning of a living organism. Drugs are widely used for the prevention, diagnosis and treatment of disease and for the relief of symptoms. The term medicine is sometimes preferred for therapeutic drugs in order to distinguish them from narcotics and other addictive drugs that are used illegally."
> *Oxford Medical Dictionary, 1996*

Clearly it can be seen that there are different categories of drugs for differing purposes. There are soft drugs (cannabis) and hard drugs (heroin, cocaine, crack cocaine). These may be used to relax or feel good but used in such a way can actually reduce performance, not to mention tarnishing the image of sport. Performance enhancing drugs (anabolic steroids and amphetamines) may be used to enhance performance or to improve body image. Medications (cough and cold preparations, painkillers) are intended to treat illness or injury. The drug culture abounds in today's society, especially amongst the younger generation. With the increased use of supplementation in sport and the unknown effects on the mix of such substances, together with the increased use of drug testing in sport, questions such as those previously raised now provide the basis for discussion, debate and test cases for the judicial bodies. The list of banned substances gets ever longer.

> "There is absolutely no anabolic-androgenic steroid that affects an athlete anabolically without also affecting him or her androgenically...There isn't an anabolic-androgenic steroid an athlete can take to increase muscle mass, endurance or speed without risking dangerous hormonal side-effects."
> *Faster, Higher, Stronger, 2000*

Sports Nutrition and Supplementation

The early 90's and into the new millennium has been characterised by a greater interest in sports nutrition as well as long, complex, legal appeals, lodged by competitors against charges of cheating and doping, to gain an unfair advantage. Don MacLaren highlighted the fact that in the last decade the number of sports nutrition research papers has risen from approximately 400 to approximately 5,000.

Research into the area of amino acids, vitamins, herbs and minerals has been carried out over the last twenty to thirty years and much has been applied to the increasing benefits to athletes. But the purpose of this chapter is not to review such studies or prepare cases for the defence and prosecution in drugs litigation but to highlight such issues, provoke/stimulate thought and to consider certain issues and topics relevant to the role of sports therapy.

As has been shown throughout this book (*see Chapter 1, Part 5; Chapter 2, Parts 3 and 8; Chapter 3, Part 4; Chapter 6, Part 4; Chapter 8, Part 3*), nutrition is a significant factor in many aspects of sport. Modern Pentathlete Stephanie Cook, who won gold in the 2000 Sydney Olympics sought nutritional advice in the form of the herb Echinacea to combat coughs, colds and fatigue (*Times, 24.10.00*). However, some performers still adopt unsatisfactory dietary regimes/eating patterns and many surveys show that few performers follow the best diets to affect optimum sports nutrition. It has also been shown that a well-balanced diet that includes adequate carbohydrates, protein and micro-nutrients, via an increased consumption of fruits and vegetables, is far more beneficial and less harmful than excessive over supplementation. **It must always be remembered that the 'balanced diet' for one athlete may contain enough vital nutrients, yet for another, the same diet may be deficient. Just as there are placebo and nocebo responders in treatment so there are such in response to dietary supplementation.**

> **"Diet in itself cannot provide fitness or championship form but a poor diet can ruin both."**
> *Torrance, A., 1988*

The use of dietary supplementation or ergogenic aids is now quite common in sports.

> **"Many performers will immediately reach for the supplements at the first sign of tiredness, a drop in performance or a persistent cold or sore throat."**
> *Griffin, J., 2000*

A survey of 113 top athletes found that 31% of them had inadvertently taken an over the counter preparation which was subsequently found to be a banned substance (*BJSM, 2000*). Whilst this can be attributed to ignorance, multivitamins, man-made natural substitutes/products, herbs and all kinds of potions, concoctions and bastardised versions of the real thing abound and for someone looking for an advantage the thought of, 'giving it a go', can be too tempting to resist. In fairness to the athlete, he/she may equate in certain instances, 'supplementary' as extra to what is naturally already there and so therefore considers the use of such aids as safe and natural and not habit forming like 'conventional' drugs. Also there is the assumption that natural is safe – but this is a false assumption as strychnine is natural! This has led to calls for not only a closer inspection of the unregulated, dietary supplement industry by the scientists but also a direct confrontation of such with the billion dollar pharmaceutical industry, who see the growth of such an industry as detrimental to their own position and development.

Clinical nutrition is the application of nutritional substances to sub-optimal conditions that can arise in the body. One interesting find amongst all of the research is, 'The principle of synergy,' when applied to herbs, vitamins and minerals that states:

> **"The combined action of two or more substances acting in concert is of much greater benefit than the sum of those coming from any of those substances alone."**
> *Melanie, A.*

The body is designed to naturally analyse and synthesise and so to develop this by taking supplements in combination may seem like a safe and natural thing to do. In fact it is suggested that the best supplements to take are those which carefully combine complementary nutrients. But even the body itself can get us into trouble, as may be the case with the banned substance nandrolone.

Nandrolone is a steroid that is similar to the male growth hormone testosterone. However, according to Dr. Mike Wheeler, a member of the expert committee appointed by UK sport to investigate the steroid, it can also be manufactured in the body by two other steroids, which have been banned by the International Olympic Committee (IOC) since 1999. This clearly raises the issue of what effect athletes are having on their bodies by jumping on the bandwagon in the pursuit of sporting perfection?

What are some of these supplements and what is the reason that makes sports people consider them for improving performance and/or reducing the time an athlete is missing training and competition as a result of injury?

Branched Chain Amino Acids (BCAAs) are leucine, isoleucine and valine, found primarily in muscle and are analysed and used for energy during exercise of more than two hours duration. Used as an ergogenic aid it has been suggested that supplementation may help replace the BCAAs, delay fatigue, effect mental and physical performance, reduce the effects of over-training and affect body composition. With regards performance the results are questionable but in general suggest that supplementation is not effective (*Williams, 1999; Davis, 1995; and Meeusen, 1995*). Gastmann and Lehmann, 1998, conclude that the hypothesis regarding over-training is inconclusive. However, some research suggests there may be some use for supplementation in affecting body composition (*Bigard, 1996; and Mourier, 1997*).

L-carnitine is involved in the transport of long chain fatty acids into the mitochondria for energy production. It may deplete after hours of work and limit the rate of fat fuel usage. The suggestion is that by increasing the amount in the diet it will burn more fat to supply energy.

Creatine or methylguanidine – acetic acid, is a naturally occurring amino acid found in fish and meat. It is also endogenously synthesised in the liver, kidneys and pancreas from glycine, arganine and methionine. Creatine supplementation may have an ergogenic effect in two ways: performance enhancement of a single bout of high intensity exercise or by repeated bouts of exercise. No ergogenic effects have been found on long duration, endurance performance. It has been touted as the most popular muscle building nutrient ever made and the research to date shows that its greatest benefit may be to those who want to put on muscle mass, especially if used with a resistance training regime. Vegetarians may have reduced creatine stores and could benefit from oral ingestion.

> **"Creatine should not be viewed as another gimmick supplement: its ingestion is a means of providing immediate, significant performance improvements to athletes involved in explosive sports."**
> *Greenhaff, P., 1995*

However, whilst creatine may have many benefits it also has shortcomings with side-effects ranging from nausea, stomach upset, dizziness or weakness and diarrhoea the most common with dosages greater than 5g daily. Muscle cramping is not as uncommon as is an increase in soft tissue injury for those who increase their workload as a result of taking the supplement. It is also thought to stress the kidneys and is contra-indicative for people with kidney disease.

> **"Creatine has many benefits but also has shortcomings."**
> *Sahelian, R., 1999*

More recent concerns were reported in *SportsCare News*, 2001, which identified, carcinogenic, digestive, muscular and cardiovascular problems associated with the use of creatine supplementation.

However, whilst these effects seem to relate to large doses and over-enthusiasm this is in contrast to other research that concludes:

> **"Short-term creatine supplementation regimes are safe, and many of the anecdotal side-effects have not occurred in clinical studies."**
> *Haff, G. G., and Kirksey, B. K., 1999*

The final words coming from Sahelian:

> **"You must be well informed before using this nutrient."**

Dehydroepiandrosterone (DHEA), is an adrenal hormone that functions as a metabolic precursor for the endogenous production of oestrogen, testosterone and other hormones. Its claimed benefits for its use in sport have ranged from increasing muscle mass and strength, affectation of body composition and fat distribution, altering mood/libido, perceived energy levels and memory function. Side-effects have been found to affect the liver, increasing the risk of uterine and prostate cancer, whilst causing all kinds of gynaecological problems. Therefore, it is no surprise that it has been subsequently banned by the IOC.

> **"Given the lack of evidence that DHEA enhances athletic performance and its potentially devastating adverse effects, DHEA supplementation is not recommended."**
> *Armsey and Green, 1997*

Echinacea, a herbal extract has been shown to shorten the duration of colds or flu because of its effect on increasing white blood cell count (*Berg, et al., 1998*).

Erythropoietin, or EPO, is a hormone secreted by the kidneys in response to hypoxia. It stimulates the bone marrow to increase the production of red blood cells. The effect is relatively quick, generally within seven days. The benefit is to increase the oxygen carrying capacity of the blood, which for endurance athletes can improve their potential. EPO has been used by athletes as an easy alternative to complex blood doping strategies. There is a risk in its use if high doses are used, especially in combination with steroids and reported side-effects can include hypertension, flu-like symptoms and hyperkalemia (*Stricker, 1998; Cowart, 1989*).

Ginkgo Biloba, is one of the world's longest living tree species. It is used to help efficient circulation, for its antioxidant function, to affect mood and to improve mental performance. To date the evidence for its use and efficacy in sport is inconclusive.

Ginseng is one of the traditional Chinese medicinal herbs and is a generic term encompassing a wide variety of compounds derived from the plant family Araliaceae. The claimed benefits of its use are that it boosts energy levels in fatigue, stress and compromised immunity. As for sport it is reputed to improve performance. However:

> **"Ginseng has been used by athletes as an ergogenic aid for many years, but there is an absence of compelling research evidence in support of its use for such purpose."**
> *Bahrke and Morgan, 1994*

Glucosamine, an amino acid, has many functions in the body ranging from water transportation, promotion of post exercise rehydration, the main source of energy for immune system cells, regulation of body pH and the stimulation of protein and glycogen synthesis. It is the major precursor of glycosaminoglycans (GAGs), which are the tissue framework onto which collagen models form. Synthesised from glutamin and glucose it is the body's rate-limiting step in GAG production and consequently the rate-limiting step in re-modelling of the connective tissues. Following soft tissue injury this limit does not allow the body to make sufficient glucosamine for optimal healing. Also as we get older, the body's ability to synthesise glucosamine declines because of the reduction in the level of the converting enzyme glucosamine synthetase. The combined effects of these is that connective tissue repair declines. Man-made glucosamine bypasses the rate limit in the GAG production system, increases GAG levels and increases connective tissue synthesis.

> **"Evidence at present is not strong enough to warrant recommending an athlete to use this supplement, but there are some suggestions of a possible role in stimulating the anabolic process."**
> *Maughan, Professor R., 2000*

However, research reviews by McAlindon, et al., 2000; Reginster, 2001 and Towheed, et al., 2001, into its effect in the treatment of osteoarthritis shows that evidence continues to build, illustrating a clear disease-modifying effect as well as showing improvements in pain and functioning with no evidence of long-term harm.

Glutamine is the most abundant, non-essential amino acid found in human muscle and plasma and is utilised for rapidly dividing cells such as white cell lymphocytes and considered essential for proper immune function. There is some evidence that endurance athletes taking glutamine recover quicker from periods of intense exercise and suffer less infections compared to those that don't (*Budgett, 2000*).

Glycerol is a three carbon alcohol occurring naturally in the body. Its use in sport is as a pre-event supplement to prolong endurance and improve thermoregulation. However, there is limited evidence that it in fact improves these things and more research is needed to fully justify its use (*Robergs and Griffin, 1998*).

HMB, (beta – hydroxy – beta – methyl butyrate) is a metabolite of the branched chain amino acid, leucine, which is found in catfish and certain citrus fruits. It claims to increase strength and endurance, increase muscle mass and minimise protein analysis. The research to date is limited and questionable and whilst no side-effects of **HMB** supplementation have been reported, its safety is still unknown (*Armsey and Green, 1997*).

Inosine, the end product in its metabolism being uric acid, is a nucleoside that has various metabolic functions. Its promotional hype for athletes claims to:

> **"Support the body in the production of short bursts of energy during intense, aerobic exercise increases the body's ability to handle rigorous exercise without inducing fatigue.....will increase the body's ability to carry oxygen."**
> *Sports Care News, 2000*

However, authors from three studies during the 90's conclude that inosine supplementation has no benefit to athletes and could actually be detrimental to health through the production of waste products. (*McNaughton, L., Dalton, B., and Tarr, J., 1999; Starling, Trapp, T. A., and Short, K. R., 1996 and Williams, M. H., Kreider, R. B., and Hunter, D. W., 1990*).

Pycnogenol, is a water soluble, bioflavonoid extracted from the bark of a French pine tree. Targeted at the treatment of injuries market, its promoters claimed it to be a natural anti-inflammatory with no side-effects; as an anti-oxidant it claims to be 50 times more effective than Vitamin E and 1000 times more effective than Vitamin C. It binds to collagen improving the strength of arteries, veins, capillaries and the skin; it improves circulation and is completely safe, non-toxic and doesn't interact with other drugs. However, one of the most serious handicaps of the bioflavonoids is the fact that bioavailability is not documented and information on humans is lacking. Furthermore metabolism of bioflavonoids is unknown (*Christie, S., 1995*).

Vespa Mandarina Japonica, may be the answer to all our prayers!

> **"Olympic star runs on hornet stomach juice…..The women's marathon winner at the Sydney Olympics has revealed the secret of her success: she drank the stomach juices of giant, killer hornets that fly 60 miles a day at up to 20 mph."**
> *Telegraph International News, 15th October, 2000*

On the question of vitamin supplementation, The New Scientist, 27.2.99, published a comprehensive review of current research findings on the dangers of vitamin supplements but Mervyn Waldman (*1999*) commenting on such said:

> **"It seems we have ignored some fundamental principles of Naturopathic Medicine viz., that one cannot extract substances from their complex, natural food source without danger."**

Upon closer inspection it is also found that the review was designed to highlight the possible dangers of megadose supplementation and did not present a balanced argument regarding general usage.

Substantial scientific evidence (*Food and Nutrition Board of the Institute of Medicine, 1998*) shows that there can be valuable benefits to health from sensible supplementation with appropriate nutrients in addition to a well-balanced diet. The relevance of this to sport needs closer examination. What is always needed is a comprehensive, research-based review that is unbiased and independent of commercial interests. Only then will the facts or fallacy argument be truly resolved (*see Chapter 1, Part 5*).

Smoking, Alcohol and Caffeine – The Social Drugs – A Few Known Facts

Smoking

A cigarette can be considered as a 'chemical cocktail' and one of the most damaging substances contained in cigarettes is tar. It literally clogs up and irritates the respiratory system. Tobacco smoke also contains carbon monoxide that pollutes the system. Nicotine is a powerful, addictive drug that together with carbon monoxide affects the heart, blood vessels and nervous system. Nicotine also depresses the nervous system, appetite and reduces the haemoglobin capacity of the blood to carry oxygen, which will obviously affect energy levels. What makes it such a powerful drug is that its effect is almost immediate, taking about seven seconds to reach the brain, which it stimulates releasing noradrenalin, which is related to the stress mechanism. It is also extremely addictive and once 'hooked' it is with you possibly for life. Smoking also has antisocial implications. Twenty per cent of smoke exhaled can be re-circulated by passive smoking. Finally as with all drugs, its use can always be justified by the user.

A trawl of the literature highlights the following:

Short-term Problems

- It can take up to 21 days for nicotine to clear the system.
- A smoker's sense of smell and taste are soon lost.
- Appetite is reduced.
- Smokers are more susceptible to colds and chest infections.
- It reduces 'peak flow' output (output during exhalation).
- It reduces exercise tolerance.
- It paralyses cilia in the bronchial tubes therefore preventing them from removing harmful irritants whilst breathing. This in turn causes the alveoli in the lungs to become congested.
- It destroys Vitamin C.
- Whilst many 'hard-drugs' can have serious psychological effects on the user, nicotine affects a person far more physically, which presents problems for those who wish to 'kick the habit', e.g. withdrawal symptoms.
- Pain responses and expectation have been found to be different in smokers than non-smokers.
- Certain personality traits can sometimes be associated with smokers, e.g. selfishness, arrogance and not truthful/realistic. Smokers do tend to understate how many cigarettes they smoke and may not accept that the inherent risks actually apply to them as well as other smokers.

Long-term Problems

- Lung/heart damage. Nicotine and carbon monoxide damage the heart and blood vessels.
- Smokers are almost certain to suffer from bronchitis, blood pressure and coronary heart disease at some stage in their lives.
- Smokers are up to 20 times more likely to contract lung cancer and 10 times more likely to contract cancer of the throat and lungs. They are twice as likely to die of heart disease as non-smokers.

Peripheral Damage

- Long-term damage can lead to peripheral vascular disease culminating in necrosis and gangrene.

- Smoking can be the cause of stomach ulcers.
- Smokers are four times more likely to suffer mental decline/cognitive impairment (*SportEX, 2000*).

The moral and ethical arguments surrounding tobacco and its advertising, especially related to sport, continue. Should a health-related industry associate itself with such a product?

Alcohol

This is one of the oldest known drugs. The alcohol we drink is called ethanol or ethyl alcohol and is obtained via fermentation or distillation. Fermentation allows enzymes in fruit juice or grain plus water to act on carbohydrates in the mixture turning it into alcohol. This is achieved in the absence of oxygen, i.e. anaerobic metabolism. Distillation, is when the products of fermentation are boiled and the alcohol evaporates and is collected separately. Distilled alcohol is much stronger than fermented, i.e. beer and wine is fermented whilst spirits are distilled. Again a review of the literature provides us with the following information:

- A can of beer has less nutritional value than a slice of bread.
- It can provide energy but muscles cannot use it so it is stored as fat.
- Alcohol is known to depress the nervous system.
- In small doses it is good as a relaxant.
- Alcohol deprives the body of its natural water and flushes out essential minerals.
- It destroys certain minerals, especially Vitamin C and lowers the blood glucose levels.
- It is a powerful vasodilator and so therefore going to the bar after traumatic injury, to drown your sorrows, may not be a good idea.
- It impairs performance and reaction time.
- It can act as a diuretic in hot weather, therefore risking dehydration. It inhibits the release of the anti-diuretic hormone that retains body fluid (see side-effects of caffeine).
- In cold weather it can reduce body temperature by dilating peripheral blood vessels leading to hypothermia.
- Sensible and irresponsible levels of consumption are suggested for the general public.

What these levels should be for an athlete range from nil to those suggested. Although some would argue the social aspects of certain sports are just as important as the game!

- Sensible weekly levels of alcohol:10/11 pints for males (20–22 units) and 7 pints for females (14 units).

- Silly weekly levels of alcohol: More than 18 pints for males (36 units) and 11 pints for females (22 units).

Short-term Problems

- Reaction times slow and concentration and motivation are reduced.
- Judgement, balance, speech and hearing become increasingly affected as more alcohol is consumed.
- Personality becomes affected.
- It can depress blood vessels of the skin resulting in heat loss.
- It lowers blood glycogen levels, therefore alcohol 24 hours before an endurance event wouldn't help. This also stops exercise sooner and makes for a longer recovery.
- It increases weight.
- It reduces fitness levels.
- It can irritate the stomach lining causing vomiting.
- It constricts arteries to the heart increasing the pulse rate and blood pressure.

Long-term Problems

- Liver damage.
- Kidney damage. These have to work harder causing cirrhosis of the liver.
- Heart damage.
- Brain cell damage.
- Gastritis in the stomach can develop.
- Malnutrition and diabetes.

Clearly the issues of smoking and alcohol are contentious ones if we compare health risks against advantages against social implication. What people should and should not do in a democracy touches on moral, ethical, social and political issues. However, sports therapists will need to address such issues.

Caffeine

Caffeine is a very common part of the diet but it is not a nutrient but a biologically occurring drug. In the world of athletics it is clearly a powerful ergogenic aid. The frequency of its use/abuse appears to be because it is socially acceptable, readily available, relatively inexpensive and can be orally ingested. In other words it is not perceived by some as 'doping'.

Caffeine has been found to be a natural constituent of over 60 plants. Coffee beans and tea leaves are the most obvious natural sources although it is found in cola, cocoa and lucozade drinks as well as in chocolate.

There is also a vast array of prescription and pharmaceutical remedies that contain caffeine, e.g. cold and pain relief tablets, drinks and stimulants such as *Pro-plus*. (One can of coke, 46mg caffeine per can = 2/3 cups of coffee – One cup tea/coffee = 100mg caffeine. This translates to a level of 1.5 mcg/ml in the urine after 2/3 hours). *Solpadeine* (30mg caffeine per capsule), a painkiller also contains paracetamol and codeine, with the caffeine being added to enhance their combined actions. Obviously its effects/side-effects depend very much on individual susceptibility and quantity.

Effects

The beneficial effects can be considered in certain people who ingest large doses, i.e. in excess of 1,000mg per day. Upon reaching the brain, via the blood, caffeine stimulates nerves in both the brain and spinal cord. It also affects the heart, lungs, kidney and certain gland functions.

- It increases awareness, vigilance, clarity of mind, ability to concentrate, intellectual performance when taken in small doses (doses 1–5 mg per kg of body weight).
- Heart rate is increased, in both speed and strength.
- It increases the rate at which the kidneys work.
- It increases breathing rate.
- It increases metabolic rate.
- It can enhance the effects of painkillers by 40%.
- It prolongs endurance by decreasing the amount of glycogen, burned by muscles.
- It stimulates the release of fats from tissues, sparing the glycogen which allows the muscles to work longer, therefore delaying the onset of fatigue.
- It increases muscle contractility.

Considerations/Value of/on Athletic Performance

Caffeine can have the effect of increasing:

- Reaction time.
- Co-ordination.
- Vision.
- Mental alertness.
- Endurance. Marginal improvements have been noted in long-term endurance exercise (more than 45 minutes sustained effort).
- It can increase strength and/or power and speed.

This is why it is classified as an illegal stimulant and is included in the IOC banned list of drugs for sports people. However, it must be found in a urine sample above 12mg/ml which equates to eight cups of coffee. As so many other things contain caffeine, this limit can inadvertently be exceeded.

Side-effects

These can range from being unpleasant to fatal and can be pretty well assured if up to 1,000 mg are ingested per day. The following side-effects have been noted:

- In large doses, trembling in the hands.
- There can be a diuretic effect, increasing the need to go to the toilet. This leads to dehydration and increased irregular heart contractions. Caffeine and alcohol take more than their own volume of liquid with them, depleting the body of vital vitamins and minerals.
- 'Caffeinism' is a state said to be similar to alcoholism and is habit forming. Doses of 15mg per kg of body weight can lead to this state.
- Nausea.
- Insomnia.
- Headaches.
- Jitteriness and muscle twitching.
- Restlessness.
- Irritability.
- Tinnitus.
- Arrythmia – irregular heartbeat.
- Palpatation – increased heart rate.
- Tachycardia – an excessively, rapid heartbeat.
- Research during the last decade has demonstrated that coffee brewed without a filter contains a fat derivative that can be detrimental to cardiovascular health.
- Mild delirium, coma, seizures and death (doses that would require a man to drink 50–160 cups of strong coffee in 30 minutes!).
- Stimulates gastric acid secretion in the stomach.
- Withdrawal symptoms are not uncommon which can include minor to severe headaches, drowsiness, fatigue and anxiety.
- Diarrhoea.
- Decreased iron intake by a third if taken with meals.
- Increased metabolic rate.
- Increased blood cholesterol levels.

Indications

Doctors in 1995 suggested no more than six strong cups daily. Obviously this depends on individual tolerance and today two cups of 'real' or four cups of 'instant' would be considered moderate.

Contra-indications

None to just one or two cups daily if there is evidence or suspected:

- High blood pressure.
- Heart problems.
- Kidney disease.
- Pre-menstrual syndrome.
- Migraine.
- Pregnancy.
- Breast-feeding.

Part 2

The Sports Injury Clinic

With the upsurge in interest, courses and qualifications in sports medicine/therapy has come the inevitable questions:

1. **What constitutes a sports injury clinic?**
2. **What qualifications, knowledge, skills and expertise should the people possess who run them?**
3. **What type of person attends them and what facilities should they offer?**

Research by the Sports Council and cited by Kingsley, 1987, found that 32% of people who attended such clinics at that time had previously had unsuccessful treatment, were from lower, middle class backgrounds and the treatment offered tended to reflect a bias towards which sport the local community supported. As for the knowledge, skills and expertise of the personnel involved most tended to be run by chartered physiotherapists or masseurs/masseuses who may or may not have had postgraduate training in sports medicine but who recognised a niche in the market.

As mentioned previously, many therapies are now leaping on the bandwagon of sports medicine, e.g. osteopathy, chiropractic, sports therapists, sports trainers, podiatrists etc. The therapist, educational establishments and training institutes, either through arrogance and/or ignorance, upon completion of 'a course' are opening so called sports injury clinics. This is sometimes on the strength of a few weekend seminars on sports injury management and/or the fact they play sport and think they know all there is to know about sport. Can one/two people ever claim to be that good? It can also be said that astute business orientated people see anything to do with sport as an ideal environment to work in/be associated with. Sports people as we know, are notorious at looking for a 'quick fix' and will often search out any establishment that offers a sympathetic ear as well as pertaining to offer a service for sports people. In the author's experience 'butterfly patients' will flit from one therapist to another until they find one who tells them what they want to hear unless the therapist identifies such people early during the consultation. This is no slight on the therapist but a reflection of the sporting mentality of certain sports people not wanting to accept responsibility for their own problems (*see Chapter 5, Part 2*).

For the therapist, just having a little knowledge, a massage couch, a spare room at home and a bucketful of bravado, is not justification for calling your premises a sports injury clinic. Sadly and naively this is all some may offer! This does not mean that a suitably qualified therapist shouldn't offer their particular knowledge, skills and expertise in treating sports people. However, it should be accepted that the range of treatment offered may be limited and referral should be made to other therapists where there is limited practical knowledge. In terms of cost effectiveness to the patient it can be argued that a few accurate diagnoses/treatments given by a therapist qualified to give such are probably better than a lot of cheaper 'hit and miss' ones. The pertinent issue here is what constitutes qualified?

So what should constitute a sports injury clinic? Dr. Malcolm Read, 1989, and the author's own views may give a good guide as to what facilities, personnel and structure, should be offered. Obviously international sports people would/should expect access to a whole range of knowledge, skills and expertise and facilities that perhaps a recreational sports person wouldn't. But if the sporting population is to receive the best possible service to which they are entitled then there should be no discrimination as to who gets what. The knowledge, skills and expertise of staff should include and offer:

- An understanding, interest and personal experience in/of sport and sporting mentality.
- A qualified physiotherapist with a qualification/interest in sports medicine.
- A qualified osteopath/chiropractor with an interest in sports medicine.
- A qualified sports therapist (*see Chapter 1, Part 1*).
- A qualified podiatrist/chiropodist with an interest/qualification in sports medicine.
- A qualified dentist, orthodontist with an interest/qualification in sports medicine.
- A qualified sports nutritionist.

- A qualified sports psychologist.
- A qualified sports physiologist/scientist.
- A specialist in rehabilitation and remedial training if not offered by any other practitioner.
- A qualified masseur/masseuse with knowledge of and an interest in sport.
- A doctor with an interest/qualification in sports medicine.

Facilities that should be offered or easily accessed/available within a few days:

- Diagnostic facilities, e.g. X-ray, blood test, ultrasound, CT scan, MR scan, isokinetic muscle assessment and exercise cardiogram facilities.
- Physiological equipment, e.g. treadmill and bike ergometer with sports-related ergometers to monitor VO_2 max, lactic acid, body fat and anaerobic capacity.
- Rehabilitation facilities, e.g. a rehabilitation gymnasium which has isokinetic machines, power gyms, free weights, static bikes, treadmill, rowing machine, theraband etc.
- Biomechanical assessment facilities, e.g. pressure pads and video monitoring running machine with incline for gait analysis etc.
- Therapeutic modalities, e.g. short waves, pulsed short wave or interferential, likon, laser traction, **TENS** etc. with a therapist qualified/insured to use them.
- Access to outpatients/in-patient facilities for referral.
- Use of a hydrotherapy pool.
- Research facilities.

Obviously, those running sports injury clinics will want to scrutinise such a list and those athletes attending recognised clinics should have a valid input as to what they would expect to find.

Part 3

Travelling with the Teams

It is now quite common for athletes and teams of all ages and all abilities to be involved in travel both nationally and internationally to train, compete, and tour. Travel is now an integral part of the life of a professional sports person. Travelling with 'the team' can take one of several forms:

- Escorting an athlete to a training camp/competition.
- Going to away fixtures with a squad/team on a regular basis which may involve an overnight stop.
- Being involved in a one-off special trip, lasting several days. This may be just to train and/or compete.

- Being part of a tour party/trip where there is a lot of travelling involved and many countries are visited.

For the sports therapist involved in such travel it is important that he/she is fully aware of the significance of the experience if it is to be worthwhile and enjoyable. Many issues are commonsense and are no different than preparing, planning and organising events 'at home' or if travelling in everyday life. However, in relation to a sports trip the significance of poor planning, preparation and organisation may mean the difference between an athlete/team fulfilling a lifetimes' ambition or not. The following thoughts and considerations can be altered, adjusted and modified to suit the occasion.

PRE-PLANNING, PREPARATION and **ORGANISATION** are the key to success and no amount can be too much as no one can guarantee everything will run smoothly. Trying to control the environment in which sports people find themselves before, during and after competition is the key to a safe and successful trip. Of course there will always be circumstances beyond anyone's control but with good planning, preparation and organisation, problems can be dealt with as and when they arise.

One of the first considerations is to decide which personnel need to be attached to the trip/tour. For example: manager, coach, assistant coach, skill specific coach, video analysis expert, sports psychologist, fitness trainer, co-ordinator, finance official/business manager, travel representative, physiotherapist, sports therapist, doctor, masseuse/masseur.

The next major consideration is what equipment will each of these personnel require. This obviously can be dealt with in relation to defining roles and responsibilities but the estimation of what to take and the logistics of carrying equipment from a to b can in itself prove an interesting problem to solve.

If the trip is going to be of any duration, involving visiting several countries, then **the use of a travel company who specialises in arranging this type of trip should be used**. Liaison with such people will be of tremendous benefit for deciding on the mode of transport, which hotels to use, etc. The hotel can then be informed as to the trip requirements, e.g. meal times, availability of meeting rooms, storage rooms, sleeping arrangements, etc. This will ensure that the trip/tour expectations can be met by the hotel. Perhaps using a hotel chain will overcome the need to duplicate requests/expectations. In the case of local travel (walking, public transport and using ones own transport) then the implications of transporting individual and groups of people need to be carefully considered. For example, the appropriate ratios of male to female, adults to children if transporting minors, mixed gender groups, insurance implications, meeting times, departure time, etc.

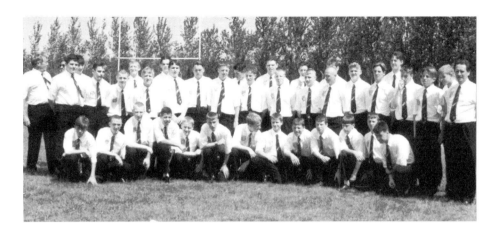

▲ *Figure 60. Which personnel need to be attached to the trip?*

Visiting the competition venue prior to the trip can be of tremendous benefit, e.g. noting the suitability of accommodation, training facilities, etc. and/or discussing the venue with someone who possesses a local knowledge has obvious advantages. Such a visit may also prove beneficial in terms of noting cultural differences. The cost of financing overseas trips is a serious consideration, perhaps not for professional sport but it maybe for the local amateur athletics club. Fund raising and sponsorship skills are now a major consideration.

Trips abroad can involve long, arduous and, at times, boring journeys, different climates, time zones, sleep patterns, customs, eating habits and cultures. All of these issues need to be considered in addition to the established practice procedures of

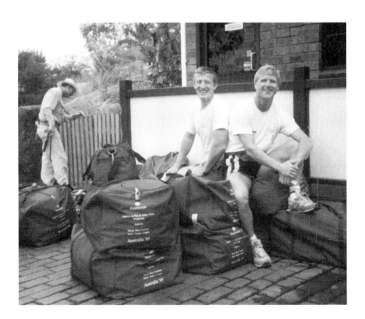

◄ *Figure 61. What equipment/luggage needs to be taken.*

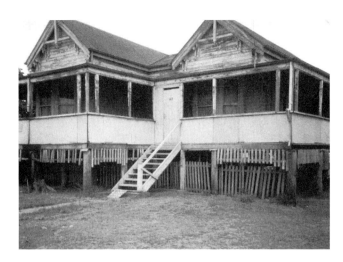

◀ *Figure 62.
Noting the
suitability of
accommodation
is clearly
important!*

looking after any sports team. **ADVICE** on **HOW** these issues could be approached **should be given as necessary before departure, with meetings and adequate documentation**, to ensure that everyone involved with the tour/trip knows exactly what to expect and what is and is not acceptable. This is very important from a legal point of view. For example, **this could involve making those on the trip/tour aware of and advising on jet lag or circadian dysrhythmia** that will affect body metabolism. Jet lag is:

> "The feelings of disorientation encountered as a result of crossing time zones.....Symptoms include fatigue and general tiredness, inability to sleep at night, loss of concentration, loss of drive, headaches and general malaise. Jet lag occurs when biological rhythms are disrupted as a result of rapid transitions across multiple time zones."
> *Reilly, T., 1999*

Its severity is affected by many factors, e.g. individuality, the number of time zones crossed, direction of travel, flight departure and arrival times. Starting with a two-hour time difference, time that will have a minimal effect, the significance of jet lag increases as the time shift increases. A shift of three hours or more can be quite substantial (*Hartmann, 1971*). The impact of jet lag may take two to three days after disembarkation before reaching a peak. Tom Reilly then indicates that after a few days:

> "There will be a window of time during the day when the period of high arousal associated with the time zone just left overlaps with the arousal high point at the new local time. This window may be predicted in advance and should be utilised for the timing of training practices in the first few days at the destination."

As a result of the earth's rotation, with the sun rising in the east and setting in the west, travelling east will have a greater effect than travelling west. Resynchronisation/adaptation from this can also be significant in that travelling west takes 30–50% less time than travelling east (*Kleinn, et al., 1971*). This is because when travelling to the east, where the countries are in front/advanced as opposed to west, where the countries are delayed/behind, the normal body clock cycle is temporarily lengthened. The body rhythms can extend in line with their natural free wheeling cycle of about 25–27 hours and then catch up (*Reilly, T., 1999*). A circadian, body clock rhythm is related to the light/dark cycle, a time span of approximately 24–27 hours, and which governs the body's physiological systems. An example of this is the body's core temperature which is slow to re-adjust after travel across time zones (*Atkinson and Reilly, 1996*). Body core temperature is at its lowest between 0700 and 0900 and then gradually increases, peaking at about 1900. Body core temperature can significantly influence nerve conduction velocity, metabolic enzyme reaction rates and psychomotor performance (*Fort, et al., 1971*). For every one-degree rise in body temperature, nerve conduction velocity increases by 2.4 m/sec. These systems follow a strict cycle with minimum and maximum occurring at certain times of the day (*Winget, et al., 1985*).

The main influences on the 'body clock' are either internal endogenous rhythms (occurring within the body) and/or 'zeitgebers' (German for time-givers), external/exogenous cues, e.g. body core temperature, rest and exercise, the amount of daylight and darkness, the time of sunrise and sunset, outside temperature, meals/diet and social influences. The internal, rhythms are synchronised or entrained to the external. It has been found that this 'body clock' is positioned in the brain, just behind the eye and is influenced by the amount of light and dark cycles of the environment (*Joseph and Knigge, 1978*). Light actually synchronises and suppresses the production of melatonin, which is secreted by the pineal gland. Melatonin and its precursor seratonin have roles in sleep regulation.

During the night their secretions are markedly higher (*Coulson, 1999*). After a journey across several time zones the body clock retains the characteristics of the point of departure before adjusting to its new environment. Such adjustment can be facilitated by activity and social contact during daylight hours (*Klein and Wegman, 1974*), but until such time as the biological clock has re-adjusted to the new time/environment, exercise performance will be affected. These effects can result in disruption of the hormonal, metabolic and renal systems (*Coulson, 1999*).

Some of these effects have been highlighted as body temperature alteration, low levels of arousal, gastro intestinal problems, disturbed sleep patterns, weakness and irritability. However, other effects can be associated with slow reaction times, muscle strength, short-term power output and muscle contractile capabilities, joint flexibility and stiffness, with the lowest levels of stiffness being recorded in the early evening (*Wright, et al., 1983*). This can obviously be of significance to sport specificity and to when to train and compete.

> **"Most components of sports performance exhibit a circadian rhythm with a peak in the later afternoon/early evening, rendering athletic performance most efficient at this time of the day....jet lag may cause a shift in the optimal circadian peak window for performance."**
> *J. Int. Med. Res. 2000*

Taking melatonin and selecting the best circadian time can result in as much as a ten per cent increase in athletic performance (*Peak Performance, 2001*).

Different chronotypes (a measure of whether a person is a morning or evening person) will adjust/resynchronise depending on the direction of travel. 'Morning larks' respond better to travelling east, as their body clocks tend to run faster, and 'evening owls' respond better to travelling west, having slower body clocks. From a practical point of view these facts can be helpful in determining the direction of travel, but the problem remains, what happens if you have different chronotypes in the travel party?

Tiredness and 'sleep deficit', can lead to a loss of skill, energy and motivation. Body resistance is lowered leading to an increased risk of injury and illness. **Rest, sleep and acclimatisation** are important to help the body recover, re-adjust and rebalance after exercise and travel. **Age and fitness play an important role in this. Children acclimatise better than adults because of a better regulation of their**

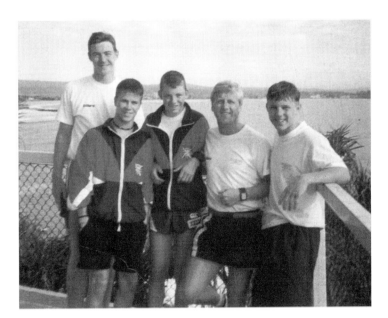

◄ *Figure 63. Down under with the boys.*

body clock, and active people are more responsive than less active. It is suggested that for every hour of time difference/time zone crossed, one day's acclimatisation should be allowed. It is also suggested that altering training times, in line with the visiting country, as well as desynchronising lifestyles in half-hour periods, prior to departure, will help acclimatisation. Also changing sleeping patterns may help, but this may be more beneficial during the journey.

Other in-flight strategies to consider during travel are setting watches to the country of destination to adjust thought patterns and adjust behaviour accordingly; missing certain meals and keeping active (stretching and isometric routines) at the appropriate times (*see also nutritional advice*).

Boredom can lead to people becoming unco-operative, sometimes aggressive and unpredictable which can lead to accidents. One of the greatest psychological influences on a trip/tour can be the effect of injuries. This applies to not only the injured party but to the support personnel. Therefore it is important on trips involving long journeys and lengthy stays away from home that athletes are kept mentally and physically active:

- Travel documentation, passports, visas, entry visas, insurance, etc. should be dealt with and scrutinised as early as possible once the trip/tour has been confirmed.
- **Legal implications must be clearly addressed**. All adults travelling with teams have a legal and moral responsibility to the people in their charge. Accountability needs to be emphasised. Everyone owes a **duty of care** to anyone whom we can reasonably foresee may be affected by their actions. Anyone responsible for the health and welfare of players and officials has a moral obligation in injury care and management to prevent further injury or worsening of the current situation. **For youngsters being away from home it is vital that 'loco parentis' (in place of the parent) issues are clearly addressed**. It must be appreciated that the younger the athlete the more responsibility will rest with the person/s responsible for organising the trip. There is also a **paramedical – legal position** to ensure the best possible care of all the athletes in their care. **Professional indemnity insurance and travel insurance should be carefully scrutinised, e.g. is bungee jumping covered?**
- Job descriptions/specifications for all personnel involved will avoid conflict as to who does what. **These should be negotiated with all personnel and then written down. Everyone must be aware of each other's role**. Trying to empathise and deal with the individuality and egos of 'the ring of influence' on the life of an athlete may be a job for the psychologist (*see Chapter 1, Part 6 and Part 7; Chapter 2, Part 8; Chapter 5, Part 2*).

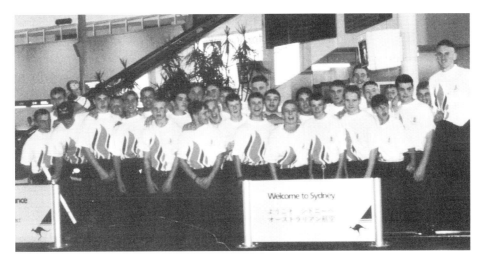

▲ *Figure 64. Agreeing a code of conduct and behaviour.*

Agreeing a code of conduct and behaviour with all concerned, as well as a selection procedure will help team building as well as maintain discipline.

Selection procedures become a major issue in team sports where selection of the key personnel to 'do the job' can be critical. In this respect it must be made clear as to why people are selected and why others are not. **Delegation of responsibility and devolution of decision-making** are vital for team spirit. Abdication of responsibility, especially self, should also be prepared for and therefore it goes without saying that rules and regulations must be enforced.

Routines must be planned in advance. A clearly thought out code of conduct will also ensure everyone is familiar with their individual and collective responsibilities and help to ensure an accident, injury free and successful trip/tour. **Tort, or civil wrong doings, can easily become an issue when dealing with minors as well as adults.** When injury occurs, **negligence** becomes an issue. Obviously words can mean different things to different people and so **it is vital that key terminology is agreed upon**, e.g. what do we mean by a successful trip – winning at all costs or everyone having a good time irrespective? (*see Chapter 7*).

- Cultural differences must also be considered with not only expected standards of behaviour but nutrition.

Getting involved as soon as possible with pre-trip fitness testing, training, and warm-up matches, etc., are vital to ensure that everyone gets to know each others idiosyncrasies.

- Being away from familiar territory and the home base will present its problems not least **'home sickness'** and the fact **that some personal things cannot be taken with you and** others **will have to be taken** with you if you want to use them. Assuming that it is always available and where it always is would be the first mistake. For the sports therapist not only do personal belongings need to be considered but how much medical and paramedical stock should be taken. **Home sickness** can become an issue for various reasons, e.g. non selection to first team, unacceptable accommodation, losing, poor performance, fatigue, missing family, friends and loved ones, personality clashes etc.

- The individual, **financial**/money management issues must also be meticulously considered, e.g. travellers cheques, local currency, the paying of bills, who pays for what, etc?

- **Nutrition** is important to avoid unnecessary illness, **e.g. adequate hydration and re-hydration** during travel, pre and post exercise, especially in extreme climates and what foods to eat and avoid. Drink plenty of fluids on long journeys and during resynchronisation, not alcohol or fizzy, and stick to fruit juice (*Reilly, Atkinson and Waterhouse, 1996*). **Start re-fuelling after competition as the muscles capacity to refuel is greatest after the first hour of training/exercise**. It can take up to 48 hours to completely replenish glycogen stores. Water, fresh fruit juice and Vitamin C after competition helps to replace electrolyte depletion (*see Chapter 1, Part 5*). **Avoid fizzy or gassy drinks and large amounts of tea and coffee as they act as a diuretic**.

Caffeine also arouses the central nervous system and is therefore not suitable prior to sleep (*see Chapter 8, Part 1*). Meals high in carbohydrates and low in protein can

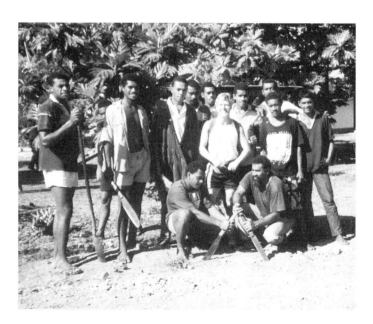

◄ *Figure 65. Cultural differences must be appreciated.*

induce drowsiness, as carbohydrates provide the substrate for serotonin, a neurotransmitter that regulates sleep. When travelling eastwards, high protein breakfasts and high carbohydrate dinners will help to build energy stores and improve alertness (*Reilly, Atkinson and Waterhouse, 1996*).

- Adequate **protection** is essential, especially regarding exposure to extremes of heat and cold, insect bites, and stings, e.g. lotions, potions and skin protectors; recommended strappings and protection for games and competition, e.g. gum shields, shin pads, shoulder pads etc.
- Also consider **medical issues**, regarding **inoculations, what medications to take, considering the banned drugs list, and familiarity with private and reciprocal health care arrangements in different countries, as well as adequate insurance cover** for all of those travelling will all need considering and acting upon. Small print on insurance policies needs to be carefully scrutinised – which countries are visited will determine the specifics. Booklets can be obtained from Health Centres and some travel companies giving advice on travel in and outside the European Community. On a visit to Los Angeles, Fiji, New Zealand and Australia some inoculations can be recommended, e.g. hepatitis A, typhoid and polio, whilst others are essential, e.g., tetanus. In terms of healthcare in 1993, Fiji had no systematic health care system, Los Angeles was private, New Zealand was reciprocal and Australia was Medicare, which was reciprocal but some facilities had to be paid for. For example, calling for an ambulance in Queensland during the course of a game as a result of an on the pitch accident/injury resulted in having to pay for the ambulance when it arrived! **In countries providing reciprocal health care arrangements, individuals need to take their NHS cards**. To avoid problems such as loss these can be kept, for safe keeping, by the medical personnel. Other areas to consider are:

- **Hygiene**, to avoid a whole host of problems but in particular fungal and viral infections, e.g. athlete's foot or groin rash.
- **First aid advice**, so that everyone travelling is aware of what to do in an emergency and acute injury situations. **It is a good idea to ensure all travelling have some kind of current first aid training**.
- **Medical records**, to ensure that amongst others, legal responsibilities are met. It is vital that adequate records are kept of each individual in the therapist's care. **Personal data should be acquired, prior to departure**, to ensure that paramedical personnel can carry out their responsibilities. **A disclaimer needs to be signed for minors** to the effect that the parent and/or legal guardian gives permission for the relevant personnel to treat any condition they are trained and qualified to treat and to act in *loco parentis* in an emergency situation (*see Appendix 4*).

- **It is also vital that clear lines of communication are established** with home whilst the tour party is away.
- **Administrative records**, to ensure all documentation is easily located, e.g. passport numbers, individual and team photographs for passes, receipts, room numbers, etc.
- **'The physiotherapy/medical bag/s, (on the field (first aid), off the field (medical) and a general, travelling supply bag may need to be considered).**

This can present one of the biggest problems/considerations for the sports therapist and can become more of an issue if the trip/tour is not accompanied by medically qualified personnel and is of any significant duration. Estimates as to how many bandages, strappings, plasters and tubs/tubes of oils and creams will be required maybe possible to base on experience or by consulting medical personnel who have travelled previously. If a sponsor can be secured then the financial constraints are reduced but there is still the question of how much one can physically carry or be allowed to take when travel baggage allowances are considered. On a trip of any duration buying in supplies as and when is an option if a supply network can be established.

If it is intended to take **electrotherapy equipment**, then small, multipurpose units, as opposed to bulky ones, will help not only with handling but also in getting it through customs with the least amount of delay, which will need clarification from the airline and carrying company. Carrying this as part of hand luggage reduces the risk of unnecessary loss or damage in transit. Upon arrival at each destination these can be categorised as:

- The need to settle into the new environment as soon as possible, with as little fuss as possible, adjusting to cultural variations.
- The need to settle into the agreed routines as soon as possible.
- The importance of resynchronising the body clock via rest, sleep, meal times, food, drink, social interaction, exercise, training, etc.
- A massage on arrival can prove therapeutic by relaxing not only the body but also the mind.

The following need to be addressed as to their availability at the sports venue:

- Training facilities, equipment etc.
- The nearest GP – address, phone number day/night/emergency.
- The nearest hospital Accident and Emergency (A & E) unit, telephone number and address.
- The nearest dentist, chiropodist, phone number and address.

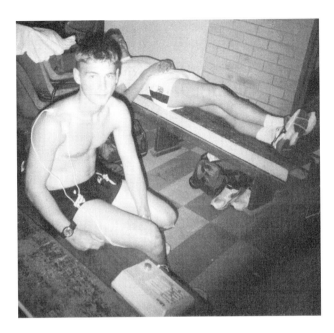

◄ *Figure 66.*
Small, multipurpose
electrotherapy
equipment is more
useful than bulky
equipment.

- Familiarity with local first aid and emergency procedures and rules regarding is what /and what is not allowed, e.g. in Queensland the physiotherapist attending to an injury on the pitch, just needs to raise his/her hand to stop the play (*J. Briggs, 1993*).

At each venue, the availability of:

- Ice and water.
- Doctor and ambulance procedure.
- First aid posts and medical room.
- Blankets.
- Couch.
- Dressing room facilities.
- Crutches, splints and stretchers.

Much of the above can and should have been dealt with during the pre-trip organisation and respective personnel can perhaps arrive early at the venue/s to prepare for the athlete/teams arrival, leaving the athlete and/or team to just concentrate on preparing for their performance. As can be seen, planning, forethought and organisation are essential if travelling with the teams is to be a successful experience. Areas such as: pre-tour/trip training schedules, fund raising, sponsorship, luggage, outfitting, travel arrangements, finance, decision-making, politics and religion, whilst equally important, haven't been dealt with in as much detail as other considerations in order to focus on the responsibility of and factors that may affect the sports therapist.

The opportunity of travelling with athletes of all ages from all spectres of the sporting world is considered one of 'the perks' of being involved in sport but as can be seen it involves more than just packing your passport and sun tan lotion.

Final Thoughts and Considerations

Which brings us to the end of the journey that started by asking what is a sports therapist and what knowledge, skills, expertise and personal qualities should they possess? At times the journey through the mind, body and spirit of the sporting world may be likened to walking through an unlit tunnel in quick sand, looking for the proverbial light, whilst sinking deeper and deeper into the mire. But for those qualified sports therapists out there, and for those wanting to be, the author hopes that in trying to answer the question, the journey has proven to be enjoyable, interesting, thought-provoking, inspirational and illuminating. When dealing with people, bodies, exercise, injury and repair the journey is, in the author's opinion, never ending. He hopes this text has laid down the foundation on which to build further knowledge, skills and expertise. Remember:

> **"You must maintain the standard of your performance by keeping your knowledge and skills up-to-date throughout your working life. In particular, you should take part regularly in education activities which relate to your branch of medicine."**
> *Webborn, Dr. N., 2000*

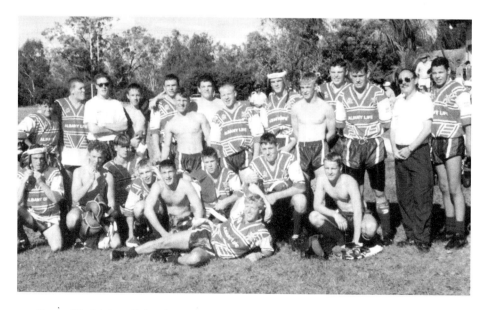

▲ *Figure 67. A job well done!*

References

1. Alfred, M. 1998: Clinical nutrition and endurance. *Mod. Athletics and Coach* (USA), 136:2, 14–15.

2. Armsey, T. D., and Green, G. A.: 1997. Nutrition supplements: science v hype. *Physician and Sports Medicine*, 25(6): 77–78, 87–92, June, 1997.

3. Association of Chief Police Officers: Drugs and sport, a factual guide for organisers of sport.

4. Atkinson, G., and Reilly, T.: 1996. Circadian rhythms in sports performance. *Sports Medicine*, 21:4, 292–312.

5. Bahrke, M. S., and Morgan, W. P.: 1994. Evaluation of the ergogenic properties of ginseng. *Sports Medicine*, 18(4), 229–248.

6. Berg, A., Northoff, H., Konig, D., et al.: 1998. Influence of Echinacin (EC31) treatment on the exercise-induced immune response in athletes. *J. of Clin. Res.*, 1: 367–380.

7. Bigard, A. X., et al.: 1996. Branched-chain amino acid supplementation during repeated prolonged skiing exercise at altitude. *International Journal of Sports Nutrition*, 6(3): 295–306.

8. Briggs, J.: 1994. Down under with the boys. Society of Sports Therapists Newsletter, 4.

9. British Journal of Sports Medicine: 2000. 34: 148–152, reported in *SportEx*, 8, Athletes Beware.

10. Budgett, Dr. R.: 2000. The unexplained, under-performance syndrome (UPS) – under-recovery and overtraining. *Faster, Higher, Stronger*, 8, July, 2000.

11. Christie, S.: 1995. Pycnogenol: the extraordinary properties of a pine bark extract. *Inter Medica*, 2:2, Spring/Summer, 1995.

12. Coulson, M.: 1999. Biological rhythms 1 and 2. *Peak Performance*, 116 and 119, April and June.

13. Davis, J. M.: 1995. Carbohydrates, branched-chain amino acids and endurance – the central fatigue hypothesis. *International Journal of Sports Nutrition*, 5(Suppl): S29–38.

14. Drugs and sport: 2000. *Faster, Higher, Stronger*, 9, 15–18, October, 2000.

15. Food and Nutrition Board of the Institute of Medicine: 1998. Dietary reference intakes for thiamin, riboflavin, niacin, vitamin B6, folate, Vitamin B12, pantothenic acid, biotin and chlorine. National Academy Press, Washington DC.

16. Fort, A., et al.: 1979. The relationship on deep-body temperature and performance on psychomotor tests. In Loat and Rhodes.

17. Gastmann, U. A. L., and Lehmann, M. J.: 1998. Overtraining and the BCAA hypothesis. *Medicine and Science in Sport and Exercise*, 30(7): 1173–1178.

18. Graham T.: 1999. Caffeine and coffee uptake. Assoc. of British Cycling Coaches. *Coaching News*, 2.

19. Greenaff, P. L.: 1995. Creatine and its application as an ergogenic aid. *International Journal of Sports Nutrition*, 5 (Supplement): S100–S110.

20. Griffin, J.: 2000. Diet and the unexplained, under-performance syndrome. *Faster, Higher, Stronger*, 8, July, 2000.

21. Haff, G. G., Kirksey, B. K., Stone, M. H.: 1999. Creatine supplementation. National Strength And Conditioning Association, 21:4, 13–23, 1998. Reported in *Strength and Cond. J.*, August.

22. Hartman, B. O.: 1989. Field study of transport aircrew and rest. In Loat and Rhodes.

23. Jackson, B. H., Kulling, F. A.: 1989. Health and ergogenic effects of caffeine. *British Journal Sports Medicine*, 23:1.

24. Journal of Neurology, Neurosurgery and Psychology 2000, 68; 622–626, May. Reported in 5, *SportEx*, June, 2000.

25. J. of Int. and Med. Res. 2000, 28 (4), 182–186, July–August, 2000.

26. Kingsley, K.: 1987. The Role(s) and whereabouts of sports injury clinics. Society of Community Medicine Conference, Manchester, 17.9.87.

27. Klein, K. E., and Wegman, H.: 1989. The resynchronisation of human circadian rhythms after transmeridian flights as a result of flight direction and mode of activity. In Loat and Rhodes.

28. Klein, K. E., et al.: 1989. Circadian performance rhythms: experimental studies in air operations. In Loat and Rhodes.

29. Loat, C. E. R., and Rhodes, C.: 1989. Jet lag and human performance. *Sports Medicine*, 8:4, 226–238.

30. Maughan, Professor, R.: 1995. Sports nutrition. Sports Science Update, Gatorade Sports Science Institute, November, 1995.

31. Maughan, Professor, R.: 2000. Sports and Exercise Nutrition Conference, Loughborough. Reported in *Sportscare News*, 19, Summer, 2000.

32. McAlindon, T. E., et al.: 2000. Glucosamine and chondroitin for treatment of osteoarthritis. A systematic quality assessment and meta-analysis. *J.A.M.A.*, 2000, 283: 1469–1473.

33. McNaughton, L., Dalton, B., and Tarr, J.: 1999. Inosine supplementation has no effect on aerobic or anaerobic cycling performance. *Int. J. of Sports Nutrition*, 9 (4): 333–334, December, 1999.

34. Meeusen, R., de Meirleir, K.: 1995. Exercise and brain neurotransmission. *Sports Medicine*, 20 (3): 160–188.

35. Mourier, A., et al.: 1997. Combined effect on calorific restriction and branched-chain amino acid supplementation on body composition and exercise performance in elite wrestlers. *International Journal of Sports Medicine*, 18(1): 47–55.

36. Oxford Concise Medical Dictionary, 4th ed., 1996.

37. Peak Performance 2001. Melatonin and Jet Lag: Issue 147, April 2001.

38. Read, Dr. M.: 1989. What to look for in a sports injury clinic. Coaching Focus, 11, Summer, 1989.

39. Reginster, J. Y., et al.: 2001. Long-term effects of glucosamine sulphate on osteoarthritic progression: a randomised, placebo-controlled clinical trial. *Lancet*, 357: 251–256.

40. Reilly, T.: 1999. Symptoms and treatment of jet lag. Association of British Cycling Coaches, *Coaching News*, 1, 11–13.

41. Robergs, R. A., and Griffin, S. E.: 1998. Glycerol: biochemistry, pharmokinetics and clinical and practical applications. *Sports Medicine*, 26(3): 145–167.

42. Slot, O.: 2001. Cheating shame of Paralympics. Sunday Telegraph, 2001.

43. Sportscare News, 2000. Ergogenic aids – inosine. 20, Autumn, 2000.

44. Starling, R. D., Trappe, T. A., Short, K. R., Sheffield-Moore, M., Jozsi, A. C., Fink, W. J., and Costill, D. L.: 1996. Effect of inosine supplementation on aerobic and anaerobic cycling performance. *Medicine and Science in Sport and Exercise*, 28 (9): 1193–8, September, 1996.

45. Sahelian, R.: 1998. Creatine – nature's muscle builder. www.labtestreview.com.

46. Tindall, Dr, N.: 1999. Health and hygiene. Society Community Medicine Conference, Manchester, 12.6.99.

47. Torrance, A.: 1988. Society of community medicine. UMIST.

48. Towheed, T. E., et al.: 2001. Glucosamine Therapy for treating osteoarthritis (Cochrane Review) In: The Cochrane Library, Issue 1, Oxford Update Software.

49. Unknown quantity: 1999. *The New Scientist*, 27.2.99.

50. Ursell, A.: 1995. The caffeine controversy. *Here's Health – Healthy Eating*, October, 1995.

51. Waldman, M.: 1999. The dangers and fallacy of vitamin supplementation. *Osteopathy Today*, October, 1999.

52. Webborn, Dr. N.: 2000. General Medical Council Guidelines. Quoted in Professional Development – CPD in Sport and Exercise Medicine: A Discussion Paper. *Sportscare News*, Autumn, 2000.

53. Werbach, M. R.: 1993. Alcohol craving, nutritional influences on illness. *International Journal of Alternative and Complementary Medicine*, July, 1993.

54. Williams, M. H.: 1999. Facts and fallacies of purported ergogenic amino acid supplements. *Clinics in Sports Medicine*, 18(3): 633–649.

55. Williams, M. H., Kreider, R. B., Hunter, D. W., Somma, C. T., Shall, L. M., Woodhouse, M. L., and Rokitski, L.: 1990. Effects of inosine supplementation on a three-mile treadmill run performance and VO2 peak. *Med. and Science in Sport and Exercise*, 22 (4), 517–22, August, 1990.

56. Williams, Professor C.: 1997. Cellular nutrition – supplements and performance in football. FA Medical Conference, Lilleshall, 4.10.97.

57. Winger, C. M., et al.: 1985. Circadian rhythms and athletic performance. *Medicine and Science in Sport and Exercise*, 17: 498–516.

58. Wright, J. E., et al.: 1989. Effects of travel across time zones on exercise capacity and performance. In Loat and Rhodes.

Bibliography

1. Branched chain amino acids. 1999. NSMI News, 17, Winter, 1999.

2. Caffeine and coffee: a useful supplement? 1998. *Sports Nutrition, Insider*, 6:2, September.

3. Caffeine – getting a buzz – out of the game. 1999. Premier Sports Medical Newsletter, May, 1999.

4. Creatine, NSMI News, 14, Spring, 1999.

5. Ginseng, NSMI News, 9, Autumn, 1997.

6. Glycerol, NSMI News, 15, Summer, 1999.

7. SportsCare News, 2001. Concerns over Creatine. Issue 22, Spring 2001.

8. Travelling and competition – a coaches' guide. 1997. *Coaching Focus*, No. 36, Winter, 1997.

9. Travelling with youngsters – a coaches' guide. 2000. *Faster Higher, Stronger*, 7, April, 2000.

Glossary of Terms

Abduction Movement away from the midline of the body.

Action Potential A large depolarisation of the membrane of a neuron or muscle cell that is conducted through the cell.

Adduction Movement towards the midline of the body.

Afferent Nerves Nerves carrying sensory input from receptors in the skin, muscles, tendons and ligaments to the central nervous system.

Angulated Fracture One end of the bone is at an angle to another.

Anterior The front or near to the front view – sometimes known as *ventral*.

Avulsion Fracture The bone is detached at the tendon attachment, usually at the epiphyseal growth plate.

Bending Loading that produces tension on one side of an object and compression on the other side. To overstress/stretch, e.g. strain/sprain.

Blood Pressure Lateral, outward pressure exerted by the blood to vessel walls as a result of ventricular contraction (systole and diastole).

Body Mass Index (BMI) A measurement of body weight determined by dividing weight (kg) by height (m) squared.

Border A ridge of bone separating two surfaces. Usually provides muscle attachment.

Cancellous Bone tissue of relatively low density.

Circadian Rhythm	24-hour biological clock.
Circumduction	Circular motion of a body segment resulting from sequential flexion, abduction, extension, and adduction, or vice versa.
Closed Fracture (Undisplaced)	No breaks in the skin and the fracture is contained in local tissue.
Comminuted Fracture	Bone is broken in more than two parts.
Complicated Fracture (Displaced)	Surrounding structures and organs are injured. These can involve a joint or a dislocation, e.g. the end of one bone breaks off and goes into the joint.
Compression	To compact/crush, e.g. haematoma.
Concentric Contraction	The muscle actively shortens and thickens as the insertions move towards the origin and the joint angle decreases. This is related to the agonist/prime mover. This kind of contraction can be considered as the accelerator.
Condyle	Rounded bulging projection of bone which participate in a joint, e.g. tibial condyle.
Connective Tissue	The most abundant tissue found in the body. It is made up of macrophages, fibroblast and mast cells surrounded by an extracellular ground matrix, which is a continuous medium that varies in density.
Contracture	Adhesions occurring in an immobilized muscle, leading to a shortened contractile state.
Contralateral	Situated on or affecting the opposite side of the body, e.g. the left and right shoulder are contralateral.
Contusion	Compression injury involving accumulation of blood and lymph within a muscle – a bruise.
Coronal/Frontal	Dividing the body into equal/unequal front and back parts.
Crushed/Compression Fracture	Usually relates to the spine or calcaneum.
Cytology	The study of cells.
Deep	Towards the inside of a part, away from the surface e.g. the muscles are deep to the skin.

Delayed Onset Muscle Soreness (DOMS)
Muscle soreness that correlates with microscopic muscle damage, oedema and loss of strength that may persist up to a week (*Burke E. R., 1997*).

Depression
Movement downwards.

Dermatome
A region of skin supplied by a single afferent neuron.

Developmental Anatomy
Anatomy that can be considered and related to scientific progress.

Diabetes
A condition in which insulin production (in the pancreas) either ceases or becomes ineffective. *Type 1* insulin dependent/diabetes mellitus, is a condition in which insulin ceases to be produced due to damage to the pancreas. *Type 2* diabetes, usually affects older people (especially those who are overweight). In this condition, insulin is produced but the system has become insensitive to it.

Diffusion
Movement not requiring mechanical force or external pressure, i.e. concentration gradients that affect small solutes such as oxygen and sugars.

Dislocation
Separation of a joint so that the bone ends are no longer in contact.

Distal
Further from the trunk or point of origin, e.g. the hand is distal to the elbow.

Dorsal
Back or posterior surface of a body part.

Dorsiflexion
Movement of the top of the foot to the anterior of the tibia.

Double Fracture
More than one break.

Eccentric Contraction
The muscle is lengthening as it develops tension. The origin and insertion are pulled apart as the muscle resists and overcomes the movement/barrier.

Efferent Nerves
Nerves carrying stimuli from the central nervous system to the muscles.

Electrotherapy
A general term applied to treatment in which sound, heat, light and other forms of electromagnetic energy, which is the simplest form of energy, are applied to the body, e.g. ultrasound, diathermy, short wave, microwave, laser etc. to assist the healing process.

Elevation	Movement upwards.
Epicondyle	Blunt projection, lateral and medial from condyles, e.g. medial epicondyle of femur.
Epithelial Tissue	Protects, secretes, absorbs and covers body surfaces, lines body cavities and forms glands.
Eversion	Turning of the sole outward so that the weight is on the inside edge of the foot.
Extension	Increase in joint angle during movement.
Flexion	Reduction in joint angle during movement.
Foramen	Hole through a bone, e.g. nutrient foramen.
Fracture	Break in the bone, resulting in the loss of continuity with or without displacement.
Full Range	The muscle works from its extreme stretched position to its extreme contracted position.
Functional Anatomy	Anatomy found in reality, with everyone being different.
Glands	Groups of epithelial tissues that produce specialised secretions onto the epithelial surface of an organ directly or through a duct – exocrine glands, or they become isolated from epithelial surfaces and discharge their secretions into the blood and lymph – endocrine glands (ductless). Their secretions are called hormones (chemical messengers).
Greenstick Fracture	Incomplete fracture of the diaphysis of a long bone – usually found in children.
Groove	Furrow on a bone eminence.
Haemarthrosis	Collection of blood within a joint or cavity.
Haematoma	Localized mass of blood and lymph confined within a space or tissue.
Histology	The study of tissues.
Hypermobility	Where there is mobility at a 'joint' beyond the normally acceptable range of movement, (*hyper* – means more than the norm; *hypo* – means less than the norm).

Hyperthermia	Elevated body temperature.
Hypothermia (Heat Loss)	Peripheral blood vessels are dilated giving signs and symptoms of cold, shivering, slow thoughts, clumsiness leading to unconsciousness.
Impacted Fracture	Fragment of bone has impacted into another.
Inferior (Caudal/Caudad)	Towards the tail, away from the head. Usually with reference to the trunk, e.g. the stomach is inferior to the head.
Inflammation	Pain, swelling, redness, heat, and loss of function that accompany musculoskeletal injuries.
Insulin	A hormone necessary for carrying glucose into the working cell and its absence causes blood glucose levels to rise (hyperglycaemia).
Interstitial Pressure	Minor pressure exerted by fluid that has 'seeped out' into the interstitial, cellular spaces and which will eventually be taken up by the lymphatics.
Inversion	Turning of the sole inward so that the weight is on the outside edge of the foot.
Ipsilateral	Situated on or affecting the same side of the body, e.g. the left shoulder and heart can be considered as ipsilateral.
Isokinetic Contraction	Related to muscular contraction at a constant speed over the full range of movement, (*iso* – means same/unchanged; *kinetic* – is related to movement energy).
Isometric Contraction (Active/Static)	A muscle does not need to alter its length when it contracts, (*iso* – means same/unchanged; *metric* – means length). There is no movement at the joint but the muscle develops tension.
Isotonic Contraction (Active/Dynamic)	The length of a muscle does change and there is movement at the joint, (*iso* – means same/unchanged; *tonic* – means tone). The tone remains constant.
Lateral	Situated away from the midline and is related to the side, e.g. the eyes are lateral to the nose. Used with reference away from the mid-sagittal plane.

Ligaments	From the Latin *'ligare'*, meaning to bind or tie, possess a fibre arrangement in different directions to allow multidirectional movement within limits. Not only are they used at joints where there is obvious movement but in many other parts of the body.
Lordosis	Excessive convex curve in the lumbar region of the spine.
Malleolus/Malleoli	Rounded projections found at the distal end of the tibia and fibula.
Medial	Situated towards the midline of the body or a structure, e.g. the eyes are medial to the ears. Used with reference towards the mid-sagittal plane.
Median	The midline dividing the body equally into left and right.
Membranes	Made of either connective or epithelial tissue and line the cavities and hollow organs of the body; cover and protect body surfaces and anchor organs and structures to each other. Their cells form sheets which secrete fluid of varying viscosity and have various characteristics and functions.
Microtubules	Allow the passage of fluids in and out of cells.
Mid–Inner Range	The muscle works from a position which is halfway between its two extremes of movement to its fullest contracted position. It is in this position that the muscles are working in their most contracted position which is the true position of strength.
Mitochondria	Barrel-like structures that are responsible for energy production within a cell.
Morphology	The study/science of the structure and form of organisms.
Myositis Ossificans	Rare process of ossification in the traumatised area of muscle following haematoma.
Myotome	A group of muscles primarily innervated by a single nerve root.

Nervous Tissue	Co-ordinates and controls together with the hormonal/endocrinal (chemical) system bodily functions by initiating and transmitting nerve impulses.
Neurotransmitter	A chemical substance which transmits impulses across a synaptic cleft.
Oblique Fracture	Bone is fractured at an oblique angle.
Open Fracture (Compound)	A break in the skin as well as the bone.
Organelles	Found in cells, collections of molecules organised in such a way as to perform an individual function.
Outer Range	The muscle works from its extreme stretched position to a point which is half way between its two extremes of movement. This doesn't so much strengthen as stretch/lengthen fibres which benefits over tight muscles. Overworking a muscle in this range may cause injury as it is usually at its most vulnerable in this position.
Passive Movement	Limb of the client/patient moved by the therapist, which tests the integrity of the joint capsule/ligament.
Pathology	The study, by scientific methods, which deals with the causes of and changes produced in the body by disease.
Physiology	The study of the functioning of body parts. Its Greek derivation comes from two words, *physics*, meaning 'nature' and *logos*, meaning science or study.
Physiotherapy	Treatment by physical means and as such embraces treatment by; massage, exercise, light, heat, cryotherapy, electrotherapy, hydrotherapy etc.
Plantar Flexion	Movement of the sole of the foot downwards.
Posterior	The body back or near to the back view – sometimes known as *dorsal/dorsum*.
Pronation	Movement of the palm face downwards.
Prone	Lying face down, a position of relative security.

Protraction	Movement of the scapulae forwards.
Proximal	Nearer to the trunk or point of origin, e.g. the shoulder is proximal to the elbow.
Resistive Movement	Related to the end feel and is the ability of the joint to protect itself during static and dynamic activity at the limit of range available.
Retraction	Movement of the scapulae backwards towards the midline.
Rotation	To compress and twist beyond the 'norm' causing soft tissue spasm.
Sagittal	Dividing the body into unequal left and right, parallel to the median plane.
Scoliosis	Lateral rotational spinal curvature.
Shearing	To compress and tension, e.g. torn menisci.
Spines/Spinous Processes	Sharp ridges, e.g. iliac crest.
Spiral Fracture	Bone is fractured creating a spiral pattern.
Splanchnology	The study of the viscera and organs within the cavities of the body.
Sprain	Injury to ligamentous tissue.
Strain	Amount of deformation with respect to the original dimensions of the structure.
Superficial	Towards the outside of a part, towards the surface, e.g. the skin is a superficial organ.
Superior (Cephalad)	Towards the head. Mostly used in reference to structures in the trunk, e.g. the head is superior to the stomach.
Supine	Lying face up, a position of relative vulnerability.
Synovial Fluid	A dialysate of blood plasma containing some protein. It has a viscous consistency, like egg white. Its main role is to lubricate the articular surfaces as well as supplying nutrients to much of the avascular cartilage.

Tendons	From the Greek '*tendu*' meaning to stretch, possess a very parallel fibre arrangement with little or no give. They vary in length, width and thickness depending on where they are located. Flattened tendons are known as aponeurosis.
Tension	To pull apart, e.g. strain/sprain.
Tissues	Organisations of large numbers of similar cells with varying amounts of non-living substance between them (intercellular), performing a specific function.
Transverse	Dividing the body into upper and lower body parts.
Transverse Fracture	Fracture where the break is straight through at right angles to the diaphysis – this fracture is a poor healer.
Traumatic Anatomy	Anatomy found when the body has been misused, overused and abused.
Trochanter/Tuberosity/ Tubercle	Broad roughened bony projections usually for the attachment of muscles or ligaments. Trochanters and tuberosities are larger, e.g. greater trochanter or femur ischial/tibial tuberosity.
Scar Tethering	Adherence of scar tissue to the underlying tissue resulting in loss of mobility and suppleness for such tissues.
Synapse	The non-physical gap/barrier found periodically along the efferent and afferent neural pathways, where the sensory and motor impulses are interrupted.
Synaptic Cleft	The space between the dendrites and the cell body of the next neuron.
Valgus	An abnormal turning away from the midline of the body, or, as in the case of *genu valgum* (knocked knees), an abnormal turning inwards.
Varus	An abnormal turning inwards towards the midline of the body or, as in the case of *genu varum* (bow legs), an abnormal turning outwards.
Vasoconstriction	Narrowing of blood vessels.

Vasodilation	Increased diameter of the blood vessels.
Viscoelasticity	The overall mechanical property of connective tissue.

Useful Addresses

Organisations, Professional Bodies, Suppliers and Website Information Related to Sports Therapy

The following information has been given in good faith but is not to be considered as endorsing any one organisation, professional body, supplier or product in favour of another. Apologies go to those who feel left out! Please telephone the publisher on 01243 539106 if you wish to be represented in any future edition or if your current address details are incorrect in this edition.

Training Organisations and Professional Bodies

Academy of Sport and Exercise Sciences
Cottswood House
Ridgemond Training College
Telford Avenue
Stevenage
SG2 0AU
Tel: 01438 722742

Arthritis Research Campaign
Copeman House
St. Mary's Gate
Chesterfield
S41 7TD
Tel: 01246 558033
www.arc.org.uk

Association of Chartered Physiotherapists in Sports Medicine (ACPSM)
Station Street
Long Eaton
Nottingham
NG10 1GJ
Tel: 0115 972 1319

Back Care
16 Elm Tree Road
Teddington
Middlesex
TW11 8ST
Tel: 020 8 977 5474

British Association of Sport and Exercise Medicine
Tel: 01744 28198

British Association of Sport and Exercise Sciences (BASES)
114 Cardigan Road
Headingley
Leeds
LS6 3BJ
Tel: 0113 289 1020

British Association of Sports Rehabilitators and Trainers (BASRAT)
Tel: 01925 229841

British Chiropractors Sports Council (BCSC)
Carlton Road
Carlton Miniott
Thirsk
YO7 4NJ
Tel: 01845 522242

British Orthopaedic Sports Trauma Association (BOSTA)
Tel: 01273 890316

Chartered Society of Physiotherapy
14 Bedford Row
London
WC1 4ER
Tel: 020 7306 6661/2 (course notices);
020 7306 6633

F. A. Medical Education Centre
Lilleshall
near Newport
TF10 9AT
Tel: 01952 605928

Institute for Optimum Nutrition
Blades Court
Deodar Road
London
SW15 2NU
Tel: 020 8877 9993
e-mail: info@ion.ac.uk

London School of Sports Massage
28 Station Parade
Willesden Green
London
NW2 4NX
Tel: 020 8452 8855

National Coaching Foundation
114 Cardigan Road
Headingley
Leeds
LS6 3BJ
Tel: 0113 274 4802
e-mail: coaching@ncf.org.uk
www.ncf.org.uk

National Osteoporosis Society
Camerton
Bath
BA2 0PJ
Tel: 01761 471771

National School of Sports Massage
16a St. Joseph's Parade
Dorset Street
Dublin 7, Ireland
Tel: 00 353 1 8307063
www.sportsmassage.ie

National Sports Medicine Institute
32 Devonshire Street
London
W1G 6PU
Tel: 020 7251 0583

National Training Organisation for Sport Recreation and Allied Occupations (SPRITO)
Tel: 029 2033 6737

Northern Institute of Massage
14–16 St. Mary's Place
Bury
BL9 0DZ
Tel/fax: 0161 797 1800
www.nim56.co.uk

National Coaching and Training Centre
University of Limerick, Limerick,
Southern Ireland
Tel: 00 353 6 1202024

Organisation of Chartered Physiotherapists in Private Practice (OCPPP)
PhysioFirst is a name that can only be used by members of the above organisation
Tel: 01327 354441, www.physiofirst.org.uk

Osteopathic Sports Care Association
P. O. Box 221
Sunbury-on-Thames
TW16 6RW
Tel: 0870 6010037

The Pain Society
9 Bedford Square
London
WC1B 3RE
Tel: 020 7636 2750
www.staff.ncl.ac.uk/r.j.hayes/
painsoc.html

Premier Training and Development Limited
Parade House
70 Fore Street
Trowbridge
BA14 8HQ
Tel: 01225 353574

Raworth College
20–26 South Street
Dorking
RH4 2HQ
Tel: 01306 742150
www.raworth.com

Scottish Massage Therapists Organisation (SMTO)
70 Lochside Road
Bridge of Don
Aberdeen
AB23 8QW
Tel: 01224 822960

Scottish National Sports Centre
Glenmore Lodge
Aviemore
PH22 IQU
Tel: 01479 861256

SMAE Institute
149 Bath Road
Maidenhead
SL6 4LA
Tel: 01628 621100

Society of Sports Therapists
45c Carrick Street
Glasgow
G2 8PJ
Tel: 0141 221 3660
www.s-s-t.org

The following universities in
co-operation with the Society of Sports
Therapists run degree courses in sports therapy:
North London, Teesside, Hertfordshire,
Chichester

Sports Nutrition Service
Department of Physical Education and
Recreation Management
Loughborough University
Loughborough
LE11 3TU
Tel: 01509 228183

Sports Rehab and Education
45c Carrick Street
Glasgow
G2 8PJ
Tel: 0141 221 1494

International/European

**International Federation of Sports Medicine
(IFSM)**
www.IFSM.com or .org

**International Society of Sports Psychology
(ISSP)**
www.ISSP.co or .org

**European Federation of Sports Psychology
(EFSP)**
www.IFSP.com or .org
www.psychology.Iu.se/FEPSAC

**National Strength and Conditioning
Association (NSCA)**
www.NSCA.com or .org

America

American Academy of Orthopaedic Surgeons
will give information on patient and public
education.

**American Athletic Trainers Association
(AATA)**
AATA.com or .org
see also **NATA and Athletic Trainers**

American College of Sports Medicine (ACSM)
www.ACSM.com or .org

**American Medical Society for Sports
Medicine (AMSSM)**
www.AMSSM.com or .org

**American Orthopaedic Society for Sports
Medicine**
http://www. sportmed.org will provide
information to health care professionals and the
general public as well as giving access to the
American Journal of Sport and Sports Medicine.

American Psychological Association
www.apa.org

American Sports Medicine Institute
http//www.asmi.org/ will provide information
on research and education regarding sports
injury prevention and treatment as well as access
to journals etc.

Athletic Trainers
http//athletictrainer.com is an informative
website specifically for athletic trainers, giving
information on journals etc.

**National Athletic Trainers Association
(NATA)**
http://www.nata.org/

Australia

Australian Association for Exercise
and Sports Science
www.aaess.com.au

Exercise and Sport Psychology
Div47APA
www.psyc.unr.edu/apadiv47

Australian Institute of Sport
Leverrier Crescent
Bruce Act 2617
PO Box 176
Belconnen Act 2616
Tel: 02 214 1578

Germany

German Association of Sports Psychologists
www.uni-leipzig.de/~asp/english

Suppliers

Advance Performance
110–114 Fulbridge Road
Peterborough
PE1 3LE
Tel: 01733 891111
Fax: 01733 891202

Alexandra Workwear
3 Hanover Square
London
W15 1HD
Tel: 020 7723 9906

Allsport Medical
15-17 The Garrick Centre
Irving Way
London
NW9 6AQ *or*
Freepost LON 12024
London
NW9 9YR
Tel: 0800 358 9991 *or*
020 8203 1441
e-mail: @allsportmedical.com.uk

Coachwise Limited
Units 2/3 Chelsea Close
off Amberley Road
Armley
Leeds
LS12 4HW
Tel: 0113 231 1310

Duffield Medical
4/6 Knowsley Road
Haslingden
Rossendale
BB4 4RX
Tel: 01706 210297
e-mail: sales@rothband.co.uk

Houghton's Books
St. Mary's Old School
Gundry Lane
Bridport
DT6 3RL
Tel: 01308 420494

Osteopathic Supplies Limited
70 Belmont Road
Hereford
HR2 7JW
Tel: 01432 263939

Physio Med-Services
7–11 Glossop Brook Business Park

Surrey Street
Glossop
SK13 7AJ
Tel: 01457 860 444
www. physio-med.com *or*
www.physiomed@physio-med.com

Physique Management Company Limited
Jackson Close
Grove Road
Drayton
Portsmouth
PO6 1UP
Tel: 0870 60 70 381
e-mail: @physique.co.uk
www.physique.co.uk

Procare/Medipost Limited
100 Shaw Road
Oldham
OL1 4AY
Tel: 0161 678 0233

Russell Medical
PO Box 3
Hanley Castle
WR8 0DJ
Tel: 01684 311 444
Fax: 01684 311 555
e-mail: thetallguy@russellmedical.co.uk

Sportscare/Medisport
100 Shaw Road
Oldham
OL1 4AY
Tel: 0161 633 5333

Sportspages
Caxton Walk
94–96 Charing Cross Road
London
WC2H OJG
Tel: 020 7240 9604
also at:

Barton Square
St. Anne's Square
Manchester
M2 7HA
Tel: 0161 832 8530

St John's Supplies
PO Box 707B
Friend Street
London
EC1V 7NE
Tel: 020 7278 7888

Trimilin (UK) Limited
Unit 16, St. James Industrial Estate
Westhampnett Road
Chichester
PO19 4JU
Tel: 01243 784488/0800 0644848
e-mail: sales@trimilin.com
www.trimilin.com

Databases/Websites

With over 60 million sites worldwide, many
originating from the USA, the following are just
a random sample of various 'search engines'
extra to the ones already listed that are useful to
not only sports therapy but sports medicine.

The **SPORT** database was developed in Canada
and contains information covering the sports
fitness and recreation industry, e.g. sports
medicine, psychology, exercise physiology,
biomechanics etc.

Sport Information Resource Centre
1600 James Naismith Drive
Gloucester
Ontario
Canada K1B 5N4
Tel: (613) 748 5658

The **MEDLINE** database, produced in the USA,
covers medical literature and is said to
complement **SPORT**. For more information
contact:

Knight-Ridder Information
Haymarket House
1 Oxenden Street
London
SW14EE

The **BANDOLIER** website is an excellent site for
a precis of most research into a given topic.

Physiobase.com is a website aimed at the
international physiotherapy community and has
a whole host of free services ranging from:

- PhysioWork for locum and
  permanent job listings.
- PhysioLibrary for research and databases.
- PhysioMail for a free e-mail service.
- Physiochat for discussion.
- Physiocourse both local and international.
- Physiodirectory a listing of clinical
  specialities.

www.healthlibrary.com is a site for information
on a wide range of complementary therapies,
diet and nutrition, fully referenced research,
natural remedies, professional bodies etc.

www.medline.com is the world's largest, medical
database.

www. findmedical.com is a website for medical
products and pieces of medical equipment,
exhibitions, conferences, workshops and
symposiums.

www.yahoo.com or .co.uk is a search engine
that lists sites in categories.

www.medweb.com and www.mspweb.com are
sites for 'link pages' of related resources to
sports medicine.

www.altavista.com is one of the most
comprehensive search engines for 'sports
medicine'.

www.medfacts.com or sprtsdoc.htm contains
video clips of operative procedures, lectures and
other events broadcast in real time as well as
'chat areas'.

www.fitnessworld.com/enth/spmed/sportsmed.
html is one of the US Sports Medicine sites.

www.enhanced-performance.com/ nideffer/
relates to sports psychology.

www.medaccess.com/fitness/fund.htm offers
advice on starting exercise etc.
www.iasi.com (International Association for
Sports Information) can be viewed in four
languages.

www.sport-medicine.com – The SportEx
database (*see publications*).

www.nsmi.org.uk – The SMART database
(*see publications*).

http://sportsci.org – An academically, sport
science-focussed site.

http://ptwww.cchs.usyd.edu.au/pedro – This
relates to the Pedro database at the Centre of
Evidence-based Physiotherapy at the University
of Sydney.

http://hanke.com/orthodoc – A site for the
study of muscles, pain and treatment.

www.sportsequipmentinsurance.com – An insurance service specifically for sports equipment.

Useful Publications

It is not the intention of the author to try and list all the publications/journals relevant to sports therapy but to provide a general, selected list that can be referred to with the references used in the text.

American Journal of Sports Medicine/American Journal of Sport and Sports Medicine
http://www.sportmed.org

British Journal of Sports Medicine
www.bmjpg.com/data/jsm.htm *or* www.bjsportsmed.com

Clinical Journal of Sports Medicine

Complementary Therapies in Medicine is a journal for health care professionals, that is published by Churchill Livingstone.
www.harcourt-international.com/journals/ctim

Gatorade's Sports Science Exchange
www.gssiweb.com/library/sse/index.html

Human Kinetic Journals
www.humankinetics.com/

INFORM. For a small annual fee the NCF will periodically send information on recent research papers related to coaching practice but very relevant to Sports Therapy.

International Journal of Sports Psychology

New Zealand Journal of Sports Medicine

Physical Therapy in Sport
The Journal of CPSM
ISSN 1466 – 853X
Harcourt Brace, Tel: 020 8308 5700
e-mail: journals@harcourt.com
www.harcourt-international.com/journals/ptsp

International Journal of Sports Psychology

New Zealand Journal of Sports Medicine
Physical Therapy in Sport, The Journal of CPSM
Harcourt Brace
Tel: 020 8308 5700
e-mail: journals@harcourt.com
www.harcourt-international.com/journals/ptsp

Peak Performance
67–71 Goswell Road
London
EC1V 7EN (Annual Subscription).

SMART (Sports Medicine and Related Topics)

A library and information service run by the NSMI and similar to the National Coaching Foundation's Inform. Tel: 020 7251 0583 ext. 228/229, Fax: 020 7251 0774
e-mail: jane.makepeace@nsmi.org.uk
http://smart.nsmi.org.uk

SportEX Medicine
Centor Publishing
Freepost LON 10827
London
SW19 1BR
Tel: 020 8287 3312
www.sportex-medicine.com

SportEX Health
The companion magazine of SportEX Medicine, details as above.

Sports Sciences Journal
www.chapmanhall.com/js/default.html

Appendices

Appendix 1

How Good a Communicator are you?

Where would you rate yourself on the following scales?

Do you:

use two-way interaction?	5 4 3 2 1	talk too much, fail to listen, or interrupt?
value what the athlete says?	5 4 3 2 1	ignore the views of the athlete?
show consistency between verbal and non-verbal language?	5 4 3 2 1	show conflict between verbal and non-verbal language?
encourage interaction by involving, questioning and respecting the athlete?	5 4 3 2 1	reduce communication channels and restrict interaction?
recognise and respect the needs/interests of each person?	5 4 3 2 1	appear disinterested, ignore some people, favour others?
send messages high on information?	5 4 3 2 1	rattle on, talk for the sake of it?
use bridging techniques and paraphrasing?	5 4 3 2 1	listen impatiently without apparent interest?
show consistency between words and actions?	5 4 3 2 1	tend to change the story during conversation?
take responsibility for the content?	5 4 3 2 1	use 'we' to share responsibility?

Appendix 2

Common Injuries of the Lower Limb and Upper Limb, Trunk and Spine

The following list has been included to show not only some of the more common injuries and conditions encountered in sport but also the enormity of the task of trying to include every conceivable problem, injury and condition a sports therapist may have to deal with. The list could have been categorised in many different ways, i.e. traumatic, inflammatory, chronic, acute, medical, adolescent etc. but has simply been listed alphabetically. The list does not profess to be definitive, nor does it intend to cover every variation on a theme. At times 'blanket terms' and syndromes are included that can cover a multitude of sins. Although the conditions are listed as lower limb; upper limb, trunk and spine it will be appreciated that many conditions apply to all areas, i.e. skin problems, sprain, strain etc.

Lower Limb

Abductor and adductor strains

Appendicitis

Arthritis/arthrosis – the most common is osteo and rheumatoid

Bruises

Bursitis

Compartment syndromes – acute and chronic

Fibromyositis

Foreign bodies

Fractures and dislocations

Groin disruption

Hallux rigidus

Hallux valgus

Hammer toe

Hamstring pulls

Hernias – inguinal, femoral, abdominal

Iliotibial band syndrome (runner's knee)

Joint sprains

Larsen-Johansson disease

Leg length discrepancy

Ligament sprains and ruptures – collaterals, cruciates etc.

Meniscus problems

Metatarsalgia

Muscle contractures, strains and ruptures

Muscle strains

Myalgia

Neuritis/neuralgia

Osgood-Schlatter's disease

Osteitis pubis

Patella conditions and injuries – e.g. chondromalacia

Patella femoral problems – e.g. osteochondritis dissecans, pathological degenerations

Periostitis

Perthe's disease

Pes cavus

Pes planus

Plantar fasciitis

Psoas spasm

Sciatic type problems

Sesamoiditis

Shin splints

Lower Limb cont...

Skin problems – viral, fungal, bacterial
   – cuts, abrasions, rashes etc.
Synovitis talipes
Talipes
Talipes calcaneus
Talipes equinus
Tendon problems –
   tenosynovitis (*also known as
   tenovaginitis*), tendonitis

Thigh (quad) strains
Tinea pedis (*athlete's foot*)
Tumours
Varus/valgus problems

Upper Limb, Trunk and Spine

Appendicitis
Arthritis/arthrosis – the most common
   is osteo and rheumatoid
Back problems!
Bruises
Bursitis
Carpal Tunnel Syndrome
Disc protrusion, prolapse,
   herniation, rupture
Dupuytren's contracture
Facet joint problems
Fibromyositis
Foreign bodies
Fractures and dislocations
Frozen shoulder
Jogger's nipple
Joint sprains
Lateral humeral epicondylitis
   (*tennis elbow*)
Ligament sprains and ruptures –
   collaterals etc.
Mallet finger
Muscle contractures, strains
   and ruptures

Myalgia
Neuritis/neuralgia
Osteoitis pubis
Pathological degeneration
Periostitis
Repetitive strain
Rib problems
Rotator cuff lesions
Skier's thumb
Skin problems – viral, fungal, bacterial
   – cuts, abrasions, rashes etc.
Spinal lesions
Spondylitis
Spondylolisthesis
Spondylosis
Spodylolysis
Synovitis
Tendon problems –
   tenosynovitis (*also known as
   tenovaginitis*), tendonitis
Torticollis
Tumours
Whiplash

Appendix 3

Training Regimes

The capacity of a muscle to move a resistance/load through a full range of joint movement is determined by many physiological factors, e.g. size of muscle, type of muscle, leverage system involved and degree of nervous system involvement. In progressive resistive exercise (PRE) the standard measure is known as 1 RM or one repetition maximum and is defined as:

> "The maximum weight that can be lifted once only through a given range."
> *Smith, G. N., 1990*

and the 10 RM is:

> "The maximum weight that can be lifted 10 times at natural speed and without rests between lifts."
> *Smith, G. N., 1990*

This usually equates to approximately two thirds of 1 RM.

However, in progressive resistive exercise, weights need to be lifted more than once to meet various training principles, i.e. the overload principle, the principle of progression and the principles of specificity and individuality. Obviously this progression needs to be carefully controlled and monitored to avoid injury. Usually 60–80% of a muscle's capacity is used, once the 1 RM has been assessed.

There are many systems that have been developed using fixed or varying numbers of repetitions, various fixed or progressive loading, in various sequences/sets and with varying rest periods between sets and repetitions. However, following simple training principles, strength requires high loads and low repetitions, endurance low loads and many repetitions are called for and with power the elements of time and speed are introduced. The following are just some of these variations.

MacQueen Regime

Designed for increasing muscle power only by using a constant high load and low repetitions.

Once the 10 RM is set and the starting position established the sequence is:

10 lifts with the full 10 RM value repeated 4 times, i.e. 4 sets of 10.
This is carried out 3 times a week and a progression of the 10 RM is made every 1–2 weeks.

De Lorme and Watkin's Regime

Here strength and endurance can be improved by using an increasing the load and low repetitions.

Once the 10 RM is set and the starting position established the sequence is:

10 lifts with half the 10 RM value.
10 lifts with three-quarters of the 10 RM value.
10 lifts with the full 10 RM value.

This therefore requires 30 lifts that are carried out 4 times a week with a progression of the 10 RM made every week.

Zinovieff or Oxford Regime

Here endurance can be improved by using low loads via a reducing weight and high repetitions.

Once the 10 RM is set and the starting position established the sequence is:

10 lifts with a full 10 RM value.
10 lifts with a full 10 RM value minus half a kilo.
10 lifts with a full 10 RM value minus a kilo.
10 lifts with a full 10 RM value minus one and a half kilos.
10 lifts with a full 10 RM value minus two kilos.
10 lifts with a full 10 RM value minus two and a half kilos.
10 lifts with a full 10 RM value minus three kilos.
10 lifts with a full 10 RM value minus three and a half kilos.
10 lifts with a full 10 RM value minus four kilos.
10 lifts with a full 10 RM value minus four and a half kilos.

This gives 100 lifts, to be carried out 5 times a week and the 10 RM progression made daily. Various forms of coloured 'rubber bands' can also be used with varying degrees of resistance and these can simply be utilised and adapted to suit a purpose.

Appendix 4

Record Keeping

The following records are given as examples of the kind of records that sports therapists need to keep and are not meant to supersede any existing records suggested by national governing bodies or sporting organisations. They are not to size or scale and can be altered and/or modified to suit the individual/circumstance.

Personal Data Record 1

NAME: _____

TEL NO: (HOME) _____ (WORK) _____

ADDRESS: _____

_____

DOB: _____ MARITAL STATUS: _____

CHILDREN: _____

EMPLOYMENT: _____

RECOMMENDED TO THE CLINIC BY: _____

REASONS FOR VISIT TO THE CLINIC: _____

NAME OF MEDICAL DOCTOR: _____

HEALTH CENTRE: _____

Are you at present under the care of a doctor or hospital? (if so give brief details/medication prescribed). You may be asked to visit your GP to rule out problems that are beyond the sphere of this practice.

Personal Data Record 2

CONSULTATION FORM FOR: _____   **DATE:** _____

PRIMARY COMPLAINT:

_____

PAIN COMPONENT:

i) Dull, deep, nagging, burning,
    tingling,crawling, electric, toothache

ii) Constant/intermittent/flitting

THERMAL COMPONENT:

i) Proximal, distal discrete

PREVIOUS TREATMENT FOR CONDITION:

(X-ray, tests, etc.)

SECONDARY COMPLAINTS:

HISTORY:

DOES THE PATIENT SUFFER FROM:

ANAEMIA:
BLOOD PRESSURE:
DIABETES:
EPILEPSY:
HEART CONDITION:
STOMACH DISORDERS +

OTHERS:

VAT TEST +/-

ASCERTAIN:

S/S, Onset/ Recurrences/
History/Rapid/ Gradual/
Insidious/ Episodic

Ant   Pain   Map   Post

Bowel Habit
Loss of Appetite
Nausea
Weight Loss
Allergies
Dietary
Dizziness/Syncope
Period Pains
Varicosity
Phlebitis
Respiratory Problems
(e.g. asthma)
DEHYDRATION/WATER

SKIN DISORDERS:
OEDEMA:
DENTAL/EYESIGHT:
HORMONAL PROBLEMS:
DRUG THERAPY:
SKINFOLD (%BODY FAT):

Biceps	Subscapularis
Triceps	Supra Illiac
Thigh	Chest
Abdomen	

WAIST/HIP RATIO:

ILLNESSES IN LAST 5 YEARS: _____

_____

_____

OPERATIONS IN LAST 5 YEARS: _____

_____

_____

GENERAL HEALTH:

LEFT OR RIGHT HANDED _____   STRESS _____

HEIGHT _____   SLEEP _____

WEIGHT _____   SMOKE _____

BMI, W/H^2 _____   ALCOHOL _____

PULSE RATING: Resting _____   HOBBIES/SPORT _____

                 After exercise _____

FAMILY HISTORY (Arthritis/cancer) _____

_____

DIAGNOSIS/RECOMMENDATIONS:

_____

_____

_____

_____

_____

_____

_____

_____

_____

_____

_____

_____

_____

In terms of devising a Personal Data Record to use and take on a tour/trip the following additional information will need to be obtained, as well as written permission from parents/guardians if accepting responsibility for minors.

Emergency telephone contact _____

NHS number/card _____

Blood group _____

Swimming competence _____

Travel sickness _____

Immunisation/vaccination history _____

Examination and Assessment

NAME: _____ DATE: _____

JOINT: _____

HISTORY: see Personal Data 1 and 2

OBSERVATION: _____

TOUCH: _____

ACTIVE MOVEMENTS: _____

PASSIVE MOVEMENTS: _____

RESISTED MOVEMENTS: _____

MUSCLES: _____

LIGAMENTS: _____

PALPATION: _____

SPECIAL TESTS: _____

JOINTS ABOVE AND BELOW: _____

FUNCTION: _____

REPEAT TO CONFIRM OR DENY: _____

OTHER COMMENTS: _____

Treatment Record

NAME: _____

Date of Assessment and Examination

First Treatment given (massage, heat, electrotherapy, exercises, etc.)

SUBSEQUENT TREATMENT REGIME:

Date _____

Progress since last visit _____
_____
_____
_____
_____

Treatment given _____
_____
_____
_____
_____
_____

Comments _____
_____
_____
_____
_____
_____
_____
_____
_____

Letter of Referral

Letterhead

Practitioner: _____   Re: _____

Date: _____   D.O.B: _____

Dear

The above patient contacted me for sports therapy treatment on _____
complaining of: _____

Relevant History: _____
_____
_____
_____
_____

Examination/assessment: _____
_____
_____
_____
_____
_____

Opinion/prognosis: _____
_____
_____
_____
_____
_____

Remarks/requests: _____
_____
_____
_____
_____

Should you wish to discuss the patient, please contact me at the above address.

Yours sincerely,

James Briggs

Appendix 5

Body Fat Assessment

The following information is supplied with due acknowledgement to: Health Related Fitness, Bill Tancred, 1987, Publisher Hodder and Stoughton, 17–19. The Nomograms used have been adapted from 'A nomogram for the estimate of percentage body fat from generalised equations' by W. B. Baun and P. E. Raven, *Research Quarterly for Exercise and Sport*, 52, 380–384.

After calculating the skinfold measurements as outlined in Chapter 4, Part 6, the following nomograms can be used to calculate the percentage body fat for boys, girls and adults by drawing straight lines between the triceps and subscapula and the age and sum of three skinfolds respectively. The results can then be related to the body fatness rating scale.

BODY FATNESS RATING SCALE

RATING	MEN % FATNESS	WOMEN % FATNESS
OBESE	20 plus	29 plus
FAT	18 – 19	24 – 28
AVERAGE	14 – 17	20 – 23
LEAN	11 – 13	16 – 19
VERY LEAN	10 and below	15 and below

Nomogram – percentage body fats (boys 13–16 years)

Nomogram – percentage body fats (girls 13–16 years)

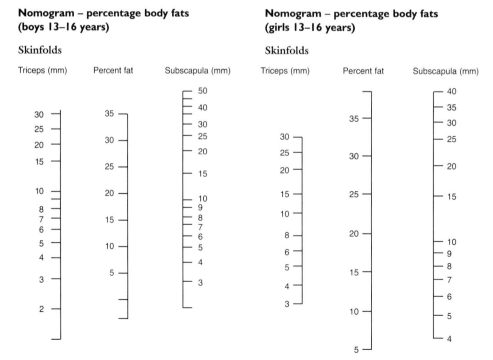

For adults, reference can be made to Clinical Sports Medicine, 2nd. ed. (2001), Brukner, P., and Khan, K., page 260, Table 33.6. Approximate mean (and range) of skinfold measurements in elite athletes of various sports.

Index

Actin 29
Action potential 231
Active 192
Adaptation 133
Alcohol 332
All-or-nothing principle 28
Analgesic 235, 272
Anatomical positions 38
Anatomy 18
Antalgic gait 206
Appendicitis 144
Asthma 140
Athlete's heart 141
Atoms 19
Avulsion fracture 177

Biological evidence 59
Biomechanical alignment 80
Blood clot 153
Body fat 71
Body mass index (BMI) 212
Body planes 38
Body shape 83
Body temperature 74
Bone 5, 174
Bony tissue 164
Bridge over break 168

Caffeine 333
Calcification 168
Callus 168
Cancellous 169
Carbohydrates 90
Carcinoma 179
Cartilage 25
Cascade effect 152, 154
Cavities 34
Cells 20
Cellular response 155
Cellulomes 235
Chemicals 19

Chemotaxis (chemotropism) 155
Central medullary cavity 26
Central nervous fatigue 70
Children 95
Chondroblasts 168
Chondrosarcoma 179
Chronic glycogen depletion 144
Chronic inflammation 157
Chronicity 157
Clinic 312
Clinical stage 283
Clothing 76, 88
Clot retraction 153
Complement 154
Compression 158, 160, 164
Connective tissue 21
Consolidation 168
Constipation 142
Contractile tissue 28
Contrast bathing 273
Cool 159, 160
Cool down 67, 85
Cramp 70, 75
Cryocuff 160
Cryotherapy 270
Cysts 180
Cytolysis 155

Deformity 176
Dehydration 75, 89, 142
Delayed onset muscle
   soreness (DOMS) 72, 128
Depolarisation 231, 233
Diabetes 145
Diapedesis 155
Diaphysis 26
Diarrhoea 142
Diet 73, 88
Diffusion 150
Digestion 142
Disability 111

Drinks — 89
Drugs testing — 140
Duty of care — 303

Early training — 134
Ease of movement — 31, 192
Ectomorph — 84
Ectoplasm — 19
Education — 78
Elastic range — 32
Electrotherapy — 266
Elevate — 159
Empirical evidence — 59
Endochrondral — 165
Endomorph — 84
Endosteum — 26
Engram — 29
Environment — 139
Epiphysis — 26
Epithelial tissue — 20
Equalisation — 150
Equipment — 76
Evidence-based medicine — 58
Exteroceptors — 289

Facilitation — 239
Fascia — 23
Fat — 90, 210
Fatigue — 68
Fibre — 91
Fibrosis replacement — 155
Fitness — 78
Fitness stage — 284
Fitness testing — 135, 287
Float phase — 205
Fluid balance — 74, 88
Footwear — 76
Fractures — 166

Gait — 176, 204
Gender differences — 92
Glands — 20
Golgi end organs — 290
Granulation *see* proliferation

Haemarthrosis — 154, 180
Haemostasis — 153
Headache — 141
Heat — 274
Heat balance — 74
Heat exhaustion — 75
Heat stroke — 75
Heel strike — 205
History taking — 189
Hydrokinetic — 150
Hypermobility — 202
Hyperthermia — 75
Hypothermia — 75

Immune system — 143
Individuality — 133
Infection — 178, 254
Inflammation — 153
Injury classification — 61
Intramembranous — 165
Isokinetic — 31
Isometric — 30
Isotonic — 30

Joint — 27
Joint fatigue — 71

Lag phase — 160
Leg length discrepancy — 196
Ligaments — 22, 176, 194
Limitation of movement — 153
Lines of gravity — 210
Lymphatic system — 143

Macromolecules — 19
Massage — 162
Maturation — 156
Medical — 140
Membrane — 34
Membrane permeability — 150
Menstruation — 144
Mesomorphy — 83
Microtubules — 19
Migraine — 141
Military posture — 209
Mitochondria — 19
Mouth to mouth resuscitation — 186
Muscle fuel — 69
Muscle pain — 70
Muscle spasms — 74
Muscle spindle — 291
Muscle type — 63
Myelination — 237
Myocarditis — 141
Myosin — 29
Myositis ossificans — 176, 254

Negligence — 303
Neoplasm — 179
Nervous tissue — 33, 164, 237
Neuron — 33, 231
Neurotransmitters — 233, 235, 236
Nutrient foramen — 25
Nutrition — 69, 88, 140, 172, 323

Pain — 74, 155, 197
Pain gate theory — 240
Pain generation — 238
Palpation — 194
Passive — 193
Pathology — 18

Periosteum 26
Personality 80
Phagocytosis 155, 168
Phenotype 81
Physiology 18
Placebo 223, 225, 252
Plastic range 32
Polarised 232
Postural check 190, 207
Pre-competition 247
Pre-discharge 134
Pre-match fitness 135
Primary gain 226
Progression 132
Proliferation 156
Proprioception 289
Proteins 90

Range of movement 31, 192
Receptors 289
Record keeping 202
Recovery 133
Regeneration (resolution) 155, 163
Relaxation 70
Remodelling 156, 164, 169
Repolarisation 233
Residual posture 210
Rest 159
Resting membrane
    potential (RMP) 232
Reversibility 132

Saltatory conduction 233
Sarcoma 179
Scar tissue 156, 177
Screening 80
Scrum pox 143
Secondary gain 226
Selection 80
Skill 85
Skin 22, 177
Skinfold-caliper 212
Sleep and rest 71
Slump posture 209
Smoking 330
Sodium-potassium pump 233
Soft tissue 15
Somatotype 81, 83
Specificity 132, 239
Sports anaemia 146
Sports massage 253
Stance phase 205
Summation 236
Super/overcompensation 131
Supperation 157
Surface markings 44
Swelling 154, 178
Swing phase 205, 206

Synapse 233, 234
Syncope 123
Synovial 27, 181
Systems 35

Technical 139
Tendons 21, 177
Tertiary gain 226
Tests 198
Thermal 269
Toe range 32
Touch 192
Training diaries 147
Training year 130
Tumour 179, 255

Under-performance
    syndrome (UPS) 126

Variation 133
Veterans 110
Vitamins 91
Volkmann's ischemic contracture 175

Waist to hip ratio 212
Warm-up 65, 85
Water 74, 89

Zeitgebers 342

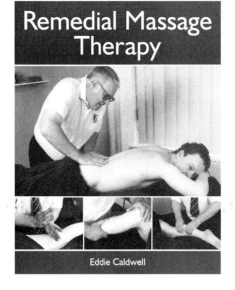

ISBN: 1 903333 02 4
Price: £15.00

Remedial massage has rocketed in popularity over the past five years. There are now more courses than ever before which offer the student the opportunity to learn this highly versatile technique which can be used on numerous conditions and in a variety of situations, from the confines of a treatment room to the sports field.

Fully illustrated with black and white photographs and line drawings, **REMEDIAL MASSAGE THERAPY** takes a comprehensive look at all aspects of remedial massage. Key areas covered include:

- The History of Massage
- Different Massage Techniques including Sports Massage
- Muscles and Joints
- Assessing and Treating the Patient
- Advertising the Practice
- A Fully Detailed Section Which Covers Treatment of Specific Areas of the Body
- Treating Children
- Origins, Insertions and Actions of Muscles

REMEDIAL MASSAGE THERAPY is full of useful, practical advice from one of the most experienced and respected practitioners in the UK, and will prove an extremely useful reference tool for any student or practitioner.

Eddie Caldwell, B.Ed. (Hons), L.C.S.P. (Phys), A.C.P., has been the Principal of the Northern Institute of Massage since 1995. Eddie qualified as a teacher of Physical Education in 1961 and gained further diplomas in Special Education at Manchester University, Sports Science at Salford College of Technology and Manipulative Therapy at the Northern Institute of Massage. The Northern Institute is accredited by the Open and Distance Learning Quality Council, and is the official training establishment for the London and Counties Society of Physiologists, established in 1919.